Current Topics in Microbiology
137 and Immunology

Editors

A. Clarke, Parkville/Victoria · R.W. Compans,
Birmingham/Alabama · M. Cooper, Birmingham/Alabama
H. Eisen, Paris · W. Goebel, Würzburg · H. Koprowski,
Philadelphia · F. Melchers, Basel · M. Oldstone,
La Jolla/California · P.K. Vogt, Los Angeles
H. Wagner, Ulm · I. Wilson, La Jolla/California

Genetics
of Immunological
Diseases

Edited by B. Mock and M. Potter

With 88 Figures

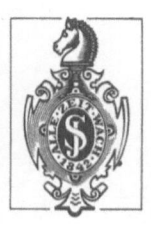

Springer-Verlag
Berlin Heidelberg NewYork
London Paris Tokyo

BEVERLY MOCK, Ph.D
MICHAEL POTTER, M.D.

Laboratory of Genetics
National Cancer Institute
National Institutes of Health
Bethesda, MD 20892, USA

ISBN 978-3-642-50061-9   ISBN 978-3-642-50059-6 (eBook)
DOI 10.1007/978-3-642-50059-6

Preface

The development of innovative molecular techniques such as pulse-field gel electrophoresis, cDNA subtraction libraries and chromosome hopping libraries coupled
with the increasing popularity in the prospect of sequencing mammalian genomes,
has triggered a resurgence of interest in finding and characterizing genes that
play a role in modifying immune processes and diseases. Genetically defined strains
of mice (e.g., inbred strains and recently derived stocks of wild mice) provide
ideal models for examining the genetic control of diseases as a result of their
syntenic relationship with man in genetic composition as well as linkage conservation. Due to the relative ease of producing a specific genotype via appropriate
breeding schedules, murine models may provide the only hope for unravelling those
complex disease processes under multigenic control.

This issue of CTMI is a collection of papers on the characterization and mapping
of genes involved in mutations and dysregulated immune responses which produce
disease phenotypes. These papers were presented at a workshop which was devoted
to examining reverse genetic approaches at localizing, cloning and characterizing
genes involved in a variety of developmental, autoimmune, neoplastic and infectious
disease processes.

In the first of three sections, a series of papers outline the most currently
used methods of mapping and isolating genes whose products are unknown. The
papers, following, are devoted to specific gene systems whose dysregulation is
likely to produce mutant or disease phenotypes. In this section, gene regulation,
ranging from evolutionary constraints on structure and function to control via
cis- and trans-acting elements, is examined in a variety of developmental and
immunological systems. The final section is devoted to a collection of elusive
disease genes involved in the control of host resistance and susceptibility.

We wish to thank Professor Dietrich Goetze, Ms. Anna Deus and the staff of Springer-
Verlag for their assistance in publishing this collection of papers, the authors
of which participated in a workshop on this subject in Bethesda, Maryland from
27-29 October, 1987. We thank the National Cancer Institute and Dr. Alan S. Rabson
for sponsoring and encouraging this workshop which brought together a diverse array
of investigators in mouse genetics. We are grateful to Ms. Victoria Rogers for
her editorial and administrative help in preparing this book.

Beverly A. Mock, Ph.D.

and

Michael Potter, M.D.
National Cancer Institute
National Institutes of Health

Table of Contents

Autoimmunity

Neoplasia

X

Indexed in Current Contents

List of Contributors

You will find the adresses at the beginning of the respective contribution

ABE, R. 177
AMARI, N.M.B. 256
ANSELL, J.D. 191
ARANT, S. 256
AVNER, P.R. 13
BALTIMORE, D. 136
BAUER, S.R. 130
BENZ, R.A. 183
BICKMORE, W. 41
BLACKWELL, J.M. 301
BLANK, R.D. 25
BLANKENHORN, E.P. 233, 264
BOSMA, G. 197
BOSMA, M.J. 197, 203
BROCKDORFF, N. 3
BROWN, S.D.M. 3, 329
BYRD, L. 268
CALAME, K.L. 100
CAMPBELL, G.R. 25
CAVANNA, J.S. 3
CHAPMAN, V.M. 18, 183, 191
COOPER, A. 301
DAWDA, P. 301
DEAN, A. 155
D'EUSTACHIO, P. 25
D'HOOSTELAERE, L. 116, 130, 276
DUNCAN, R. 264
EHRLICH, R. 148
ERHART, M.A. 70
FIBI, M. 82
FIGUEROA, F. 55
FISHER, E.M.C. 3
FLEISZER, D. 243
FORRESTER, L.M. 191
FOWLIS, D.J. 191
FREDRICKSON, T.N. 250
FULTZ, M.J. 165
GELLERT, M. 94
GIBSON, D. 116
GRAHAM, A. 87
GRANT, S.G. 18, 183
GREENFIELD, A.J. 3
GROS, P. 310
GRUSS, P. 82
GUENET, J.L. 13
HARTMAN, A.B. 211
HASTIE, N.D. 41
HEESE, J.E. 94
HERRMANN, B.G. 77

HEYNINGEN, V. van 41
HICKEY, W.F. 233
HILGERS, J. 116, 243
HODES, R.J. 177
HOGAN, B.L.M. 87
HOLLAND, P.W.H. 87
HUPPI, K. 116, 268, 276, 289
HYNES, R. 310
ISHIZAKA, S.T. 240
ISLAM, M.Q. 33
JANEWAY, C.A. 171, 329
JAY, G. 140
KAKKIS, E. 100
KASAHARA, M. 55
KESSEL, M. 82
KIM, M.G. 203
KING, M. 301
KLEIN, J. 55
KOZAK, C.A. 250
KRUMLAUF, R. 87
KWASNIEWSKI, M. 316
LaFUSE, W. 316
LEHRACH, H. 47, 77
LEVAN, G. 33
LIEBER, M.R. 94
LILLY, F. 240
LUMSDEN, A. 87
LYON, M.F. 3
MacKENZIE, C. 191
MALLETT, C. 116, 211
MARCU, K.B. 203
MASSIE, M. 316
MAULE, J. 41
MELCHERS, F. 130
MERUELO, D. 256
MICKLEM, H.S. 191
MILLER, D.R. 183
MIZUUCHI, K. 94
MOCK, B. 116, 268, 276, 289, 295, 329
MORSE III, H.C. 227, 329
MULLINS, L.J. 18
NADEAU, J.H. 39, 70
NASIR, J. 3
NATH, J. 316
NESBITT, M.N. 310, 325
NOTKINS, A.L. 211
O'REILLY, A.J. 18
OWEN, F.L. 155

PAMPENO, C.L. 256
PARSHAD, R. 289
PETERMAN, G.M. 155
PETERSON, C.L. 100
PHILLIPS, S.J. 70
PILLAI, S. 136
POLLAK, M. 25
PORTEOUS, D.J. 41
POTTER, M. 116, 264, 268, 276, 289, 295, 329
POUSTKA, A. 47
PRABHAKAR, B.S. 211
REINER, A.H. 39
RIBLET, R. 107
ROACH, T.I.A. 301
ROHME, D. 47
RUSSELL, L.B. 47
SANFORD, K.K. 289
SCANDALIS, S. 256
SCHRICKER, P. 276
SCHULER, W. 197, 203
SCHURR, E. 310
SCHWEITZER, P.A. 223
SCOLESE, A.E. 18
SELDIN, M.F. 227
SHULTZ, L.D. 216, 223
SILVER, L.M. 64
SIMON-CHAZOTTES, D. 13
SINGER, D.S. 148
SINGHAI, R. 155
SKAMENE, E. 243, 310, 325
SMITH-GILL, S.J. 211
SRINIVASAPPA, J. 211
STEINBERG, A.D. 227
STEPHENSON, D.A. 18, 183
STEVENSON, M.M. 325
STUBBS, L. 47
SZPIRER, C. 33
SZPIRER, J. 33
TEUSCHER, C. 233, 264
TOOLE, S. 301
TSAO, B. 100
TUTTER, A. 107
VESPA, L. 316
VILLAR, C.J. 250
VINCEK, V. 55
VOGEL, S.N. 165
WEBER, J.S. 140
ZHANG, D. 256
ZWILLING, B.S. 316

I. Localizing and Cloning Genes

The Long-Range Mapping of Mammalian Chromosomes

S.D.M. Brown, N. Brockdorff, J.S. Cavanna, E.M.C. Fisher, A.J. Greenfield, M.F. Lyon[1], and J. Nasir

INTRODUCTION

Very little is known of the long-range sequence organisation of mammalian chromosomes; or of the relationship of long-range sequence organisation to the physical and genetic properites of. mammalian chromosomes. While the organisation of sequences of varying repetition in individual DNA clones of limited size (< 50 kb) is well documented, the detailed physical and genetic relationships of unique and repeat sequences over long distances on the mammalian chromosome is poorly characterised. In order to allow us to determine the physical and genetic relationships of individual DNA sequences over long distances it has been necessary to construct long-range genetic and physical maps that encompass chromosome regions much greater in size than the average DNA clone. At the same time such long-range genetic and physical maps can determine the genetic and physical limits on the chromosome of a number of genetic loci of known phenotype and unknown gene product and provide a number of molecular start-points for the isolation of such genes, which are not approachable by classical genetic engineering techniques.

Recently, a number of novel techniques have become available to obtain clones from specific chromosomal regions that can be used as markers in the long-range mapping of mammalian chromosomes. Coupled with advances in methods for the rapid long-range genetic and physical mapping of DNA clones on mammalian chromosomes, many chromosome regions are mapped in fine detail. We describe here the detailed long-range mapping of two mouse chromosomes, the X and 7, that has enabled us not only to determine the genetic relationships of a number of interesting loci but has also uncovered novel long-range sequence organisations that would have remained undetectable by classical techniques.

LONG RANGE MAPPING OF MAMMALIAN CHROMOSOMES

The Mouse and Human haploid genomes each contain of the order of 3×10^9 bp of DNA. Given the genetic length of the mouse genome as 1600 cM, it is easy to calculate that on average every 1 cM of the mouse genome corresponds to 1.7 megabases (Mb).

Department of Biochemistry and Molecular Genetics, St. Mary's Hospital Medical School, London W2 1PG, U.K.

[1] MRC Radiobiology Unit, Chilton, Didcot, Oxon OX11 0RD, U.K.

From ENU mutagenesis experiments (Shedlovsky et al., 1986) a conservative estimate of 10,000 genes in the mouse genome has been arrived at and would indicate that genes are spaced every 0.1-0.2 cM, or every 300 kb approximately. However, it has been suggested (Dove, 1987) that the frequency of transcribed regions is probably more frequent by a factor of 3-5 indicating a spacing of genes, on average, every 100 kb or less. The presence of ~30,000 methylation-free or HTF islands (CpG clusters 500-2,000 bp long that are highly undermethylated) in the mouse genome, many of which appear to be highly associated with transcribed sequences, would support this (Bird, 1986; Lindsday & Bird, 1987). The assumption is that any molecular map that could analyse the rich diversity of sequence organisation in the mammalian genome would need molecular map information spaced at least as frequently as the simplest functional sequence module we have so far observed - the gene. This implies that molecular maps would require markers every 100 kb or every 0.06 cM in genetic terms. Genetic mapping in mice to the level of 0.06 cM would require the analysis of at least 1,000 progeny from a suitable cross. Such experiments can only be performed on a limited basis.

However, new technologies which allow us to construct long-range physical restriction maps up to 5 Mb (see below) have meant that in preparing long-range molecular maps it has been sufficient to space clones genetically at the order of 1 cM and then to link them by physical means. Genetically-mapped clones provide start-points for the examination of neighbouring regions by physical mapping and the process of physical mapping itself identifies the HTF islands that are indicative of genic sequences and links the map into a coherent, continuous whole. The exact physical relationship of sequences, e.g. repeat sequences, in this map will allow us to pursue the nature of their interactions and the relationship of interaction to physical position.

Although we have assumed that our maps should be at least as detailed as the average gene spacing, this is not to imply that all the hierarchical sequence organisations are to be found at this level. The calculations above are merely averages and the absence of knowledge of their standard errors reflects our ignorance of the overall long-range organisation of mammalian chromosomes. But we have some hints. For example, it is known that a single human gene at the Duchenne muscular dystrophy locus extends over at least 1 Mb (Monaco & Kunkel, 1986) and, as we will see below, there appear to be very large (~1 Mb) euchromatic regions of the mouse genome highly saturated with non-genic repeat sequences.

<u>Microdissection and Microcloning of Clones for the Genetic</u>

<u>Mapping of Mouse Chromosomes</u>

In order to map a particular region of a mammalian chromosome, we require a set of molecular clones from that region of the chromosome. Molecular clones specific to an individual

chromosome have in the past been produced by flow-sorting of
chromosomes (Davies et al., 1981); species-specific repeat
screening of a library of clones from a somatic cell hybrid
containing the chromosome on a background of unrelated
chromosomes (Bishop et al., 1983); similar analyses of DNA
libraries produced from selected chromosome mediated gene
transfectants of somatic cells (Pritchard & Goodfellow, 1987).
However, the most direct technique is that of microdissection and
microcloning (Brown, 1985). Microdissection involves the direct
physical dissection of the pertinent chromosome region and
microcloning of the DNA isolated from the collected chromosome
fragments utilising special microprocedures. A number of
mammalian chromosome regions have been microcloned by us and
others, notably the mouse t-complex on chromosome 17 (Rohme et
al., 1984); a proximal region of the mouse X chromosome (Fisher
et al., 1985; see Fig. 1); a proximal region of mouse chromosome
7 (Greenfield & Brown, 1987) and the distal half of the short arm
of human chromosome 2 (Bates et al., 1986). In order to
genetically map the clones from chromosomes 7 and X in the mouse
we have taken advantage of the ability to perform an
interspecific backcross utilising wild Mus spretus mice and
inbred Mus domesticus strains (Robert et al., 1985). The high
level of divergence between domesticus and spretus allows the
detection of abundant restriction fragment length variants
between the genomes of the two species. Domesticus females mated
with spretus males produce fertile female progeny which can be
backcrossed to domesticus males and the segregation of spretus
and domesticus variants scored. Incorporation of known coat-
texture or coat-colour mutations in the cross provides a ready
system for positioning microclones on the genetic map. On the
mouse X chromosome (see Fig. 1) microclones have been mapped with
respect to the Tabby (Ta) and Harlequin (Hq) mutations
(Brockdorff et al., 1987a, b) and on mouse chromosome 7 (see Fig.
2) with respect to the pink-eye (p) and chinchilla (c^{ch})
mutations (Greenfield & Brown, 1987). In addition, the genetic
linkage of microclones with respect to each other is determined
and, by utilising a simple multipoint analysis the genetic and,
of course, the physical order of clones is uncovered. In this
way on the mouse X chromosome (Fig. 1) a large number of clones
have been mapped and ordered to the proximal region.

The genetic mapping of a number of microclones and other DNA
probes to the proximal region of the mouse X chromosome and mouse
chromosome 7 has already begun to delineate some interesting
genetic relationships. On the mouse X, an exonic probe from the
human Duchenne muscular dystrophy gene (DMD, Fig. 1) maps
provocatively close to a mouse X-linked muscular dystrophy
mutation (mdx) and surprisingly distant from spf, the mouse
homologue of the OTC (ornithine transcarbamylase) gene
(Brockdorff et al., 1987a). On the human X chromosome OTC and
DMD are closely-linked. Whether or not DMD and mdx are
homologous genetic loci, on the mouse X chromosome there appears
to be some clustering of genes involved in muscle phenotype: DMD
and mdx, Phk (a locus controlling expression of phosphorylase
kinase in skeletal muscle) and the mouse homologue to Emery-

6

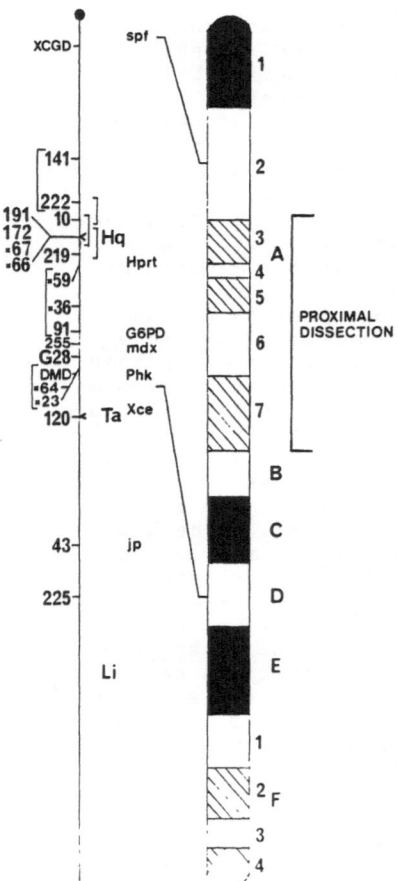

Fig. 1. Molecular map of the mouse X chromosome.
The genetic map positions of microclones and gene probes on the
mouse X chromosome are illustrated to the left of the genetic
map. To the right of the genetic map is shown the relative
positions of the Hq and Ta loci used in the interspecific cross.
The concordance between the physical and genetic maps of the   X
chromosome is indicated in two instances.

Dreifuss muscular dystrophy which likely maps in the mouse-human conserved linkage group Hprt-G6pd. On mouse chromosome 7, it has been reported that a Na,K-ATPase subunit gene (Atpa-2) maps to the proximal region (Kent et al., 1987). We have confirmed this mapping: the gene must map close to the pudgy locus - a locus involved in somitogenesis. Pudgy mutants show defective segmentation during somite formation and the ensuing adults have a fused, chaotic vertebral skeleton. Interestingly, it has been reported that ATPase antagonists can interfere with proper somite segregation (Gruneberg, 1961).

PFGE Mapping - Long Range Physical Mapping of Chromosomes

On the mouse X chromosome, 17 clones have been mapped over a proximal region of some 30 cM that extends from 141 to Ta (Fig. 1). On average the clones are spaced less than 2 cM apart and at a distance whereby the clones may be physically linked by Pulse Field Gel Electrophoresis (PGFE) mapping.

As a result of the extensive CpG methylation in mammalian genomes, a number of restriction enzymes, particularly those with recognition sequences rich in CpG, cut infrequently in the genome and mainly at the HTF islands associated with genes (see above). These so-called rare cutter enzymes produce very large restriction fragments ranging from 100 kb to >5 Mb. The large rare cutter restriction fragments are separable on agarose gels by PFGE. In this way, restriction maps can be constructed over very large genetic distances (Burmeister & Lehrach, 1986). The density of microclones mapped on the mouse X chromosome means that there is a good possibility of physically linking these clones by PFGE and incorporating them into a long-range, genetically-orientated, physical map of the mouse X chromosome. This work has already begun to identify unusual long-range sequence structures on the mouse X chromosome.

A REPEAT SEQUENCE ISLAND ON THE MOUSE X CHROMOSOME

One of the microclones, 141, mapped to the X chromosome (Fig. 1) detects a novel sequence organisation - a repeat sequence island: a small family of repeat sequences that is genetically and physically localised to a small euchromatic region of the X chromosome. The 141 sequence is itself part of a longer complex repeat unit of which there are approximatley 50 copies in the Mus domesticus genome. All fifty copies are inherited as a single Mendelian locus in the interspecific backcrosses used for X-chromosome mapping indicating they are genetically finely-localised on the mouse X. In addition, pulse-field restriction mapping of the 141 sequences indicates they are physically finely-localised on the X chromosome. All 141 sequences are localised within a single SacII restriction fragment less than 1 Mb in size (Fig. 3). Three other rare cutter restriction enzymes also fail to cut within the island (Fig. 3) - all 141 sequences are contained within single large (>1 Mb) restriction fragments.

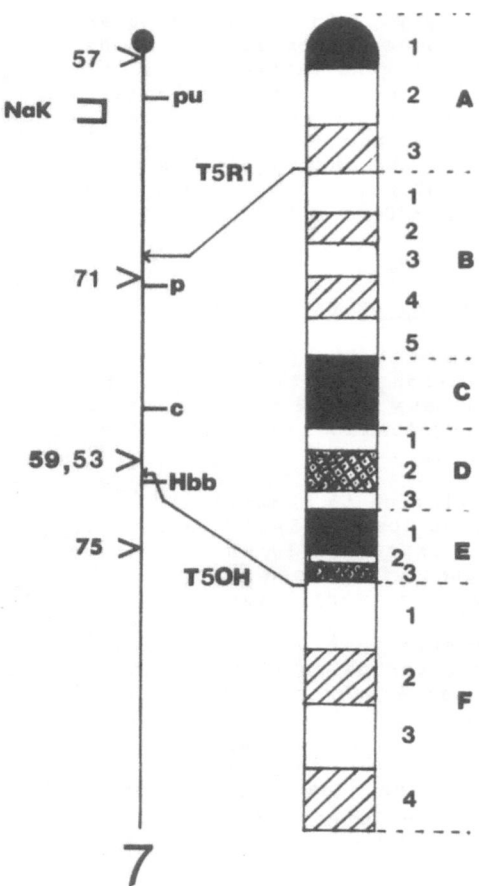

Fig. 2. Genetic and physical maps of mouse chromosome 7.
The positions of microclones and other mapped probes are
indicated on the left-hand side of the genetic map (NaK = Na,K-
ATPase probe). The translocation breakpoints T5R1 and T5OH offer
a comparison between the physical and genetic maps.

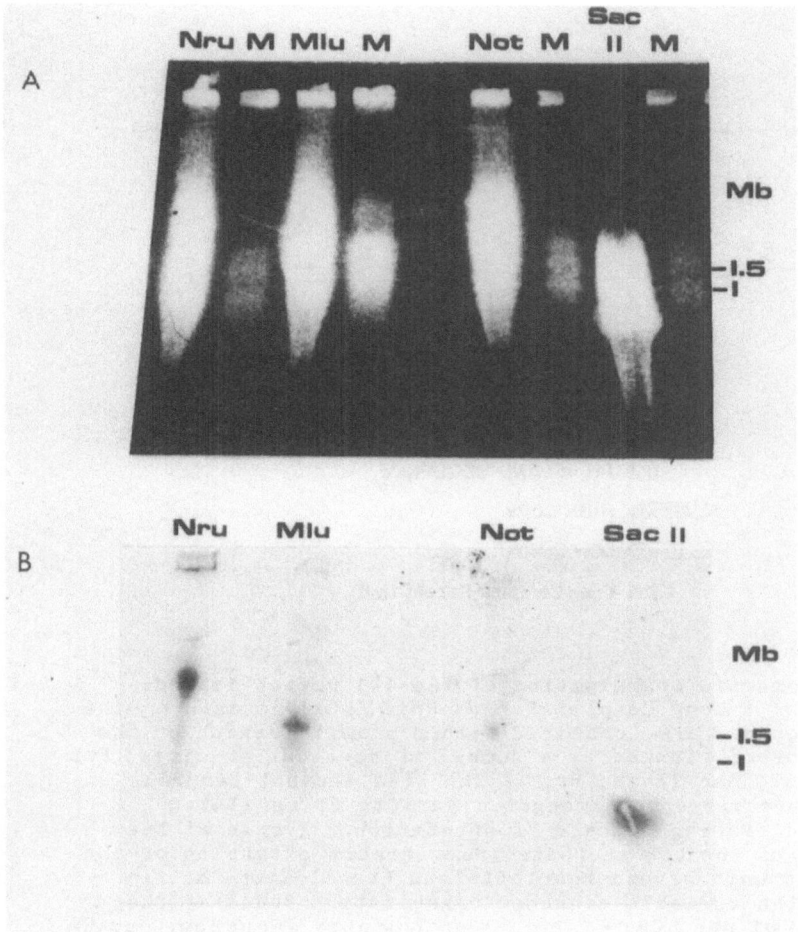

Fig. 3. a) **Pulse-field gel electrophoresis of four rare cutter digests (Nru I, Mlu I, Not I, Sac II) of mouse C57B1/10 high molecular weight DNA.** Large restriction fragments (>500 kb) were separated in an agarose gel on an orthogonal field gel electrophoresis apparatus using a long pulse time (1 hour). Marker tracks (M) carry yeast chromosomes from H. wingei. Three groups of chromosomes are observed - the two larger groups of approximately 1 Mb and 1.5 Mb in size.
b) **Southern hybridisation of the 141 microclone to Nru I, Mlu I, Not I and Sac II digests of C57B1/10 DNA separated by PFGE as shown above (Fig.2a).** In each case, only a single hybridising band is observed.

There appears to be a low abundance of rare cutter sites within the repeat island and therefore an absence of detectable HTF islands that is in contrast to the calculated average separation of transcribed sequences and HTF islands on the genome of 100 kb (see above) suggesting this is a relatively large, euchromatic region of the mouse genome devoid of expressed sequences.

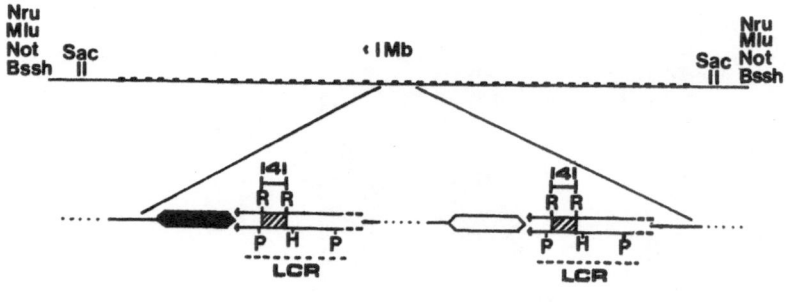

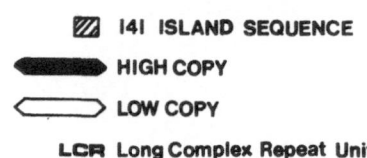

▨ 141 ISLAND SEQUENCE

◆ HIGH COPY

◇ LOW COPY

LCR Long Complex Repeat Unit

Fig. 4 Diagrammatic organisation of the 141 repeat island.
Fifty copies of a Long Complex Repeat Unit (LCR) containing the
141 island sequence are localised within a small region of the
mouse X chromosome flanked by a number of rare cutter sites: Not
I, Mlu I, Nru I, Sac II and Bssh. The LCRs are not tandemly
repeated but are dispersed amongst a variety of unrelated
sequences of differing degrees of repetition. Arrows at the
left-hand end of the LCR indicate the variable extension of the
complex repeat unit beyond the left-hand Pvu II site that is
reflected in the variable sequence organisation found at the
left-hand end of the LCR: high copy or low copy sequences can be
found in restriction fragments directly adjacent to the LCR. The
limits of the LCR in the other direction are not established
(indicated by dashes).

Interestingly, in the _spretus_ genome only a few copies of the
homologous sequence are present again entirely at the same X
chromosomal locus. No 141 homologous sequences are found in the
chinese hamster or human genomes indicating that the repeat
island has arisen recently in evolutionary time.

The long complex repeat unit that contains the 141 sequence is
not tandemly organised within the repeat island but dispersed
within the island amongst a variety of sequences of differing
degrees of repetition (Fig. 4). However, the close physical
proximity of the complex repeat units suggests that the 141
island may have arisen by a process of unequal crossing-over.

Nevertheless, the dispersion of 141 sequences amongst other unrelated sequences suggests that a concommitant scrambling process of integration or transposition is occurring within the island. In support of this, it appears that there is considerable variability amongst the members of the repeat family at one end of the complex repeat unit, and this is in contrast to the relatively conserved organisation at the core of the repeat unit (Fig. 4). This suggests that during evolution of the repeat island there may have been frequent encroachment or rearrangement of sequences at one end of the unit.

What has predisposed this sequence region to such rapid amplification is not yet clear. Whether it is the 141 sequence itself or other sequences within the long complex repeat unit or, alternatively, unrelated sequences within the island is not known. Perhaps a comparison with sequences at the homologous locus in spretus may yet resolve this point and also identify what consequences the amplified domesticus island has for chromosome structure. The genetic consequences to the chromosome of such a repeat sequence organisation are unclear at present.

CONCLUSIONS

Long range genetic and physical mapping of the mouse genome has not only begun to define the genetic and physical relationship of a number of genetic loci but has also delineated unusual organisations of small localised families of complex repeat units. It is clear that this fresh panoramic view of the genome has begun to uncover long-range chromosomal properties previously unobserved by classic DNA studies.

ACKNOWLEDGEMENTS

Much of the work was supported by grants from the Medical Research Council of Great Britain, the Nuffield Foundation and Birthright.

REFERENCES

Bates, G.P., Wainwright, B.J., Williamson, R. and Brown, S.D.M. (1986) Microdissection of and microcloning from the short arm of human chromosome 2. Mol. Cell Biol. 6: 826-3830.
Bird, A.P. (1986) CpG-rich islands and the function of DNA methylation. Nature 321: 209-213.
Bishop, C.E., Guellaen, G., Geldwerth, D., Voss, R., Fellous, M. and Weissenbach, J. (1983) Single-copy DNA sequences specific for the human Y chromosome. Nature 303: 831-832.
Brockdorff, N., Cross, G., Cavanna, J., Fisher, E.M.C., Lyon, M.F., Davies, K.E. and Brown, S.D.M. (1987a) The mapping of a cDNA from the human X-linked Duchenne muscular dystrophy gene to the mouse X chromosome. Nature 328: 166-168.

Brockdorff, N., Fisher, E.M.C., Cavanna, J., Lyon, M.F. and
   Brown, S.D.M. (1987b) Construction of a detailed molecular map of
   the mouse X chromosome by microcloning and interspecific crosses.
   EMBO J. 6: 329-13297.
Brown, S.D.M. (1985) Mapping mammalian chromosomes: new
   technologies for old problems. Trends Genet. 1: 219-220.
Burmeister, M. and Lehrach, H. (1986) Long-range restriction map
   around the Duchenne muscular dystrophy gene. Nature 324: 582-
   585.
Davies, K.E., Young, B.D., Elles, R.G., Hill, M.E. and
   Williamson, R. (1981) Cloning of a representative genomic library
   of the human X chromosome after sorting by flow cytometry.
   Nature 293: 374-376.
Dove, W.F. (1987) Molecular genetics of Mus musculus; point
   mutagenesis and millimorgans. Genetics 116: 5-8.
Fisher, E.M.C., Cavanna, J.S. and Brown, S.D.M. (1985)
   Microdissection and microcloning of the mouse X chromosome. Proc.
   Natl. Acad. Sci. USA 82: 5846-5849.
Greenfield, A.J. and Brown, S.D.M. (1987) Microdissection and
   microcloning from the proximal region of mouse chromosome 7:
   isolation of clones genetically linked to the pudgy locus.
   Genomics, in press.
Gruneberg, H. (1961) Genetical studies on the skeleton of the
   mouse XXIX Pudgy. Genet. Res. 2: 384-393.
Kent, R.B., Fallows, D.A., Geissler, E., Glaser, T., Emanuel,
   J.R., Lalley, P.A., Levenson, R. and Housman, D.E. (1987) Genes
   encoding α and β subunits of Na,K-ATPase are located on three
   different chromosomes in the mouse. Proc. Natl. Acad. Sci. USA.
   84: 5369-5373.
Lindsay, S. and Bird, A.P. (1987) Use of restriction enzymes to
   detect potential gene sequences in mammalian DNA. Nature 327:
   336-338.
Monaco, A.P. and Kunkel, L.M. (1987) A giant locus for the
   Duchenne and Becker muscular dystrophy gene. Trends Genet. 3:
   33-37.
Pritchard, C.A. and Goodfellow, P.N. (1987) Investigation of
   chromosome-mediated gene transfer using the HPRT region of the
   human X chromosome as a model. Genes and Development 1: 172-178.
Robert, B., Barton, P., Minty, A., Daubos, P., Weydert, A.
   Bonhomme, F., Catalan, J., Chazottes, C., Guenet, J-L. and
   Buckingham, M. (1985) Investigation of genetic linkage between
   myosin and actin genes using an interspecific mouse backcross.
   Nature 314: 181-183.
Rohme, D., Fox, H.J., Herrmann, B., Frischauf, A-M., Edstrom,
   J.E., Mains, P., Silver, L.M. and Lehrach, H. (1984) Molecular
   clones of the mouse t complex derived from microdissected
   metaphase chromosomes. Cell 36: 783-788.
Shedlovsky, A., Guenet, J.L., Johnson, L.L. and Dove, W.F. (1986)
   Induction of recessive lethal mutations in the T/t-H-2 region of
   the mouse genome by a point mutagen. Genet. Res. 47: 135-142.

The Use of Interspecific Mouse Crosses for Gene Localization: Present Status and Future Perspectives

J. L. Guénet[1], D. Simon-Chazottes[1], and P. R. Avner[2]

INTRODUCTION

The advent of recombinant DNA technology has suggested a new way
to define a very large number of polymorphic marker loci using
restriction endonucleases and specific DNA probes.
DNA restriction enzymes recognize specific DNA sequences and
catalyze endonucleolytic cleavages yielding fragments of various
(defined) lengths which may be visualized after size separation
by electrophoresis in agarose gels.
Using the method first reported by SOUTHERN et al (1975) the
fragments encoding specific sequences can be detected within a
large and complex population of DNA fragments by hybridization
with DNA probes labelled to very high specific radioactivity
allowing identification of single copy sequences in mammalian
DNA.
Restriction fragments are inherited as simple Mendelian
codominant markers and thus can be used for the purpose of
cartography.
For a specific endonuclease the restriction fragments produced
are, by definition, invariant within a given inbred mouse strain
whilst polymorphism sometimes occurs between two or more
different inbred strains. This results from many kinds of
genotypic differences: one or more individual bases can differ
resulting in loss of a cleavage site or, on the contrary,
formation of a new one ; alternatively insertion or deletion of
blocks of DNA (such as retroviruses, pseudogenes, etc..) within
a fragment can alter its size.
In the mouse, Restriction Fragment Length Polymorphisms (RFLP's)
can be detected in recombinant DNA's of different origins. DNA
from individual Recombinant Inbred Strains, for example, have
been studied in several laboratories where appropriate
polymorphisms exist between the two parental strains. The
quality of the information collected depends upon the number of
Recombinant Inbred Strains available.
This number unfortunately is generally not very large and, as
for a given set, the number of strains is generally small the
technique is of rather limited value.
"Sweeping" a much greater length of the chromosome by the use of
interstrain mouse backcrosses has proven more useful for the
localization of new probes especially when the parental strains
have been preselected for the existence of suitable RFLP's.
Unfortunately interstrain genetic divergence within laboratory

[1] Unité de Génétique des Mammifères, Institut Pasteur de PARIS.
25 Rue du Dr Roux 75724 PARIS Cedex 15 FRANCE
[2] Unité d'Immuno-génétique Humaine, Institut Pasteur de PARIS.
25 Rue du Dr Roux 75724 PARIS Cedex 15 FRANCE

Current Topics in Microbiology and Immunology, Vol. 137
© Springer-Verlag Berlin · Heidelberg 1988

animals is limited to such an extent (BONHOMME *et al* 1987)that some probes cannot be mapped using laboratory mouse strains while others require the use of rare (and expensive!) enzymes to produce useful RFLP's.
For this reason, we and others, have developed a new approach to cartography using both RFLP's and interspecific mouse crosses.

DIVERSITY WITHIN THE GENUS *Mus*.

Based on studies of the genetic variability of wild mice, and using both DNA and biochemical markers, the genus *Mus* can be divided up into a complex of species containing the four major biochemical groupings *Mus m. domesticus, Mus m. musculus, Mus m. castaneus* and *Mus m. bactrianus* (all of which can be treated as sub-species) and at least eight other species including three European species, the mound building mouse *Mus spicilegus*, the western Mediterranean mouse *Mus spretus* and the eastern Mediterranean short tailed mouse known as *Mus spretoides*.
The degree of fertility between the various groupings is correlated to the degree of taxa divergence, and ranges from complete sterility to reduced fertility.
None of the mice belonging to the different groupings within the complex species containing *Mus m. musculus* and *Mus m. domesticus* ever produce hybrids in the wild with mice belonging to other species even though, for example, *Mus m. domesticus* and *Mus spretus* mice can be found living sympatrically in France, Spain, Portugal, and North Africa. *Mus m. domesticus* and, of course, laboratory mice are however able to produce viable hybrids under laboratory conditions (natural matings or artificial insemination) with *Mus spretus, Mus spicilegus* and *Mus spretoides* mice.
This last observation has opened up the way for exploiting the considerable polymorphism and genetic variation accumulated in each of these species for genetic studies and particularly for the purpose of cartography.

INTERSPECIFIC BACKCROSSES INVOLVING *Mus spretus*

The major part of genetic analysis carried out using interspecies crosses has centered around *Mus spretus* derived strains since, compared to the other species or sub-species allowing the production of viable and fertile hybrids under standard laboratory conditions, *Mus spretus* shows the greatest degree of allelic variation when compared to laboratory mouse strains.
Interspecies crosses involving *Mus spretus* and laboratory mice are, for reasons of efficiency, normally set up using the laboratory mouse as female, although progeny can be obtained in both cross configurations. While the F1 females resulting are fertile and used to produce the backcross generation, F1 males are sterile.
Segregating backcross progeny born to such F1 females are first typed for all known and localized markers segregating, such as coat color alleles, cell surface antigens, biochemical markers and unique or anonymous cloned DNA fragments. A "Species Distribution Pattern" of the segregating polymorphism is then established by analogy with the <u>Strain</u> Distribution Pattern established for the Recombinant Inbred Strains (R.I.S.) of laboratory mice.

The RFLP obtained with a given probe and a given endonuclease is, in the same way, translated in terms of + or - according to whether the segment of DNA characteristic of the *Mus spretus* species is present or not. The +/- distribution pattern is matched to that of the already existing panel and with the help of a computer program, linkage with other loci eventually detected.

As increasing numbers of loci are placed on each individual chromosome, the entire haplotype of any given backcross animal becomes known and, with it, a knowledge of the recombination breakpoints having occurred on each chromosome during the single round of meiosis the animals have gone through.

VALIDITY AND ADVANTAGES OF THE MAPPING SYSTEM USING *Mus* INTERSPECIFIC CROSSES.

Over 50 different autosomal genes have been localized, in our laboratory, using a DNA panel obtained from 75 C57BL/6 X *Mus spretus* mice or 50 BALB/c X *Mus spretus* mice DNA panel. Each chromosome is now covered by at least one marker and certain autosomes such as chromosome 1,7,11,12,13,17 by considerably more. The chromosome which has been most extensively mapped using the *Mus spretus* system is however the X chromosome (AVNER *et al*, BROWN *et al*, CHAPMAN *et al* etc..) where over a 60 probes have been localized.

The mapping system using *Mus spretus* Hybrids seems to be very reliable. We, and others, have accumulated evidence that it probably does not introduce any widespread bias into gene localization. We have found, for example, that genes known to be syntenic on the basis of intraspecific genetic crosses also show cosegregation in interspecific crosses. Moreover the estimated genetic distances computed between certain loci using interspecific mouse crosses closely parallel those observed using classical crosses or R.I.S. analysis. CHAPMAN and coworkers have focussed on the use of known genetic markers on the X chromosome to map genes in inter- specific hybrids using both C57BL/6 x *Mus spretus* F1 females and C57BL/6 x *Mus musculus* F1 females. These markers include cDNA probes for ornithine transcarbamylase (*Otc*), tissue inhibitor of metallo-proteinases (*Timp*), hypoxanthine phosphoribosyl transferase (*Hprt*), coagulation factor IX (*Cf-9*), coagulation factor VIII (*Cf-8*), red-sensitive visual pigment (*Rsvp*), a genomic fragment closely associated with the human glucose-6-phosphate dehydrogenase (*G6pd*) locus, and an enzyme activity variant for alpha-galactosidase (*Ags*). The gene order for the 8 markers used did not differ between the two crosses and the overall frequency of recombination was the same in both backcrosses, with the established map distance of 52 cM between the two most distant markers (*Otc* and *Ags*) in both crosses.

Despite these results, the presence of localized and limited recombination "hot spots" in the *Mus spretus* genome, absent from laboratory mice, and affecting genetic distance evaluation cannot be totally excluded.

Mapping using *Mus spretus* hybrids is almost universally applicable. It can be applied in all circumstances where a probe is available since the discovery of a suitable restriction polymorphism is generally not a problem even with the cheapest and most common restriction enzymes. Moreover results collected from former analysis substantiate future ones.

The mapping system using *Mus spretus* hybrids is <u>easy to apply</u> since it only requires repetitive use of a single simple technique. DNA "blots" can be used over and over as long as hybridization is not impaired by repeated washings.

The mapping system using *Mus spretus* hybrids moreover has <u>no upper limit</u> since results from experiment n can be added to those of experiments n-1, n-2, etc… It must be kept in mind however that the resolution of the genetic map depends <u>exclusively</u> upon the total number of cross-overs collected within the backcross genomes. Ordering loci on a map requires, by definition, that at least one recombination event split the parental arrangements.

DRAWBACKS OF THE MAPPING SYSTEM USING *Mus* INTERSPECIFIC CROSSES.

The mapping system using *Mus spretus* hybrids, aside from its several advantages, has however a few drawbacks that must be mentioned here.

It must be noted first that, F1 males being sterile, it is not possible to investigate meiotic products produced by them. The genetic distances computed thus results exclusively from analysis of the female gametes.

For the same reason it is not possible to analyze the X-Y pairing region and it is not possible to develop efficiently, at least with *Mus spretus* as a sexual partner, Recombinant Inbred Strains in order to preserve and propagate forever the "scrambled" genomes that geneticists are so fond of.

Finally the main drawback concerning the use of the mouse interspecific hybrids for the purpose of mapping is due to the fact that DNA stocks prepared from the backcross progeny are limited in amount and become exhausted precisely when the "Species Distribution Pattern" characterizing a set of animals is extensively documented.

POSSIBLE IMPROVEMENTS TO THE MAPPING SYSTEM USING *Mus* INTERSPECIFIC CROSSES.

While *Mus spretus* interspecific hybrids are regularly male sterile and sometimes relatively difficult to produce under laboratory conditions it must be kept in mind that several highly inbred lines of *Mus musculus musculus* are available. These lines represent an interesting source of polymorphism which should be borne in mind, even if hybrid sterility problems can again occur, for making R.I.Strains the DNA of which would be available in unlimited quantities.

Technical "tricks", like developing extensively re-usable blots, simultaneously hybridizing with several non-overlapping DNA probes on the same blot, using moderately repeated DNA sequences dispersed within the mouse genome or using *Mus spretus* specific DNA sequences on "dot-blots" may be considered as valuable improvements aimed at saving DNA particularly when a rough localization is sufficient.

We have recently undertaken the production of embryos,trisomic for specific chromosomes that are compatible with a long lifespan, the triplicated chromosome having three different origins (*Mus spretus, Mus m.musculus, Mus m. domesticus*), with the idea that it should be possible to use these unbalanced genomes for the detection of chromosomal syntenies.

CONCLUSIONS

The technique of cartography using *Mus spretus* hybrids does not represents the sort of breakthrough in mouse mapping methodology that the discovery of RFLP's did seven years ago. It should be considered more as an improvement taking advantage of a favorable situation, which may be specific to the mouse: the possibility to obtain viable and fertile interspecific hybrids. It has nevertheless opened the way for considerable refinements in establishing the mouse genetic map since, due to considerable evolutionary divergence, the genetic polymorphism between this species and laboratory strains is very great.

REFERENCES

Avner PR, Amar L, Arnaud D, Hanauer A, and Cambrou J (1987): Detailed ordering of markers localizing to the Xq26-Xqter region of the human X chromosome by use of an interspecific *Mus spretus* mouse cross Proc. Natl. Acad. Sci 84:1629-1633

Avner PR, Amar L, Dandolo L, Guénet JL: The impact of interspecific *Mus spretus* crosses on knowledge of the Mouse X chromosome and autosomes Trends in Genetics in Press January 1988

Bonhomme F, and Guénet JL (*in press*) The wild house mouse and its relatives in Genetic variant and strains of the laboratory mouse Ed. LYON MF and SEARLE AG Oxford University Press

Botstein D, White RL, Skolnick M, Davis RW (1980): Construction of a genetic linkage map in man using restriction fragment length polymorphisms Am. J. Hum.Genet.32:314-331

Brockdorff N, Fisher EMC, Cavanna JS, Lyon MF and Brown SDM (1987): Construction of a detailed molecular map of the mouse X chromosome by microcloning and interspecific crosses The EMBO Journal Vol.6 number 11

Chapman V (1987) Private communication Mouse News letter

Guénet JL (1986) The contribution of wild derived mouse inbred strains to gene mapping methodology Current topics Microbiol. Immunol. 127:109-113.

Robert B, Barton P, Minty A, Daubas P, Weydert A, Bonhomme F, Catalan J, Chazottes D, Guénet JL, Buckingham M (1985): Investigation of genetic linkage between myosin and actin genes using an interspecific mouse backcross Nature 314:181-183

Southern EM (1975): Detection of specific sequences among DNA fragments separated by gel electrophoresis.J. Mol. Biol.98:503-517

X-Chromosome Gene Order in Different *Mus* Species Crosses

D.A. Stephenson, S.G. Grant, L.J. Mullins, A.E. Scolese, A.J. O'Reilly, and V.M. Chapman

INTRODUCTION

The advent of molecular genetics heralds a new era in linkage analysis. It is now possible to map any locus and define its linkage relationship within the mammalian genome using a single set of informative offspring. This new mapping methodology, which has been used successfully to map both autosomal genes (Roberts et al., 1985; Bućan et al., 1986; Heidmann et al., 1986; Nadeau et al., 1986; Reeves et al., 1987; Seldin et al., 1987) and sex-linked loci (Amar et al., 1985; Avner et al., 1987a; Avner et al., 1987b; Brockdorff et al., 1987; Chamberlain et al., 1987; Heilig et al., 1987), utilizes naturally occurring polymorphisms at the level of the nucleotide sequence between inbred strains of mice and those derived from the wild species *Mus spretus* and *Mus musculus* (Brown, 1985; Guénet, this publication).

In their study of chromosome 4, Nadeau et al. (1986) suggested there was a potential rearrangement in gene order between the laboratory mouse and wild-derived M. spretus. Additional data now suggests that there may also be a difference in the arrangement of genes within the t-complex on chromosome 17 (Silver, this publication). The t complex, however, is quite unusual in that inversional rearrangements have been reported even among closely related M. musculus and M. domesticus populations in the wild (Klein et al., 1984). If rearrangements in gene order have occurred between the more evolutionary divergent Mus species it may limit the usefulness of interspecific crosses for ordering genes within the mouse genome. Structural rearrangements in the genome may be an important mechanism for the maintenance of speciation since they (i) inhibit illegitimate recombination which might otherwise lead to a loss or duplication of information and (ii) affect normal chromosomal assortment. Presumably the more divergent the species the greater the probability of structural rearrangements in the organization of genetic information. If there are such rearrangements among the Mus species they are not cytogenetically detectable, since karyotypic analysis suggests that there is little if any difference in the physical appearance of chromosomes between diverse Mus species (Hsu et al., 1978). In fact, the inversional events associated with the t complex escape cytogenetic detection (Womack and Roderick, 1974). The inbred and wild-derived genomes also differ at the molecular level in the number, type and placement of repeated sequence families (Sutton and McCallum, 1972; Siracusa, 1983), perhaps to the extent that they may interfere with normal synaptonemal pairing during meiotic prophase. This reduced homology could affect chromosome pairing at meiosis, and produce significant changes in the frequency of recombinations, leading to alterations in map distances across a chromosome.

In an attempt to address the issues of (i) interspecies variation in gene order, and (ii) possible differences in relative recombination frequencies within interspecific crosses, such crosses were constructed between the inbred laboratory strain C57BL/6JRos and two different wild-derived Mus species: M. musculus and M. spretus. The M. musculus stock was an outbred colony originally established from three trapping locations in Denmark (Nielsen and Chapman, 1977). These mice readily interbreed with laboratory strains in reciprocal crosses, and both sexes of the resulting F_1 progeny are fertile. Analysis of major and minor satellite sequences and dispersed repeated elements shows no qualitative differences between these mice and laboratory strains (Siracusa, 1983). The M. spretus stock was an outbred colony originally trapped in Spain and France (Chapman et al., 1983). Interbreeding with laboratory strains is restricted in these mice, and only the F_1 females are fertile. Furthermore, M. spretus differs from laboratory strains in the relative abundance of

Department of Molecular and Cellular Biology, Roswell Park Memorial Institute, 666 Elm Street, Buffalo, NY 14263, USA.

centromeric major and minor satellite sequences (Brown and Dover, 1980; Siracusa, 1983), and in the cross-reactivity of dispersed repeated sequence probes from laboratory strain genomic DNA.

For reasons of historical interest, we began our study by examining markers on the mouse X chromosome. The region examined in our study extends from the most proximal marker ornithine transcarbamoylase (Otc/spf; sparse-fur) to alpha-galactosidase (Ags), spanning an estimated 60 cM of the mouse X chromosome (Lyon, 1987), with the intervening markers hypoxanthine phosphoribosyl transferase (Hprt), clotting factor-9 (Cf-9), clotting factor-8 (Cf-8), glucose-6-phosphate dehydrogenase (G6pd) and red-sensitive visual pigment (Rsvp).

In excess of one hundred males (with an equivalent number of females) were generated in each backcross study between F_1 females and C57BL/6JRos males (Figure 1). Genomic DNA from the spleen of each mouse was prepared for analysis. The DNA was digested with a restriction endonuclease which revealed species-specific polymorphisms for Otc, Hprt, Cf-9, Cf-8, G6pd, Rsvp and Ags upon Southern analysis (Mullins et al., manuscript submitted). Restriction fragment length polymorphisms were detected in both wild-derived Mus species using a battery of five commonly available restriction endonucleases. Enzyme activity and stability assays were also used in the classification of the Ags locus, and Hprt results were confirmed by isozyme analysis (Chapman et al., 1983). Males were used exclusively in this instance to provide unequivocal characterization of each locus.

FIGURE 1: Breeding protocol used in the generation of backcross progeny involving the inbred strain C57BL/6JRos and either M. spretus or M. musculus.

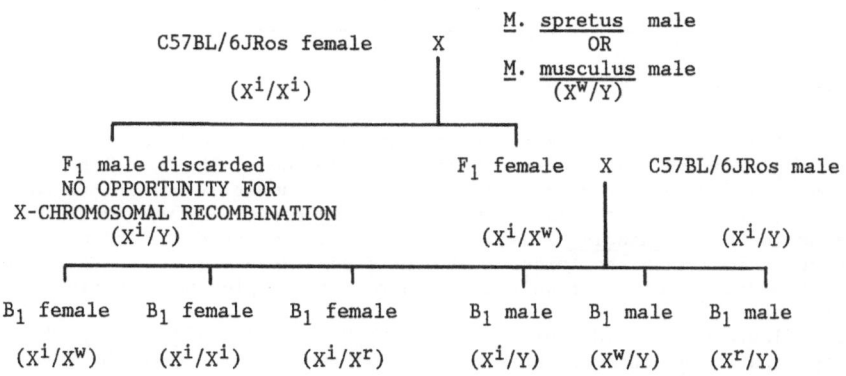

X^i,X^w,X^r: inbred, wild-derived, and recombinant X chromosomes respectively

SEGREGATION OF ALLELES

It is important to assure that proper segregation of alleles is occurring in these interspecific crosses, because any deviation from the expected Mendelian mode of inheritance would suggest a selective bias in the sample, as is frequently seen with certain t haplotypes (Lyon and Meredith, 1964). Such a distortion could, if unrecognized, have a significant impact on both gene order and estimated map distances. Although it is difficult to perceive that the loci examined in our study would have an impact on the segregation of alleles, the use of wild-derived mouse species could introduce factors, as yet undefined, which in turn could lead to the selection of a biased sample. A reduction in fecundity, as seen in some crosses involving M. spretus, such as BALB/cJ x M. spretus (unpublished observations), may be indicative of such selection factors.

As demonstrated in Table 1, no significant deviations from the expected Mendelian segregation ratios were observed for any of the seven loci examined in either backcross, suggesting there was no overt bias in the mice sampled. Furthermore, no distortion in sex ratio was detected in the progeny of either cross. Similarly, segregation of alleles for loci spanning an estimated 30 cM on chromosome 6 involving a M. spretus backcross (Bućan et al., 1987) are consistent with a Mendelian mode of inheritance. Analysis of a limited number of autosomal loci encompassing chromosomes 2, 7 and 8 suggest that chromosomal assortment may also be occurring normally (unpublished data). We conclude, therefore, that there is little evidence to suggest that the use of the wild-derived Mus species have any significant impact on sample bias.

TABLE 1: Segregation of sex-linked genes in backcrosses using wild-derived M. spretus and M. musculus.

Locus	M. spretus	χ^2	M. musculus	χ^2
Otc	50	0.00	50	0.09
Hprt	52	0.16	54	0.24
Cf-9	55	1.00	58	1.64
Cf-8	58	2.56	57	1.17
G6pd	58	2.56	57	1.17
Rsvp	58	2.56	57	1.17
Ags	49	0.04	58	1.64
	N = 100		N = 103	

X-CHROMOSOMAL GENE ORDER

The gene order for all seven X-linked marker loci was determined by minimizing the number of multiple recombinant events across the chromosome. The most likely gene order was the same for both crosses, and minimized the number of multiple recombinant events to four double recombinations in the M. spretus cross and two double recombinations in the M. musculus cross. With this gene order there are no triple or greater recombinations in either cross. Alternate gene orders greatly increased the number of double recombinations required, or introduced triple recombinations.

Our results indicate a gene order of Otc, Hprt, Cf-9, (Cf-8/G6pd/Rsvp), Ags for both the M. spretus and the M. musculus backcrosses. No recombinants were observed between G6pd, Cf-8 and Rsvp in either cross, which precludes the assignment of a gene order for these loci. The absence of recombination between these three loci in both crosses indicates either that they are tightly linked on the X chromosomes of both wild-derived species, or that there may be some undetermined factor, such as a small chromosomal rearrangement, impairing recombination in this region. The identical ordering of loci along the length of the chromosome, however, indicates that no major rearrangements in X-chromosomal genetic material has taken place since the divergence of the two wild-derived parental species.

RECOMBINATION DISTANCES

A comparison of overall recombination across the X chromosome between our two crosses demonstrates that the frequency of recombination between the two most distant markers tested, Otc and Ags, does not significantly differ (χ^2=2.264). Indeed, there were no significant differences apparent in any pairwise comparison between the two crosses, suggesting that the overall pattern of recombination was the same in both systems

(Table 2). A statistical treatment of certain intervals is given in Table 3. Thus, not only do our two crosses yield the same absolute gene order, but, based on recombination frequencies, these genes are similarly spaced along the chromosome. We can therefore detect no evolutionary alterations between the M. spretus and M. musculus X chromosomes. It must be noted that we can make no such conclusions about either wild-derived X chromosome and that of the inbred C57BL/6JRos laboratory strain. Indeed, if the clustering of the three loci for G6pd, Cf-8 and Rsvp is due to a small chromosomal rearrangement, then the two wild-derived stocks must have similar rearrangements in this region.

TABLE 2: Frequency of recombinants between marker loci.

Interval	M. spretus	M. musculus
Otc-Hprt	12	15
Hprt-Cf-9	3	6
Cf-9-G6pd*	9	7
G6pd-Ags	28	22
	N = 100	N = 103

* G6pd/Cf-8/Rsvp cluster

PERSPECTIVE AND CONCLUSIONS

The use of two diverse Mus species, M. musculus and M. spretus, in crosses with a single inbred strain, C57BL/6JRos, has resulted in backcross progeny which provide identical X-chromosome gene orders and very similar gene maps. No evidence was found to suggest the selection of a biased sample in either backcross. These findings suggest that the basic order of X-chromosome genes is similar between evolutionarily distinct Mus species.

The map order of Otc, Hprt, Cf-9, (Cf-8/G6pd/Rsvp), Ags was established by minimizing the number of multiple recombinant events. Any other combination merely served to increase the frequency of multiple recombinants. This approach is only feasible following complete analysis of the data set, as it provides unequivocal evidence for the appropriate order, without resorting to statistical estimations of "best-fit". Moreover, multilocus characterization of each recombinant establishes a valid secondary linkage testing scheme to place additional loci on the X chromosome relative to other genes. In that sense, these are cumulative resources which can contribute to the eventual establishment of a fully delineated X chromosome.

The order defined for Otc, Hprt, G6pd, and Ags in these backcrosses is consistent with that on the current linkage map of the mouse (Lyon, 1987). Similarly, the relative position of Cf-9 between Hprt and G6pd in our studies is in agreement with that reported by Avner et al., (1987a), also employing M. spretus in a backcross study. Thus our observations, in which all genes were mapped concurrently in the same set of animals, substantiate the putative gene order obtained from the compilation of data generated by many independent mapping studies, using two, three and four point crosses among inbred strains. Although gene order appears to be maintained within our two crosses, it should be emphasized that genetic information may be specifically conserved across species barriers on the X chromosome (Ohno, 1969; Lalley and McKusick, 1985), and as such, rearrangements in gene order may be less likely to occur on this chromosome than on the autosomes.

Comparison of the recombination fractions with those observed in both backcrosses of the present study suggest that they are consistent with published data (Table 3).

The Hprt-Cf-9 and Hprt-G6pd comparisons were again based upon data presented by Avner et al., (1987a), using M. spretus in a backcross study, and therefore would not be expected to yield very different results, unless there were significant differences between the two M. spretus stocks. The fact that the data are comparable demonstrates the cumulative nature of these two independent interspecific crosses, making it possible to amalgamate the data and thus generate a better estimate of map distance for the common loci. Similarly, the Hprt-Ags recombination fractions were in concordance with the published data using congenic strains carrying enzymic polymorphisms for these two loci (Chapman et al., 1983). Whilst this might be perceived as evidence supporting the use of wild-derived species in mapping studies of the mouse genome, it should be noted that the allelic variants used by Chapman et al., (1983) were originally derived from feral stocks, and as such do not necessarily constitute a significant deviation from the crosses used in the present study.

TABLE 3: Comparison of the number of recombinants between Hprt and Ags.

INTERVAL	PRESENT STUDY		χ^2	PUBLISHED DATA	χ^2
	M. spretus	M. musculus			
Hprt-Ags	40/100	35/103	0.789	27/82[b]	1.210
Hprt-Cf-9	3/100	6/103	0.405[a]	3/98[c]	1.382
Hprt-G6pd	12/100	13/103	0.018	21/186[c]	0.116

[a] with Yates' correction
[b] Chapman et al., (1983) d.f. 2
[c] Avner et al., (1987a) d.f. 2

Our results suggest that the relatively greater period of separation between M. spretus and C57BL/6JRos compared with M. musculus or other laboratory strains does not impair meiotic recombination to a significant degree. Whether this is true of the entire X chromosome, particularly the X:Y pairing region, remains to be tested.

While in our study we have confined ourselves to an examination of gene order and recombination on the X chromosome, these backcross animals should be equally polymorphic for autosomal markers. Numerous examples exist, in both mouse (Davisson & Roderick, 1981) and man (Donis-Keller et al., 1987), of differences in the recombination frequency between loci depending upon the gender of the informative heterozygote. Why this should be is a matter for speculation, but it may well reflect differences in gametogenesis between the two sexes. Such observations emphasize the importance of performing reciprocal crosses for mapping autosomal loci. Such considerations are not important for X-linked genes, since recombination between X chromosomes can only occur in the female. Thus far only M. spretus has been used extensively in interspecific crosses to map a large number of genes. This species was chosen because of its evolutionary distance from the laboratory derived mouse strains, thus increasing the possibility of sequence divergence (Brown, 1985). In our hands, M. musculus has proven equally useful, yielding as much detectable sequence polymorphism with common restriction enzymes as M. spretus (unpublished observations). M. musculus is potentially more closely related to M. domesticus, from which the inbred strains are purported to be derived (Marshall, 1981; Ferns et al., 1982) than M. spretus (Bonhomme et al., 1984). It has been suggested, however, that laboratory mice may in fact be "multi-racial", in that they are derived from several different Mus species, including M. musculus (Blank et al., 1986). Unlike M. spretus, M. musculus interbreeds freely with the laboratory derived mouse strains. Thus, M. musculus may prove as useful as M. spretus for mapping studies, if not more so, because of the possibility of performing reciprocal crosses.

This work was supported in part by NIH grants GM 33160 and GM 24125.

REFERENCES

Amar LC, Arnaud D, Cambrou J, Guenet J-L, Avner PR (1985) Mapping of the mouse X chromosome using random genetic probes and an interspecific mouse cross. EMBO J 4:3695-3700

Avner P, Amar L, Arnaud D, Hanauer A, Cambrou J (1987a) Detailed ordering of markers localizing to the Xq26-Xqter region of the human X chromosome by use of an interspecific Mus spretus mouse cross. Proc Natl Acad Sci USA 84:1629-1633

Avner P, Bucan M, Arnaud D, Lehrach H, Rapp U (1987b) A-raf oncogene localized on mouse X chromosome to region some 10-17 centimorgans proximal to hypoxanthine phosphoribosyltransferase gene. Somat Cell Mol Genet 13:267-272

Blank RD, Campbell GR, D'Eustachio P (1986) Possible derivation of the laboratory genome from multiple wild Mus species. Genetics 114:1257-1269

Bonhomme F, Catalan J, Britton-Davidian J, Chapman VM, Moriwaki K, Nevo E, Thaler L (1984) Biochemical diversity and evolution in the genus Mus. Biochem Genet 22:275-303

Brockdorff N, Cross GS, Cavanna JS, Fisher EMC, Lyon MF, Davies KE, Brown SDM (1987) The mapping of a cDNA from the human X-linked Duchenne muscular dystrophy gene to the mouse X chromosome. Nature 328:166-168

Brown SDM (1985) Mapping mammalian chromosomes: new technologies for old problems. Trends Genet 1:219-220

Brown SDM, Dover GA (1980) Conservation of segmental variants of satallite DNA of Mus musculus in a related species: Mus spretus. Nature 285:47-49

Bucan M, Yang-Feng T, Colberg-Poley A, Wolgemuth DJ, Francke U, Lehrach H (1986) Genetic and cytogenetic localisation of the homeobox containing genes on mouse chromosome 6 and human chromosome 7. EMBO J 5:2899-2905

Chamberlain JS, Grant SG, Reeves AA, Mullins LM, Stephenson DA, Hoffman EP, Monaco AP, Kunkel LM, Caskey CT, Chapman VM (1987) Regional localization of the murine Duchenne muscular dystrophy gene on the mouse X chromosome. Somat Cell Mol Genet 13:671-678

Chapman VM, Kratzer PG, Quarantillo BA (1983) Electorphoretic variation for X chromosome-linked hypoxanthine phosphoribosyl transferase (HPRT) in wild-derived mice. Genetics 103:785-795

Davisson MT, Roderick TH (1981) Recombination percentages. In: Green MC (ed) Genetic variants and strains of the laboratory mouse. Gustav Fischer Verlag, Stuttgart, p 283

Donis-Keller H, and many others (1987) A genetic linkage map of the human genome. Cell 51:319-377

Ferns SD, Sage RD, Wilson AC (1982) Evidence from mtDNA sequences that common laboratory strains of inbred mice are descended from a single female. Nature 295:163-165

Heidmann O, Buonanno A, Geoffroy B, Robert B, Guenet J-L, Merlie JP, Changeux J-P (1986) Chromosomal localization of muscle nicotinic acetylcholine receptor genes in the mouse. Science 234:866-868

Heilig R, Lemaire C, Mandel J-L, Dandolo L, Amar L, Avner P (1987) Localization of the region homologous to the Duchenne muscular dystrophy locus on the mouse X chromosome. Nature 328:168-170

Hsu TS, Markvong A, Marshall JT (1978) G-band patterns of six species of mice belonging to subgenus Mus. Cytogenet Cell Genet 20:304-307

Klein J, Sipos P, Figueroa F (1984) Polymorphism of t-complex genes in European wild mice. Genet Res 44:39-46

Lalley PA, McKusick VA (1985) Report of the committee on comparative mapping. Cytogenet Cell Genet 40:536-566

Lyon MF (1987) Mouse chromosome atlas. Mouse News Lett 78:12-38

Lyon MF, Meredith R (1964) The nature of t alleles in the mouse. I. Genetic analysis of a series of mutants derived from a lethal allele. Heredity 19:301-312

Marshall JT (1981) Taxonomy. In: Foster HL, Small JD, Fox JG (eds) The Mouse in Biomedical Research. Academic Press, New York, p 17

Nadeau JH, Berger FG, Kelley KA, Pitha PM, Sidman CL, Worrall N (1986) Rearrangement of genes located on homologous chromosomal segments in mouse and man: the location of genes for alpha- and beta-interferon, alpha-1 acid glycoprotein-1 and -2, and aminolevulinate dehydratase on mouse chromosome 4. Genetics 114:1239-1255

Nielsen JT, Chapman VM (1977) Electrophoretic variation for X-chromosome-linked phosphoglycerate kinase (PGK-1) in the mouse. Genetics 87:319-325

Ohno S (1969) Evolution of sex chromosomes in mammals. Ann Rev Genet 3:495-524

Reeves RH, Gallahan D, O'Hara BF, Callahan R, Gearhart JD (1987) Genetic mapping of Prm-1, Igl-1, Smst, Mtv-6, Sod-1, and Est-2 and localization of the Down syndrome region on mouse chromosome 16. Cytogenet Cell Genet 44:76-81

Robert B, Barton P, Minty A, Daubas P, Weyder A, Bonhomme F, Catalan J, Chazottes D, Guenet J-L, Buckingham M (1985) Investigation of genetic linkage between myosin and actin genes using an interspecific mouse back-cross. Nature 314:181-183

Seldin MF, Morse HC, D'Hoostelaere L, Britten JL, Steinberg AD (1987) Mapping of alpha-spectrin on distal mouse chromosome 1. Cytogenet Cell Genet 45:52-54

Siracusa LDA (1983) A molecular and genetic analysis of satellite DNA in the mouse. Ph.D. Thesis, State University of New York at Buffalo

Sutton WD, McCallum M (1972) Related satellite DNA's in the genus Mus. J Mol Biol 71:633-656

Womack JE, Roderick TH (1974) T-alleles in the mouse are probably not inversions. J Hered 65:308-310

Bayesian Multilocus Linkage Mapping

R.D. Blank, G.R. Campbell, M. Pollak, and P. D'Eustachio

INTRODUCTION

The construction of mammalian genetic maps entails finding solutions
to a number of distinct but interrelated problems. First, linkage to
the correct chromosome and chromosomal region must be established, and
linkage to other chromosomal regions must be excluded. Second, the
map distances separating a new marker from a set of previously mapped
markers must be calculated. Third, all the markers must be ordered
correctly. Fourth, during the above operations, the effects of
interference must be assessed and, if significant, corrected for.
Finally, in cases which do not allow unambiguous maps to be
constructed, it is useful to know how much additional data must be
gathered. In solving these problems, it is desirable that the data be
used efficiently and that the analysis proceed rapidly.

Here, we describe a package of computational tools which satisfy these
objectives. These materials are based on the algorithm BAYLOC, which
performs Bayesian multilocus linkage analysis. The FORTRAN programs
described below are available on request.

ASSIGNMENT TO CORRECT LINKAGE GROUP

Determination of genetic linkage depends on the fact that unlinked
loci will assort randomly, while linked loci will cosegregate more
than 50% of the time. Inference about linkage is based on the
observation of a statistically significant correlation between the
segregation of a test locus and one or more markers. Silver and
Buckler (1986) have argued that the appropriate statistical question
is framed in terms of conditional probability and is therefore
amenable to analysis through the use of Bayes' theorem. The
consequence of this analysis is that establishment of linkage at the
95% confidence level requires that the observed data have a binomial
probability of less than ~10^{-4} of being drawn from a sample in which
a test locus and a marker are assorting independently. The Bayesian
approach also allows correlation of the map distance between a test
locus and a marker and the number of informative chromosomes needed to
establish linkage at a given confidence level. Use of Bayes' Theorem
provides a straightforward method for deciding on the degree of
superiority of the best order to the second best order (see also
Bishop 1985), unlike another rapid multilocus mapping strategy (Lander
and Green 1987; Lander et al. to be published).

Multilocus mapping solves two important practical problems. The first
is construction of maps from limited data (Lathrop et al. 1985). Use

Department of Biochemistry and Kaplan Cancer Center, New York
University School of Medicine

Current Topics in Microbiology and Immunology, Vol. 137
© Springer-Verlag Berlin · Heidelberg 1988

of a multilocus rather than a pairwise strategy requires fewer informative individuals for establishing linkage or limiting a locus's position to a small range. The second is elimination of some kinds of false positive linkages. Due to the large number of mapped markers a new test locus may, by chance alone, cosegregate with an unlinked marker well enough to satisfy the statistical test of linkage. Multipoint mapping is of significant help here because the test locus must then not only cosegregate frequently with the markers, but must also find a position within the map defined by the markers.

We maintain a number of files containing typing data from recombinant inbred (RI) (Taylor 1978) and backcross mice. These files store the data as a 2-dimensional matrix, with one dimension representing individuals and the other representing loci, sorted by chromosome and with loci assigned to each chromosome listed in tentative map order. As additional loci are typed and maps are revised, the appropriate matrix can be modified as required. Loci that cannot be mapped to a chromosome are assigned to 'chromosome 21' and listed in alphabetical order.

After gathering typing data for a new locus, the first step in mapping it is to seek an obvious chromosomal assignment. We do this using the program LINKBOD, which is based on the BAYLOC algorithm. LINKBOD contains routines for computing the probability of linkage (both Bayesian and binomial) for two loci, given input numbers of discordant and informative mice; for two loci, using marker data in files; for one locus vs. all loci with typing data in files (LINKALL option); or for one locus vs. all pairs of loci on a single chromosome (LINKPR option). The initial efforts are best carried out using the LINKALL option. Early in a mapping project definitive assertions are unnecessary. Rather, the goal is to direct further analysis to the most promising regions of the genome and to proceed in a systematic manner to refine the analysis. Initial confidence limits should therefore be lenient (e.g. pairwise BOD scores $\geq$ 0.20 are generally worth saving).

As an example, Table 1A shows summary data of running the LINKALL option of LINKBOD for the locus Mtv-9 in seven RI panels. These data resemble the output of a sequence homology search. While there is a strong suggestion that Mtv-9 resides on chromosome 12, the best pairwise comparison fails to reach even the 90% confidence level. Indeed, five chromosomes carry markers satisfying the conditions of the search. As in homology searches, a strongly favored relationship and several weaker relationships are uncovered between the test object and the database entries.

Table 1A.

LOCUS (CHROMOSOME)	DISCORDANT / INFORMATIVE	BAYESIAN LINK PROB	BINOMIAL LINK PROB	NOMINAL MAP DIST
D12-ny8 (12)	2 / 17	87.707	99.883	3.57
c-Fos (12)	2 / 15	72.190	99.631	4.17
B2m (2)	13 / 44	50.034	99.522	13.27
H1s (13)	10 / 35	40.825	99.166	12.50
H3f2 (?)	2 / 11	28.897	96.729	6.25
Il1a (2)	30 / 82	25.793	99.009	20.27
Bmn (3)	6 / 22	24.292	97.376	11.54
Fcs-2 (12)	6 / 22	24.292	97.376	11.54
MLC1,3*F (1)	7 / 24	20.228	96.804	12.96

A total of 337 loci were tested for linkage to Mtv-9 at 20.0% confidence.

Table 1B.

CHR	I	J	BAYES % PROB	BINOM % PROB
12	D12-ny1	D12-ny8	93.79	91.18
12	D12-ny5	D12-ny8	92.01	93.17
12	D12-ny5	Igh-Cf	90.82	98.23

Given the failure to establish linkage of Mtv-9 to any chromosome unambiguously using this data set and pairwise analysis, we then use the LINKPR option of LINKBOD to investigate chromosomes 2 and 12, the two yielding multiple presumptive matches. The results are displayed in Table 1B. These results illustrate the power of the multilocus approach, as it is now possible to map Mtv-9 to three pairs of chromosome 12 loci at a confidence level of >90%. No pairs of chromosome 2 loci meet even this degree of confidence. Of course, if linkage to a particular chromosome is established by pairwise analysis, the three locus comparisons may be omitted. At this point, it is appropriate to proceed to calculations using BAYLOC or its automated version, AUTOBLOC, to construct a genetic map.

CONSTRUCTION OF A CHROMOSOMAL GENETIC MAP

The BAYLOC program (Blank and D'Eustachio to be published) can be summarized briefly. The program calculates multilocus Bayesian genetic maps for a test locus given recombination data between it and a set of previously mapped markers. The results are tabulated as probabilities of the test locus's residence at each 1 cM interval along the length of the chromosome given the positions of the markers and the actual recombination data. The results of a single run of BAYLOC are in effect a Bayes' Theorem transformed version of the maximum likelihood multilocus method (Lathrop et al. 1984). The transformation normalizes the distribution of probabilities of a test locus's map position to a sum of 1 over the entire genome. This transformation is useful in that it allows the confidence intervals, exclusion intervals, and assessments of marker order to be calculated explicitly. Confidence intervals are found by summing the best positions' probabilities until the confidence criterion is exceeded. Exclusion ranges are calculated in similar fashion, starting from the worst positions and proceeding until the confidence criterion is exceeded.

Detailed maps are constructed by sequential addition of loci to a preexisting framework of linked loci. The strategy leading to the most complete maps is to begin with a trio of loci whose linkage is well-established but are nevertheless separated by an appreciable distance. Appreciable distance, in this context, means 15 - 20 % recombination fractions for backcrosses and ~5 cM apparent map distance for RI's. In such cases, the central marker will be linked to both outside markers, while the outside markers will be approximately unlinked to each other. Loci believed to reside very close to previously mapped markers should be added late, as these most often result in ambiguity as to order.

There are several advantages to using a sequential approach. First, many potential locus orders need never be considered. For a map of n distinguishable loci, n!/2 locus orders are possible. Multilocus strategies that require systematic evaluation of all possible orders thus become unwieldy even for small (~10) numbers of loci (>1.8 x

10^6 orders), even if the unit steps in the procedure are rapid. The sequential approach considers only $\Sigma(i=3,n)i = (n - 2)(n + 3)/2$ orders (52 for 10 loci), a far smaller number than $n!/2$. Second, sequential map construction allows the adequacy of the map to be assessed as each locus is added. Third, when order fails to be determined with certainty, BAYLOC can be used to estimate the data needed to resolve the ambiguity. The necessary data can take two general forms: the number of individuals required with the loci already included in the map, or the approximate location of a marker not yet included in the map whose segregation with the unorderable locus would provide sufficient information for unambiguous mapping. Thus failure to map a locus successfully leads to a prescription for future experiments.

Many of the steps outlined above have been automated in AUTOBLOC. This program optimizes each marker's position as each new locus is added to the map, assigning each to its maximum BOD location. For each marker after each addition to the map, the conditional probability of the marker's lying between its nearest flanking informative markers given the remainder of the data is computed. Nearest informative markers are those which in addition to being typed for both the test locus and the flanking marker, also display at least 1 recombination event between the marker and the test locus. We generally use a 99% confidence as to marker order as the criterion for establishing order.

An eight marker map of chromosome 12 based on a C57BL/6J x SWR backcross illustrates the use of AUTOBLOC. The mapping strategy and the results of adding each locus are shown in Fig. 1. Panel B was included to illustrate failure to establish order at 99%, our criterion for continuing to add to the map. In the remaining panels, additional markers are added successfully, ending with D12-ny4, the locus that failed to map earlier. This once again demonstrates the practical import of the multilocus approach, as addition of markers to the map rather than enlargement of the sample allowed the locus to be placed. Figure 1 also shows 95% and 99% confidence intervals for the loci. These become narrower as markers are added to the map and are discontinuous when order is not established at that confidence level.

ASSUMPTIONS ABOUT INTERFERENCE

BAYLOC and AUTOBLOC use data expressed as recombinants/informative chromosomes. The calculation does not attempt to distinguish even-numbered crossover events from noncrossovers nor to distinguish higher odd-rank crossovers from single crossovers. This approach is taken consciously, as it considers the data without asserting an implicit assumption about order. The practical consequence of this simplification is threefold. First, running of the program is greatly accelerated. Second, the final optimized maps generated are slightly compressed compared to maps generated by pairwise mapping. Third, multilocus mapping can be carried out for data sets in which it is impossible to reconstruct the haplotypes generated at a single meiosis. This is particularly useful for RI strain analysis and incomplete backcross data, such as those obtained by pooling several 2- and 3-point crosses.

At the final stages of map construction, however, it is desirable to be able to reconstruct the distribution of chromosomes generated during the experiment so that the frequency of multiple crossover events can be compared with the map. We have developed a version of

A. Optimal 3-point map including <u>D12-ny2</u> (2), <u>D12-ny1</u> (1), and <u>Fos</u> (F)

B. Add <u>D12-ny4</u> (4)

C. Remove <u>D12-ny4</u> and add <u>Pre-1</u> (P)

D. Add <u>D12-ny3</u> (3)

E. Add <u>Mtv-9</u> (M)

F. Add <u>Igh-Ca</u> (C)

G. Add <u>D12-ny4</u> (4)

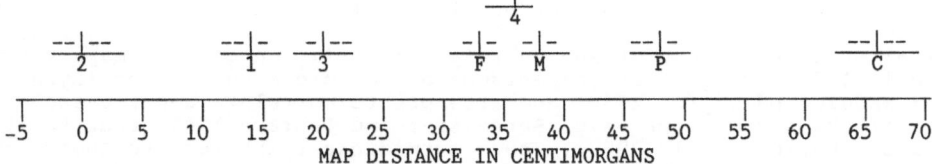

H. Recalculate counting recombination events as inferred by marker order

-5   0   5   10   15   20   25   30   35   40   45   50   55   60   65   70
MAP DISTANCE IN CENTIMORGANS

Fig 1. Construction of a linkage map from a chromosome 12 C57BL/6J x SWR/J backcross informative for all 8 marker loci. Each panel shows addition of a locus, as noted. Up to 316 mice were informative for any pair of loci. Vertical lines show best locations for the markers, double horizontal lines show 95% confidence intervals for those locations, and single horizontal lines show 99% confidence intervals. Discontinuous confidence intervals result when the marker order is ambiguous.

BAYLOC which does this. It is important when using this program to have a very high level of confidence in the marker order, as the program assumes the order to be correct. The program works by recalculating the data as crossover events/informative chromosomes in a genetic interval defined by each pair of loci and finding the maximum BOD for the test locus. By counting events rather than recombinants, the compression of the BAYLOC map relative to the pairwise map is reversed. The event-based map is shown in Fig. 1H.

The versions of BAYLOC and AUTOBLOC now in use allow the user to invoke either the Haldane(1919) or Kosambi(1944) mapping functions. Various other mapping functions have also been devised (e.g. Carter and Falconer 1951; Rao et al. 1977) and could be incorporated into the programs.

CONCLUSIONS AND PROSPECTS

We have described a package of computer programs for generating high resolution linkage maps rapidly. The central calculation is a multilocus Bayesian mapping routine, BAYLOC. We have illustrated the application of these computational tools to several cases using actual data.

Experimental study of interference in a chromosome 12 multipoint backcross is currently underway in our laboratory. This is but one of several biological questions whose answers depend on complete, accurate maps. Our preliminary results suggest that the occurrence of crossovers is significantly nonrandom, as there are too few noncrossover and multiple crossover chromosomes and too many single crossover chromosomes. Similar calculations using others' M. domesticus x M. spretus backcross data (e.g. Bucan et al. 1986; Robert et al. 1985) indicate that this is a common phenomenon in this breeding system. Biological characterization of interference in this setting may yield clues as to the differences in chromosomal structure or genomic organization which exist between sibling species. The issue of genomic organization also bears on attempts to understand the origins of inbred mice (Blank et al. 1986; Bonhomme et al. 1984; Figueroa et al. 1987; Fitch and Atchley 1985; Rice and O'Brien 1980). We speculate that inbred mice differ not only at genetic points, but that numerous small insertions, deletions, and other rearrangements exist between the genomes of various inbred mouse strains.

Several other avenues of research rely critically on genetic maps. These include phylogenetic comparisons of genomic organization (Lyon 1987; Nadeau and Taylor 1984) and attempts to correlate genetic and physical chromosome maps (e.g. Burmeister and Lehrach 1986; Poustka et al. 1986; Barlow et al. 1987). These formidable tasks require that genetic data be available in useful form and amenable to rapid, efficient, and accurate analysis.

ACKNOWLEDGEMENTS

We thank Dr. P.R. Smith, Dep't of Cell Biology, NYU Medical Center, for helpful advice and for access to a VAX750 computer. This work was supported by research award 1-1018 from the National Foundation - March of Dimes, and by grant GM32105 from the NIH. R.D.B. is a predoctoral trainee of the NIH Medical Scientist Training Program.

REFERENCES

Barlow DP, Bucan M, Lehrach H, Hogan BL, Gough NM (1987) Close genetic and physical linkage between the murine haematopoietic growth factor genes GM-CSF and Multi-CSF(IL3). EMBO J 6:617-623

Bishop DT (1985) The information content of phase-known matings for ordering genetic loci. Genet. Epidem. 2: 349-361

Blank RD, D'Eustachio P (to be published) Construction of Genetic Maps Using Bayesian Location Scores.

Bonhomme F, Catalan J, Britton-Davidian J, Chapman VM, Moriwaki K, Nevo E, Thaler L (1984) Biochemical diversity and evolution in the genus Mus. Biochem Genet 22: 275-303

Bucan M, Yang-Fen T, Colberg-Poley AM, Wolgemuth DJ, Guenet J-L, Francke U, Lehrach H (1986) Genetic and cytogenetic localisation of the homeo box containing genes on mouse chromosome 6 and human chromosome 7. EMBO J 5: 2899-2905

Burmeister M, Lehrach H (1986) Long-range restriction map around the Duchenne muscular dystrophy gene. Nature 324: 582-585

Carter TC, Falconer DS (1951) Stocks for detecting linkage in the mouse and the theory of their design. J Genet 50: 307-323

Figueroa F, Kasahara M, Tichy H, Neufeld E, Ritte U, Klein J (1987) Polymorphism of unique noncoding DNA sequences in wild and laboratory mice. Genetics 117: 101-108

Fitch WM, Atchley WR (1985) Evolution in inbred strains of mice appears rapid. Science 228: 1169-1175

Haldane JBS (1919) The combination of linkage values, and the calculation of distances between the loci of linked factors. J Genet 8: 299-309

Kosambi DD (1944) The estimation of map distances from recombination values. Ann Eugen 14: 172-175

Lander ES, Green P (1987) Construction of multilocus genetic linkage maps in humans. Proc Natl Acad Sci USA 84: 2363-2367

Lander ES, Green P, Abrahamson J, Barlow A, Daly M, Lincoln S, Newburg L (to be published) Mapmaker: an interactive computer package for constructing primary genetic linkage maps of experimental and natural populations. Genomics

Lathrop GM, Lalouel JM, Julier C, Ott J (1984) Strategies for multilocus linkage analysis in humans. Proc Natl Acad Sci USA 81: 3443-3446

Lathrop GM, Lalouel JM, Julier C, Ott J (1985) Am J Hum Genet 37: 482-498

Lyon MF (1987) Mouse chromosome atlas. Mouse News Letter 78: 13-33

Nadeau J, Taylor BA (1984) Length of chromosome segments preserved since the divergence of man and mouse. Proc Natl Acad Sci USA 81: 814-818

Poustka A, Pohl T, Barlow DP, Zehetner G, Craig A, Michiels F, Ehrich E, Frischauf AM, Lehrach H (1986) Molecular approaches to mammalian genetics. Cold Spring Harbor Symp. Quant. Biol. 51: 131–139

Rao DC, Morton NE, Lindsten J, Hulten M, Yee S (1977) A mapping function for man. Hum Hered 27: 99–104

Rice MC, O'Brien SJ (1980) Genetic variance of outbred Swiss mice. Nature 283: 157–161

Robert B, Barton P, Minty A, Daubas P, Weydert A, Bonhomme F, Catalan J, Chazottes D, Guenet J-L, Buckingham M (1985) Investigation of genetic linkage between myosin and actin using an interspecific mouse backcross. Nature 314: 181–183

Silver J, Buckler CE (1986) Statistical considerations for linkage analysis using recombinant inbred strains and backcrosses. Proc Natl Acad Sci USA 83: 1423–1427

Taylor BA (1978) Recombinant inbred strains: use in genetic mapping. In: Morse HC (ed) Origins of inbred mice. Academic Press, New York, pp 423–438

The Rat Gene Map

C. Szpirer, J. Szpirer, M.Q. Islam[1], and G. Levan[1]

INTRODUCTION

Rat genetics is much less developed than mouse (or human) genetics.
Since the rat is used as an experimental animal in several fields,
such as cancer research, this lack of genetic information is often
frustrating. It would thus be helpful to extend the knowledge of the
rat gene map. In addition, such data would allow comparisons with
the gene map of other species and favor the study of chromosome
evolution.

During the last few years, in collaboration with other groups, we
have been able to map about 30 rat genes, on 14 of the 22 different
rat chromosomes (see Levan et al., 1986). These assignments were
obtained by the methods of somatic cell genetics, using a panel of
mouse hepatoma – rat hepatocyte hybrids that segregate rat
chromosomes (Szpirer et al., 1980). The rat chromosomes retained in
the hybrid clones or subclones were identified by G-banding and most
genes mapped were sought for in DNA extracted from the hybrids, by
Southern blot analysis.

GENE ASSIGNMENTS AND CONSERVED SYNTENY

Our data, including unpublished results (IGL, ORM, NEU, MIS1, ALDOB,
A2UG) are summarized in Tables 1, 2 and 3. Some of these
assignments are briefly commented below. These localizations,
combined with results obtained by other authors (using somatic cell
hybrids or in situ hybridization; for references, see Levan et al.,
1986; Cramer, 1987; Lalley and O'Brien, 1987) have led to new
knowledge of conserved synteny between man, mouse and rat; these
data are summarized in Table 4.

Among the first rat genes we mapped are the albumin and
alpha-fetoprotein (AFP) genes, that we assigned to chromosome 14
(see Table 1). In man and mouse (for references on mouse and human
gene localizations, see Mouse News Letter, 78, 1987; Lalley and
O'Brien, 1987; McAlpine et al., 1985, and HGM9, Cytogenet Cell
Genet, in press) these genes are closely linked on chromosomes 4 and
5, respectively. We also assigned to rat chromosome 14, the gene
coding for the vitamine D binding protein (VDBP, or Gc globulin),
the third member of the albumin-AFP family; in man, the VDBP (GC)
gene is linked to to the albumin-AFP cluster, in the region q11-13
of chromosome 4. Interestingly, the structural genes coding for the
fibrinogen (FB) chains are also on the long arm of human chromosome
4, in the region q26-28. In the rat, these genes are not syntenic
with the albumin-AFP-VDBP genes: the FB genes were assigned to rat

Département de Biologie Moléculaire, Université Libre de Bruxelles,
Rue des Chevaux, 67; B-1640 Rhode-St-Genèse, Belgium
[1]Department of Genetics, University of Gothenburg, Box 33031,
S-400 33 Goteborg, Sweden.

Current Topics in Microbiology and Immunology, Vol. 137
© Springer-Verlag Berlin · Heidelberg 1988

chromosome 2 by in situ hybridization and by the analysis of our
mouse - rat hybrids (Szpirer et al., 1987). The localization of the
rat FG genes is one of the few rat gene assignments that are
confirmed (i.e. made by two independent laboratories).

Table 1. Rat Ig and plasma protein genes, and comparative mapping.

Locus	RNO	MMU	HSA
IGH	6q32(LGVIII)	12	14q32
IGK	4	6	2p12
IGL	11	16	22q11
ALB	14(LGIX)	5	4q11-13
AFP	14	5	4q11-13
VDPB(GC)	14	-	4q11-13
FGA	2q31-34	-	4q26-28
FGB	2q31-34	-	4q26-28
FGG	2q31-34	-	4q26-28
TF	8	9	3q21-26
C3	9	17	19p13
ORM(AGP)	5	4	9q34

RNO = rat chromosomes; MMU = mouse chromosomes; HSA = human
chromosomes. LG = linkage group.

Several rat oncogenes have been mapped; our localizations are
summarized in Table 2. The HRAS1 oncogene assignment (RNO 1) is one
of the confirmed rat gene assignments. The MYC oncogene is
particularly interesting. Indeed, this oncogene is known to be
involved in specific chomosome rearrangements in B- and T-cell
tumors. In most cases of B-cell neoplasia (human Burkitt's lymphomas
and murine plasmacytomas), the MYC oncogene (on HSA 8 and MMU 15) is
transposed to the chromosome that carries the immunnoglobulin heavy
chain (IGH) locus (HSA 14, MMU 12; for a review, see Cory, 1986).
In the rat, immunocytomas of spontaneous origin show a reciprocal
translocation between chromosomes 6 and 7 (Wiener et al., 1982). The
rat MYC oncogene was assigned to chromosome 7 and the rat IGH locus
to chromosome 6. In addition, the MYC oncogene is generally
rearranged in rat immunocytomas (Sumegi et al., 1983), and
juxtaposition of MYC to IGH has been demonstrated in such tumor
cells (Pear et al., 1986). Chromosomal translocations juxtaposing
MYC and immunoglobulin DNA sequences thus occur in three types of
B-cell tumors, of different etiology, and in three species, man,
mouse and rat. The assignments of MYC to rat chromosome 7, and of
IGH to rat chromosome 6 is in line with banding homology between RNO
7 and MMU 15, and between RNO 6 and MMU 12 (see Fig. 1 and Nesbitt,
1974; Yoshida, 1978).

T-cell neoplasia can be induced in the mouse by retrovirus
integration in the vicinity of Myc, at a site called Pvt-1 (Graham

Table 2. Rat oncogenes and common MoMuLV integration sites, and comparative mapping.

Locus	RNO	MMU	HSA
HRAS1	1(LGI)	7	11pter–15
HRAS2	X	–	Xpter–q28
KRAS2	4	6	12p12
ERBA1	15	11	17q11–21
ERBB1	14	11	7p14–12
NEU(ERBB2)	10	–	17q21
MYC	7	15	8q24
MYCL	5	–	1p
MYCN	6	–	2p23–24
MLVI1	7	15	–
MLVI2	2	15	5p14
MLVI3	15	–	–
MIS1	7	15(Pvt-1)	8q24

Table 3. Rat genes: miscellaneous, and comparative mapping.

Locus	RNO	MMU	HSA
GH	10	–	17p22–24
PRL	17	–	6p23–q12
ALDOB	5	–	9q31–32
A2UG(MUP)	5(LGII)	4	–
CRYG	9(LGX)	1 (Len–1)	2q33–35
TG	7	15	8q24

et al., 1985). In the rat, thymomas are induced by the Moloney murine leukemia virus (MoMuLV), and many of them bear a retroviral insert at one of several common but distinct integration sites: MIS1 (homologous to the mouse Pvt-1 locus; Villeneuve et al., 1986), MLVI1, MLVI2 and MLVI3 (for references, see Tsichlis et al., 1985). The rat MIS1 and MLVI1 regions are localized on chromosome 7 (Ingvarsson et al., 1987; Tsichlis et al., 1985), like MYC. Provirus insertion in MIS1 or MLVI1 may deregulate MYC expression in rat thymomas, like in retrovirus-induced mouse T-lymphomas or in mouse plasmacytomas carrying Igk-Pvt-1 translocations (Graham et al., 1985). The rat MLVI2 and MLVI3 loci are located on chromosomes 2 and 15, respectively; therefore, these sites cannot be involved in cis-acting deregulation of MYC. However, since MLVI3 is syntenic with ERBA, the possibility that retrovirus integration in the MLVI3 locus could alter the expression of ERBA should be considered.

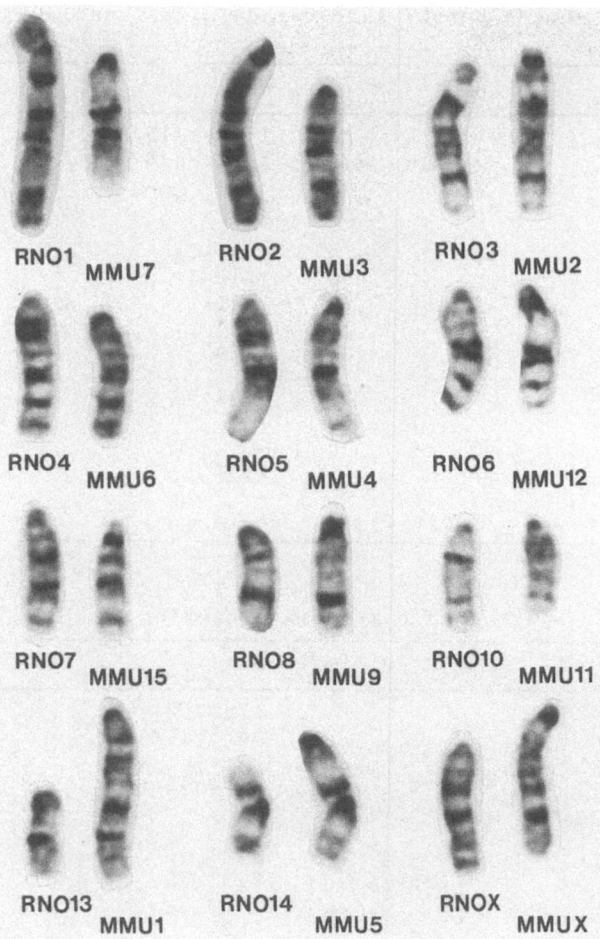

Fig. 1. G-banding
homology between
rat (RNO) and
mouse (MMU)
chromosomes.

Some mouse and rat chromosomes show striking banding homologies, as
illustrated by Fig. 1 (see also Nesbitt, 1974; Yoshida, 1978). The
present data on the rat gene map (Levan at al., 1986, and this
paper) allows us to deduce genetic homologies between these two
species. Table 4 shows a list of chromosomes that carry conserved
synteny groups containing at least two genes; this comparison
confirms, at the gene level most morphological similarities between
mouse and rat chromosomes. Comparison with the human gene map
extends, not unexpectedly, to rat chromosomes, syntenic homologies
already known between mouse and human chromosomes; in addition, the
data obtained in the rat define new regions of conserved linkage in
rodents and man, such as the MYC – thyroglobulin (TG) group (RNO 7 –
HSA 8q24), the fibrinogen genes (RNO 2 – HSA 4q26-28), and the
growth hormone – NEU (ERBB2) group (RNO 10 – HSA 17q21-24). The
available information on the known homologies between different
species, including rat, mouse and man, has recently been reviewed by
Lalley and O'Brien (1987).

Table 4: Conserved syntenyic groups in rat, mouse and man.

Locus	RNO	MMU	HSA
HPRT,HRAS2	X	X	X
INS,HRAS1,HBB	1(LGI)	7	11p
FGA,-B,-G	2		4q26-28
-	2	3	
ABL,AK1	3	2	9q34
IGK	4	6	
KRAS2,TPI1	4	6	12p
ENO1,FUCA	5	4	1p
ORM,ALDOB	5		9q
ACP1,IGK	6	12	2p25
ACP1,MYCN	6		2p
MYC,TG	7	15	8q24
TF,MPI	8	9	
TK,GALK	10	11	17q21-22
GH,ERBB2	10		17q21-24
-	13	1	
ALB,AFP	14	5	4q11-13
VDBP(GC)	14		4q11-13

This table summarizes the homologies between rat, mouse and human
chromosomes and shows the chromosomes exhibiting banding homomogy
(underlined) and/or carrying at least two genes (first column) that
are syntenic in rat, mouse and/or man

NON-RANDOM CHROMOSOME LOSS IN MOUSE HEPATOMA - RAT HEPATOCYTE
HYBRIDS.

The chromosome analysis of the mouse hepatoma - rat hepatocyte
hybrids revealed that rat chromosome loss is not random (see Szpirer
et al. 1984, 1987). The fusion of mouse hepatoma cells with normal
adult rat hepatocytes yielded proliferating hybrids at a very low
rate (about 0.001 hybrid per 100 treated cells). However 45 hybrid
clones could be isolated (LB hybrids; Szpirer et al., 1980). Most of
them (31 out 45) had doubled the number of mouse chromosomes (2S
hybrids). The remaining 14 hybrids were subjected to detailed
chromosome analysis (Szpirer et al., 1984) (and used to map rat
genes, as summarized above). This analysis revealed that the 1S LB
hybrids preferentially retained 2 unselected rat chromosomes, RNO 4
and RNO 7 (retained in 13 and 12 clones, respectively) and
preferentially lost RNO 8 (absent in 12 clones). On the other hand,
among the 31 2S clones, 13 retained rat chromosome 8 (they secreted
rat transferrin, the structural gene of which is on RNO 8; Szpirer
et al., 1980, 1987). Rat chromosome 8 is thus preferentially lost in
the mouse hepatoma - rat hepatocyte hybrids that did not double the
mouse hepatoma genome.

From these results, we conclude that rat chromosome 8 confers
specifically a growth disadvantage to the hepatoma - hepatocyte
hybrids. The non-mitotic state of the normal adult hepatocyte
appears to block proliferation of the hy.brids and the loss of rat
chromosome 8 seems to be required to allow their continuous growth;
alternatively, doubling the hepatoma genome seems to counterbalance
the negative effect of rat chromosome 8. We suppose that this
chromosome carries a growth control gene.

REFERENCES

Cory S (1986) Activation of cellular oncogenes in hemopoietic
    cells by chromosome translocation. Cancer Res 47: 189-234
Cramer DV (1987) Biochemical loci of the rat. In: O'Brien SJ (ed)
    Genetic Maps, vol 4, Cold Spring Harbor Laboratory.
Graham M, Adams JM, Cory S (1985) Retroviral inserts in the
    chromosome 15 locus for plasmacytoma variant (6:15) translocations
    in some murine T lymphomas. Nature 314: 740-743
Lalley PA, O'Brien SJ (1987) Report of the committee on
    comparative mapping. HGM9. Cytogenet Cell Genet, in press.
Levan G, Szpirer J, Szpirer C, Yoshida (1986) Present status of
    chromosome localization of rat genes. Rat News Letter 17: 3-8
McAlpine PJ, Shows TB, Miller RL, Pakstis AJ (1985) The 1985 catalog
    of mapped genes and report of the nomenclature committee. HGM8.
    Cytogent Cell Genet 40: 8-66
Nesbitt MN (1974) Evolutionary relationship between rat and
    mouse chromosomes. Chromosoma 46: 217-224
Pear WS, Ingvarsson S, Steffen D, Munke M, Francke U, Bazin H,
    Klein G, Sumegi J (1986) Multiple chromosomal rearrangements in a
    spontaneously arising t(6;7) rat immunocytoma juxtapose c-myc and
    immunoglobulin heavy chain sequences. Proc Natl Acad Sci USA 83:
    7376-7380
Sumegi J, Spira J, Bazin H, Szpirer J, Levan G, Klein G (1983) Rat
    c-myc oncogene is located on chromosome 7 and rearranges in
    immunocytomas with t(6:7) chromosomal translocation.
    Nature 306: 497-499
Szpirer J, Islam MQ, Cooke N, Szpirer C, Levan G (1987) Assignment
    of three rat genes coding for plasma proteins: transferrin, the
    third component of complement and beta-fibrinogen to chromosome 8,
    9 and 2. Cytogenet Cell Genet, in press
Szpirer J, Levan G, Thorn M, Szpirer C (1984) Gene mapping in the
    rat by mouse-rat somatic cell hybridization: synteny of the
    albumin and alpha-fetoprotein genes and assignment to
    chromosome 14. Cytogenet Cell Genet 38: 142-149.
Szpirer J, Szpirer C, Wanson JC (1980) Control of serum protein
    production in hepatocyte hybridomas: immmortalization and
    expression of normal hepatocyte genes. Proc Natl Acad Sci USA
    77: 6616-6620
Villeneuve L, Rassart E, Jolicoeur P, Graham M, Adams JM (1986)
    Proviral integration site Mis-1 in rat thymomas corresponds to the
    Pvt-1 translocation breakpoint in murine plasmacytomas. Mol Cell
    Biol 6: 1834-1837
Wiener F, Babonits M, Spira J, Klein G, Bazin H (1982) Non-
    random chromosomal changes involving chromosomes 6 and 7 in
    spontaneous rat immunocytomas. Internat J Cancer 29: 431-437
Yoshida MC (1978) Rat gene mapping by rat-mouse somatic cell
    hybridization and a comparative Q-banding analysis between
    rat and mouse chromosomes. Cytogent Cell Genet 22: 606-609

Linkage and Synteny Homologies in Mouse and Man

J. H. Nadeau and A. H. Reiner

The following map shows the chromosomal location of genes that have been mapped in both mouse and man. The chromosomal location of the homologous gene in man is indicated after each mouse gene. Chromosome arm assignment is also given when known. Highlighted are chromosome segments that are marked by two or more genes whose homologues in man are located on the same chromosome and that are not interrupted by genes whose homologues in man are located on other chromosomes. Synteny assignments are given below each chromosome.

We maintain a database of linkage and synteny data for all mammals and welcome information concerning errors of commission or omission and inquiries concerning comparative gene mapping data.

This work was supported by NIH grants GM-32461 and GM-39414.

Jackson Laboratory
Bar Harbor, Maine 04609

40

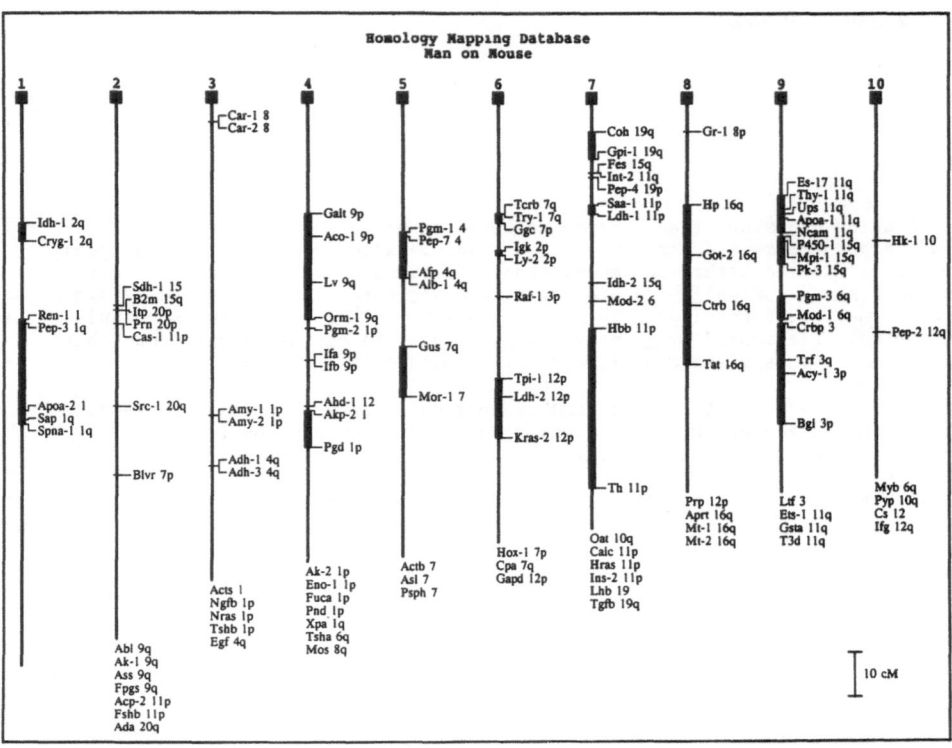

Homology Mapping Database
Man on Mouse

1
2
3

— Car-1 8
— Car-2 8

4
5
6
7
— Coh 19q
8
— Gr-1 8p
9
10

— Idh-1 2q
— Cryg-1 2q

— Galt 9p
— Aco-1 9p

— Pgm-1 4
— Pep-7 4

— Tcrb 7q
— Try-1 7q
— Ggc 7p
— Igk 2p
— Ly-2 2p

— Gpi-1 19q
— Fes 15q
— Int-2 11q
— Pep-4 19p
— Saa-1 11p
— Ldh-1 11p

— Hp 16q

— Es-17 11q
— Thy-1 11q
— Ups 11q
— Apoa-1 11q
— Ncam 11q
— P450-1 15q
— Mpi-1 15q
— Pk-3 15q

— Hk-1 10

— Sdh-1 15
— B2m 15q
— Itp 20p
— Prn 20p
— Cas-1 11p

— Lv 9q

— Afp 4q
— Alb-1 4q

— Got-2 16q

— Ren-1 1
— Pep-3 1q

— Orm-1 9q
— Pgm-2 1p

— Raf-1 3p

— Idh-2 15q
— Mod-2 6

— Ctrb 16q

— Pgm-3 6q
— Mod-1 6q
— Crbp 3

— Pep-2 12q

— Ifa 9p
— Ifb 9p

— Gus 7q

— Hbb 11p

— Apoa-2 1
— Sap 1q
— Spna-1 1q

— Src-1 20q

— Amy-1 1p
— Amy-2 1p

— Ahd-1 12
— Akp-2 1

— Mor-1 7

— Tpi-1 12p
— Ldh-2 12p

— Tat 16q

— Trf 3q
— Acy-1 3p

— Adh-1 4q
— Adh-3 4q

— Pgd 1p

— Kras-2 12p

— Bgl 3p

— Blvr 7p

— Th 11p

Acts 1
Ngfb 1p
Nras 1p
Tshb 1p
Egf 4q

Ak-2 1p
Eno-1 1p
Fuca 1p
Pnd 1p
Xpa 1q
Tsha 6q
Mos 8q

Actb 7
Asl 7
Psph 7

Hox-1 7p
Cpa 7q
Gapd 12p

Oat 10q
Caic 11p
Hras 11p
Ins-2 11p
Lhb 19
Tgfb 19q

Prp 12p
Aprt 16q
Mt-1 16q
Mt-2 16q

Ltf 3
Ets-1 11q
Gsta 11q
T3d 11q

Myb 6q
Pyp 10q
Cs 12
Ifg 12q

Abl 9q
Ak-1 9q
Ass 9q
Fpgs 9q
Acp-2 11p
Fshb 11p
Ada 20q

⊢ 10 cM

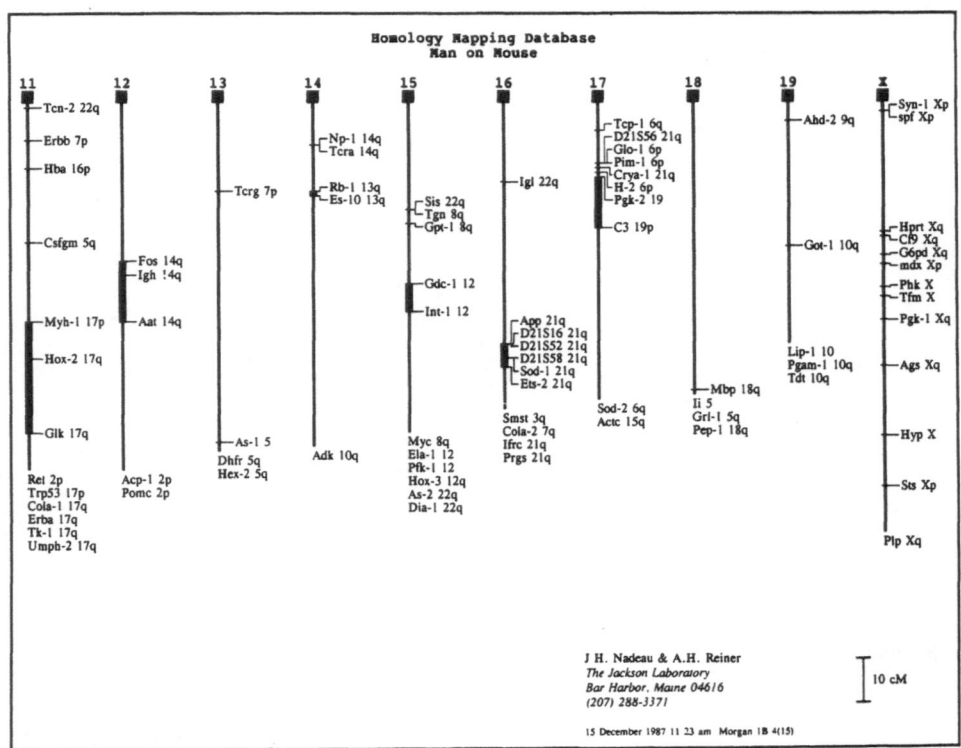

Homology Mapping Database
Man on Mouse

11
— Tcn-2 22q

12
13
14
15
16
17
— Tcp-1 6q
— D21S56 21q
— Glo-1 6p
— Pim-1 6p
— Crya-1 21q
— H-2 6p
— Pgk-2 19

18
19
X
— Syn-1 Xp
— spf Xp

— Erbb 7p

— Ahd-2 9q

— Hba 16p

— Np-1 14q
— Tcra 14q

— Igl 22q

— Tcrg 7p

— Rb-1 13q
— Es-10 13q

— Sis 22q
— Tgn 8q
— Gpt-1 8q

— C3 19p

— Csfgm 5q

— Fos 14q
— Igh 14q

— Hprt Xq
— Cf9 Xq
— G6pd Xq
— mdx Xp

— Gdc-1 12

— Got-1 10q

— Phk X
— Tfm X

— Myh-1 17p

— Aat 14q

— Int-1 12

— Pgk-1 Xq

— Hox-2 17q

— App 21q
— D21S16 21q
— D21S52 21q
— D21S58 21q
— Sod-1 21q
— Ets-2 21q

— Lip-1 10
Pgam-1 10q
Tdt 10q

— Ags Xq

— Glk 17q

— As-1 5

— Myc 8q
Ela-1 12
Pfk-1 12
Hox-3 12q
As-2 22q
Dia-1 22q

— Mbp 18q

— Hyp X

— Smst 3q
Cola-2 7q
Ifrc 21q
Prgs 21q

— Sod-2 6q
Actc 15q

Ii 5
Gri-1 5q
Pep-1 18q

Ret 2p
Trp53 17p
Cola-1 17q
Erba 17q
Tk-1 17q
Umph-2 17q

Acp-1 2p
Pomc 2p

Dhfr 5q
Hex-2 5q

Adk 10q

— Sts Xp

— Plp Xq

J H. Nadeau & A.H. Reiner
The Jackson Laboratory
Bar Harbor. Maine 04616
(207) 288-3371

⊢ 10 cM

15 December 1987 11 23 am Morgan 1B 4(15)

Molecular Analysis of the Aniridia – Wilms' Tumor Syndrome

N. D. Hastie, D. J. Porteous, W. Bickmore, J. Maule, and V. van Heyningen

INTRODUCTION

Wilms' tumor is an embryonic nephroblastoma which occurs at a
frequency of 1/10,000 children and usually manifests within the first
three years of life. 1/50 of the individuals with Wilms' tumor also
suffers from congenital aniridia (no iris), a condition which
ultimately leads to blindness if untreated. Conversely 1/2 to 1/3
children with sporadic aniridia will go on to develop Wilms' tumor.
Individuals with both these conditions are almost invariably mentally
retarded and will often have other genitourinary abnormalities such as
ambiguous genitalia, gonadoblastoma and a variety of kidney defects.
This syndrome, the WAGR syndrome (Wilms' tumor, Aniridia, Genitourinary abnormalities, Mental Retardation) is associated frequently
with a constitutional deletion of the short arm of one chromosome 11
which always involves the distal part of band 11p13 (Riccardi et al.,
1978).

There is a considerable body of genetic and molecular evidence to
support the idea that the Wilms' tumor mutation is recessive at the
cellular level (Knudson and Strong, 1972; Koufos et al., 1984). Thus
if a deletion or mutation of one copy of the gene is inherited the
second copy must undergo a similar event in the tumor tissue itself.
It seems reasonable to hypothesise that the Wilms' tumor (WT) gene
product is essential for differentiation of embryonic nephroblasts
into nephrons; if the gene product is lacking these stem cells fail
to differentiate and continue to proliferate leading to the formation
of malignant tumors which may or may not require other genetic changes
for their progression. Manifestation of aniridia on the other hand
only requires a 50% reduction in the level of the aniridia (AN) gene
product; this is an example of haploid insufficiency. It is unclear
at present whether other genitourinary abnormalities associated with
this syndrome are a direct consequence of mutations in the WT gene or
reflect mutations in different genes within 11p13.

En route to isolating these interesting genes we are first identifying
markers which map to the critical 11p13 region, as evidenced by their
absence from the deleted chromosomes. To facilitate this analysis we
have established a panel of somatic cell hybrids in which the rearranged
chromosomes have been segregated from their normal counterparts.
Translocations associated with a particular phenotype are of special
interest as they may have breakpoints which lie within the gene
itself. We are working with two reciprocal translocations with breakpoints in 11p13, one found in all the affected members of a family
segregating for aniridia (4;11 translocation), the other in a still-
born individual with renal dysplasia (2;11 translocation). Again
somatic cell hybrids containing the different parts of these translocations have been established. These panels of somatic hybrids with
rearranged chromosome 11s not only help to identify markers close to

MRC Clinical and Population Cytogenetics Unit, Western General
Hospital, Crewe Road, Edinburgh EH4 2XU, U.K.

the genes of interest but also are invaluable aids for constructing physical linkage maps of the short arm of chromosome 11. In order to enrich for markers located in the short arm of the chromosome we have exploited the technique of chromosome-mediated gene transfer (CMGT).

Establishing the Panel of Somatic Cell Hybrids Containing Rearranged Chromosome 11s

In order to identify patients who were likely to have 11p13 deletions we located individuals who had suffered from both aniridia and Wilms' tumor or patients with mental retardation and aniridia. We first identified 5 individuals determined by Giemsa and reverse banding to have deletions in 11p13 ranging in size from half the short arm of the chromosome to barely detectable deficiencies encompassing just part of the 11p13 band (van Heyningen et al., 1985). Lymphoblastoid cell lines were established from these patients by transformation of lymphocytes with Epstein Barr virus. These cell lines were fused to mouse plasmacytoma cells and individual clones resulting from the fusion were scored for the presence of the deleted or normal chromosome. In the case of the smallest detectable deletions we could only identify correctly the cell line containing the deleted chromosome by subsequent marker loss analysis. To facilitate this onerous task we have used FACS to select for hybrids containing chromosome 11 using monoclonal antibodies to cell surface markers encoded by genes located on chromosome 11 (Seawright et al., 1988). Obviously the smallest detectable deletions are most useful in pinpointing markers to the critical region of 11p13. We now have hybrids containing chromosomes with 3 such barely detectable deletions which involve only part of chromosome 11p13; these are ANX6.4, SAX3.10 and MAX15. In addition, we have established hybrids in which the different parts of the translocations associated with aniridia (SIMX hybrids) and renal dysplasia (POR hybrids) have been segregated from each other and the normal chromosome 11.

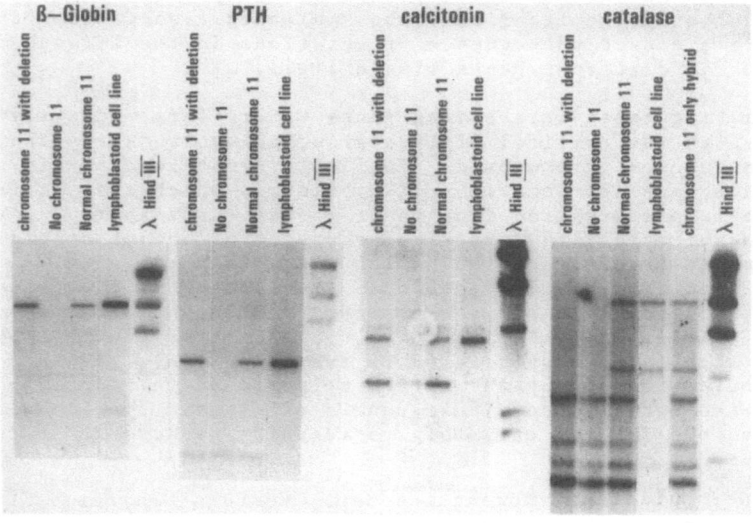

Fig. 1. Southern analysis to determine the status of 11p genes in a large deletion.

Mapping Genes to the Panel of Hybrids

We were first interested in determining whether any genes known to map on chromosome 11 are located in the 11p13 region and thus useful starting points for isolating the WT and AN genes. At the time we initiated our study the Beta haemoglobin chain (HBB) gene, the calcitonin (CALC) gene and the parathyroid hormone (PTH) gene were all known to map on chromosome 11 and probes for all these were available. Of most interest however was the as yet uncloned gene for catalase (CAT) the levels of which were reduced in many WAGR patients. We used an oligonucleotide probe predicted from the amino acid sequence to isolate the catalase gene (van Heyningen et al., 1985). Figure 1 shows the results of a Southern blot analysis in which radioactive probes for these genes were hybridised to DNA from somatic cell hybrids containing the normal (NYX5.6) or deleted (11p13 to 11p15.4; NYX3.1) chromosome 11 from one of our patients. Of these four genes

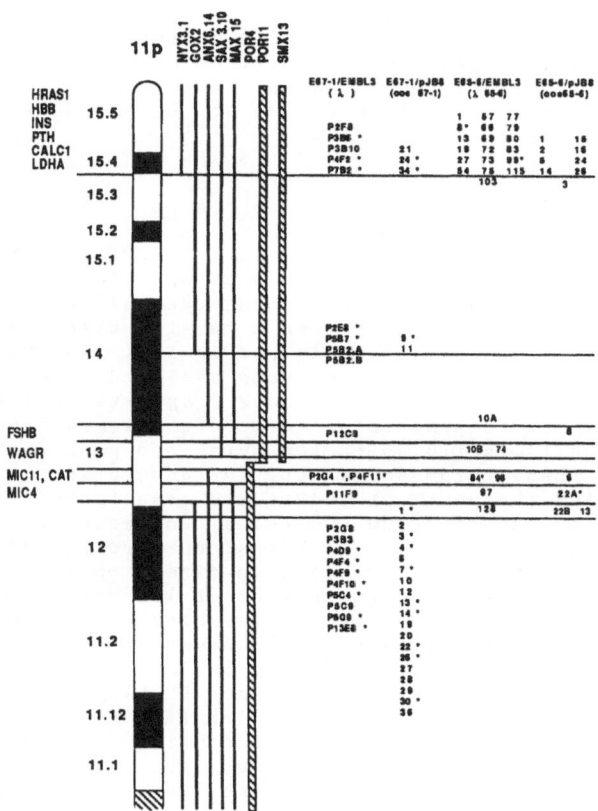

Fig. 2. A physical map of the short arm of chromosome 11 and the WAGR region. On the left hand side the positions of genes are indicated: INS is the insulin gene, MIC11 and MIC4 are the genes encoding cell surface markers. The numbers on the right hand side refer to the positions of anonymous DNA markers obtained from the chromosome transfectants E67-1 and E65-6. The narrow lines represent chromosomes with deletions, the hatched broad lines represent translocated chromosomes.

only the CAT gene is absent from the deleted chromosome. This gene
must be located between 11p13 and 11p15.4 and the other genes must map
below 11p13 or between 11p13 to 11pter. Similar data from other laboratories and in situ hybridisation analysis showed that these genes
map between 11p15.4 and 11pter. Figure 2 (left side) summarises the
mapping data for a number of genes using our panel of hybrids. Data
obtained from hybrids containing the translocated chromosomes (POR and
SIMO) is particularly helpful when combined with deletion analysis.
For example, from analysing the deletions the lactate dehydrogenase A
(LDHA) gene could map to 11p15-11pter or below 11p13. The former
alternative must be correct as the LDHA gene is located in the upper
translocated segment in each case.

We can now start to order the genes within the 11p13 band itself. For
example, the CAT gene is deleted in NYX3.1, GOX2, SAX3.10 and MAX15
but not deleted from ANX6.14. The ANX deletion extends from the
middle part of 11p13 to the 11p13-11p14 boundary. So we can say the
CAT gene is in the proximal half of 11p13 and closer to the centromere
than the WT and AN genes.

Recently the beta subunit of the follicle stimulating hormone gene
(FSHB) was shown to be located in 11p13 and deleted from all WAGR
patients studied (Glaser et al., 1986). Our analysis confirms this
location and shows that the FSHB gene must be distal to the WT and AN
genes as it is not deleted in SAX3.10 and MAX15.

H-ras Mediated Chromosome Transfer Generates New Markers for 11p13

The CAT and FSHB genes are the closest known markers to the WT and AN
genes but are still likely to be several megabases away as evidenced
by their maintenance in several chromosomes containing cytologically
detectable 11p13 deletions. Thus we had to devise a way to select for
clones which mapped to 11p and to the p13 band in particular. To this
end we chose to use the procedure known as chromosome mediated gene
transfer (for review see Porteous, 1987) to introduce fragments of 11p
into mouse cells. In brief we first prepared mitotic chromosomes from
the human bladder carcinoma cell line in which the H-ras oncogene on
chromosome 11p15 is active. These chromosomes were introduced into
mouse C127 cells by the calcium phosphate procedure and transformed
foci were obtained at the frequency of 1/500,000 cells (Porteous et
al., 1986). We then proceeded to show that the transfected cells had
taken up stably fragments of chromosome 11 ranging in size from 1 to
50 megabases. Analysis of the patterns of cotransfer of 11p markers
along with H-ras showed that in each case large scale deletions accompanied the chromosome transfer process (Table 1). However in both
transformed clones E671 (~30mb human DNA) and E656 (~5-10mb human DNA)
markers flanking the WAGR locus were transferred intact (MIC11 maps
closer than CAT) so we decided to make genomic DNA libraries from both
these transfectants with the hope that these would be enriched for 11p
and 11p13 markers. This indeed proved to be the case; phage or cos-
mids containing human inserts were isolated from these libraries using
a labeled "alu" or total human DNA probe and then mapped to our panel
of deletions and translocations (Porteous et al., 1987). All 100 or so
new markers isolated this way mapped to chromosome 11 and the majority
of these to 11p (Figure 2, right side). These markers now allow us to
distinguish the end points of the different deletions which appear to
be a nested set. The new markers establish that our panel can be used
to divide the short arm of chromosome 11 into 10 contiguous segments.
Most importantly we now have 12 new markers mapping to 11p13, at least
2 of these closer than FSHB to the WAGR genes.

CO-TRANSFER OF SYNTENIC GENE MARKERS IN HRAS1-CMGT.

HRAS1-CMGT	HRAS1	INS	HBB	PTH	CALC1	LDHA	FSHB	MIC11	CAT	MIC4	PGA	APOA1	MIC8
E65-6 +	·	·	·	·	·	+	+	+	·	·	·	·	·
E67-1 +	+	+	·	·	·	+	+	+	+	·	+	·	·
E67-4 +	·	·	·	·	·	·	+	+	+	·	·	·	·

Table 1. Co-transfer of syntenic gene markers in HRAS1-CMGT. The genes are listed according to the consensus map order. PGA is the pepsinogen-A gene, Apo-A1 is the apolipoprotein-A1 gene and MIC8 is the gene encoding a cell surface antigen.

Future Plans to Isolate the Genes

We now have 14 markers which map to the 11p13 band, a spacing on average of 300-400 kb pairs per marker. Thus some of these markers may be very close to or within one of the WAGR genes if the latter are several hundred kb in size. The clones marked with an asterisk (Figure 2) hybridise to mouse as well as human DNA and so might constitute exons of genes. We are using these to look for transcripts and using all the clones to look for rearrangements within Wilms' tumors, a property expected of the WT gene by analogy with the retinoblastoma gene (Friend et al., 1986). However before looking for genes it is perhaps best to build up a large scale map of this region using pulsed field gel electrophoresis (PFGE) (Schwarz and Cantor, 1984). We have succeeded in linking up the FSHB gene and the λPI2C9 clone. It is crucial to link markers which flank the WT and AN genes by PFGE in order to obtain an idea of the limits of the problem.

Perhaps the best way to isolate the aniridia gene is to attempt to identify clones which map to the SIMX translocation breakpoint itself. Again PFGE should allow us to pick up the translocation and deletion breakpoints at distance. The POR translocation was associated with renal dysplasia, a condition characterised by failure of nephron differentiation. This breakpoint might well be within the WT gene itself or another closely linked gene involved in kidney differentiation. If deemed practicable we will start to walk or jump (Poustka and Lehrach, 1986) from our closest markers to these translocation breakpoints. If we need to obtain more markers we will construct libraries from large fragments containing our closest markers and isolated from preparative pulsed field gels. As an alternative we have successfully carried out CMGT using, this time, antibodies to MIC4 and MIC11 to select mouse cells containing the p13 region using the FACS.

REFERENCES

Friend SH, Bernards R, Rogelj S, Weinberg RA, Rapaport JM, Albert DM and Dryja TP (1986) A human DNA segment with properties of the gene that predisposes to retinoblastoma and osteosarcoma. Nature 323: 643-646.
Glaser T, Lewis WH, Bruns GAP, Watkins PC, Rogler CE, Shows TB, Powers VE, Willard HF, Goguen JM, Simola KOJ and Housman DE (1986) Nature 321:882-887.

Knudson AG Jr and Strong LC (1972) Mutation and cancer: a model for
  Wilms' tumor of the kidney. J Natl Cancer Inst 48:313-324.
Koufos A, Hansen MF, Lampkin BC, Workman ML, Copeland NG, Jenkins NA
  and Cavenee WK (1984) Loss of alleles at loci on human chromosome 11
  during genesis of Wilms' tumor. Nature 309:170-172.
Porteous DJ, Morten JEN, Cranston G, Fletcher JM, Mitchell AR, van
  Heyningen V, Fantes JA, Boyd PA and Hastie ND (1986) Molecular and
  physical arrangements of human DNA in HRAS1-selected, chromosome-
  mediated transfectants. Mol Cell Biol 6:2223-2232.
Porteous DJ, Bickmore W., Christie S, Boyd PA, Cranston G, Fletcher
  JM, Gosden JR, Rout D, Seawright A, Simola KOJ, van Heyningen V and
  Hastie ND (1987) HRAS1-selected chromosome transfer generates
  markers that colocalize anirida- and genitourinary dysplasia-
  associated translocation breakpoints and the Wilms' tumor gene
  within band 11p13. Proc Natl Acad Sci USA 84:5355-5459.
Porteous DJ (1987) Chromosome mediated gene transfer: a functional
  assay for complex loci and an aid to human genome mapping. Trends
  in Genetics 7: 177-182.
Riccardi VM, Hittner HM, Strong LC, Fernback DJ, Lebo R and Ferrell RF
  (1982) Wilms' tumor with aniridia/iris dysplasia and apparently
  normal chromosomes. Pediatrics 100:574-577.
Poustka A and Lehrach H (1986) Jumping libraries and linking
  libraries: the next generation of molecular tools in mammalian
  genetics. Trends in Genetics 2:174-179.
Schwartz DC and Cantor CR (1984) Separation of yeast chromosome-sized
  DNAs by pulsed field gradient gel electrophoresis. Cell 37:67-75.
Seawright A, Fletcher JM, Fantes JA, Morrison H, Porteous DJ, Li SS-L,
  Hastie ND and van Heyningen V (1988) Analysis of WAGR deletions and
  related translocations with gene-specific DNA probes, using FACS-
  selected cell hybrids. Somat Cell Mol Genet (in press).
van Heyningen V, Boyd PA, Seawright A, Fletcher JM, Fantes JA, Buckton
  KE, Spowart G, Porteous DJ, Hill RE, Newton MS and Hastie ND (1985)
  Molecular analysis of chromosome 11 deletions in aniridia-Wilms'
  tumor syndrome. Proc Natl Acad Sci USA 82:8592-8596.

ACKNOWLEDGEMENTS

We would like to thank Professor H.J. Evans for his support and
encouragement throughout all phases of this work; Sheila Christie,
Judy Fletcher, Anne Seawright, Hazel Cameron and Gwen Cranston for
excellent technical assistance; Katie Browne for excellent
secretarial assistance and Sandy Bruce and Norman Davidson for
excellent photographic work.

Approaching the Mouse *Steel* Locus from Closely Linked Molecular Markers

L. Stubbs , A. Poustka*, D. Rohme**, L. B. Russell***, and H. Lehrach

INTRODUCTION

The mouse *Steel* locus is involved in a crucial step of the early development of three important stem cell types: skin melanocytes, erythropoietic stem cells, and primordial germ cells. Homozygotes of the more severe alleles are typically white with black eyes, sterile, and suffer from a severe macrocytic anemia which often results in the death of affected animals in utero, or shortly after birth (Sarvella and Russell, 1956). The effects of *Sl* mutations can first be detected during the period when the three stem cell populations begin to migrate from their distinct sites of origin to colonize specific target tissues, within which their proliferation and further differentiation will be completed. In *Sl* homozygotes, the migrating cells apparently do not reach their targets in sufficient numbers to allow continued normal development (Bennett, 1956). The stem cells themselves are not defective, and can develop normally when placed into the proper wild type environment (McCulloch et al, 1965; Mayer, 1973); instead it is the tissues with which the stem cells interact as they proliferate and differentiate, during migration and beyond, that are responsible for expression of the mutant phenotype. Although no simple plan for the isolation of *Sl* coding sequences can be currently envisioned, the extensive genetic analysis of the locus makes it a good candidate for the application of recently developed "reverse genetic" approaches. Toward the goal of the isolation and analysis of DNA sequences at *Sl*, we have initiated such a molecular approach, beginning with the mapping of the locus relative to closely linked markers, and the directed movement from the markers toward the gene using chromosome jumping (Poustka and Lehrach, 1986) and related techniques.

RESULTS AND DISCUSSION

Mapping the T(10;17) breakpoint

Our approach requires that cloned markers exist which lie relatively close to the gene in question; in practical terms, maximally within one centimorgan. Since *Sl* has been mapped to a region of chromosome 10 devoid of such closely linked markers, we have used mice carrying a 10;17 translocation which is itself a *Steel* mutation (T11Rl; Cacheiro and Russell, 1975), to bring the locus into close linkage with markers mapping within the proximal third of chromosome 17. Due to efforts by a number of laboratories over the past several years, this region of chromosome 17, containing the T/t complex and the MHC, is well saturated with closely-spaced and well-mapped molecular markers (Steinmetz et al, 1982; Herrmann et al, 1986). It was therefore likely that we might find markers lying close enough to the

---

Imperial Cancer Research Fund Laboratories, P.O. Box 123, Lincoln's Inn Fields, London W2CA 3PX UK

*Max Planck Institut fur Medizinische Forschung, Neuenheimer Feld, D-6900 Heidelberg, FRG
** University of Lund, Lund, Sweden
***Biology Division, Oak Ridge National Laboratories, Oak Ridge, Tennessee

11RI mouse fibroblasts × hamster

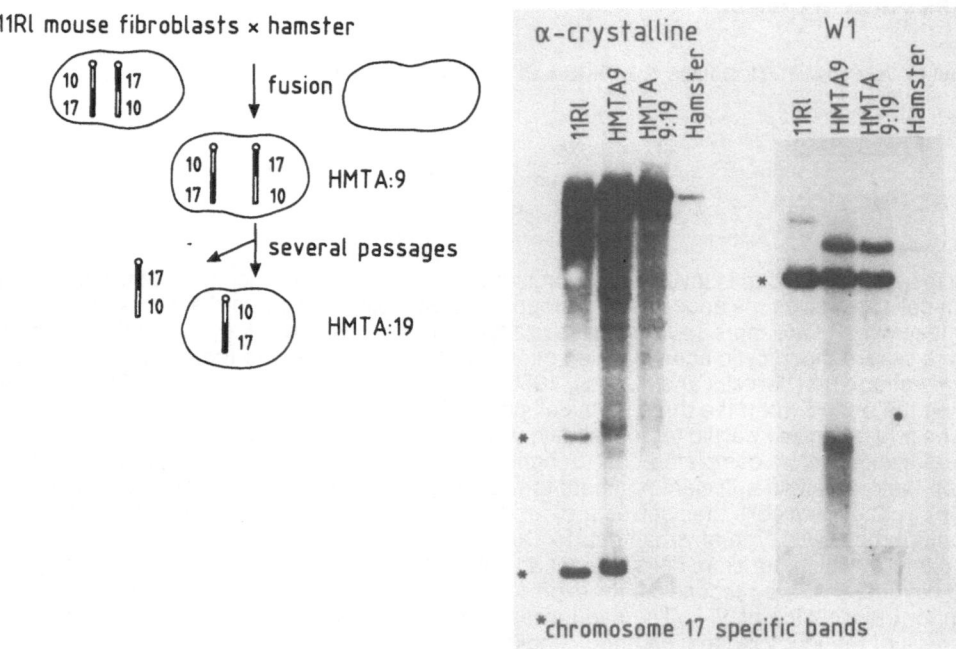

Figure 1. Schematic outline of the derivation of hybrid cell lines used for mapping, and Southern blot comparing EcoR1 digested DNA derived from T11RI mice, V79 hamster cells, and the two mouse-hamster hybrid lines, after hybridization with w1 and Crya-1 probes.

---

chromosome 17 translocation breakpoint to allow eventual access to associated sequences on chromosome 10. In order to map the site of translocation on chromosome 17, we fused lung fibroblasts derived from heterozygous T11RI /+ mice to transformed hamster cells, and passed independent clonal lines for several generations. We then screened DNA isolated from a number of lines on Southern blots with probes located either very distally or proximally on chromosome 17, in order to identify cell lines which had lost one or the other of the two reciprocal translocation chromosomes, along with the wild type copy of chromosome 17. In this way one cell line , HMTA 9:19, was identified, which carried DNA sequences derived from the distal portion of mouse chromosome 17 but not from the from the proximal region. After hybridization of a number of cloned markers to DNA derived from HMTA 9:19, we were able to locate two markers which are closely neighboring on wild type chromosome17, but separated onto different chromosomes by the T11RI translocation. Figure 1 shows a Southern blot analysis of DNA derived from a spleen of an T11RI homozygous mouse, compared with DNA from HMTA 9:19, HMTA 9 (the parent cell line of HMTA 9, containing both translocation chromosomes), and V79 hamster cells. As can be seen, the probe w1, derived from the most proximal cloned portion of the MHC (Weiss et al, 1984), detects a mouse-specific EcoR1 fragment in both of the hybrid cell lines, while the cDNA for alpha-A-crystallin (*Crya-1*; King et al 1982) recognizes mouse-specific EcoR1 fragments only in HMTA 9, and not in the HMTA 9:19 cell line. *Crya-1* has been shown to map 1 cM proximal to the *H2K* gene, which lies just 70 kb distal of the w1 probe . These results thus place the T11RI translocation breakpoint within a 1 cM region lying between *Crya-1* and the proximal end of the MHC.

A physical map of the w1 to *Crya-1* interval

Before beginning a series of jumps between flanking markers w1 and Crya-1 toward the translocation breakpoint, it was necessary to establish a long-range restriction map around the two probes. Establishment of the map was necessary for the localization of nearby sites for rare-cutting restriction enzymes, which represent the startpoints and endpoints in our jumping libraries, as well as for the determination of a minimal distance between the two markers in wild type DNA, and from the markers to the site of translocation. Cosmid clones immediately surrounding w1 show an unusual concentration of rare-cutting enzyme sites, most of which are very well cut in genomic DNA (L.Stubbs, unpublished). One cluster of sites lying 7 kb proximal of w1 provides an endpoint for many different restriction fragments, so that most fragments detected by the w1 probe on Southern blots are quite short, or extend distally toward *H2K*. The one exception is a restriction fragment generated by the enzyme Not I, which measures approximately 1.5 million base pairs (Mbp) in length; since a very well-cut Not I site lies just 20 kb proximal to w1, we can determine that this very long fragment extends away from the MHC, and toward *Crya-1* (Figure 2, figure 3). The Crya-1 probe detects a separate pair of partially cut fragments of 800-900 kbp (fig.3), and so it is possible to establish that the interval between the two neighboring probes is at least 1.5 Mbp in length. We have not yet been able to determine the position of the Crya-1 probe relative to the ends of the restriction fragments which it detects on Southern blots, nor to find fragments generated by either complete or partial digests which physically link the w1 and Crya-1 sequences. Therefore the exact distance between these two markers is as yet unknown.

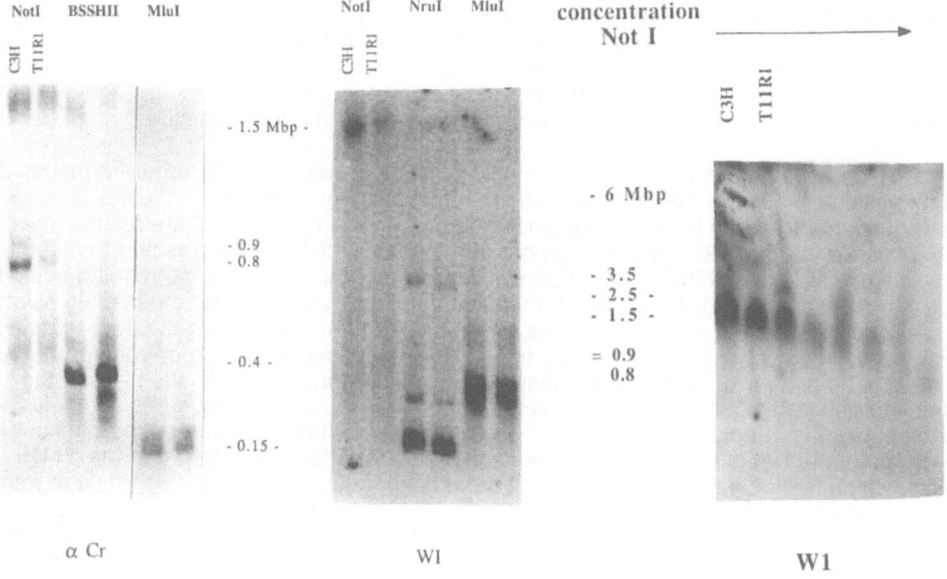

Figure 2. Southern blots comparing DNA from T11RI and C3H mice, separated on pulsed-field gels after restriction with rare-cutting enzymes. Left: Complete digests, hybridized with w1 or Crya-1 probes. Right: DNA treated with a range of concentrations of the enzyme Not I, to yeild partially cut fragments, and hybridized with the w1 probe.

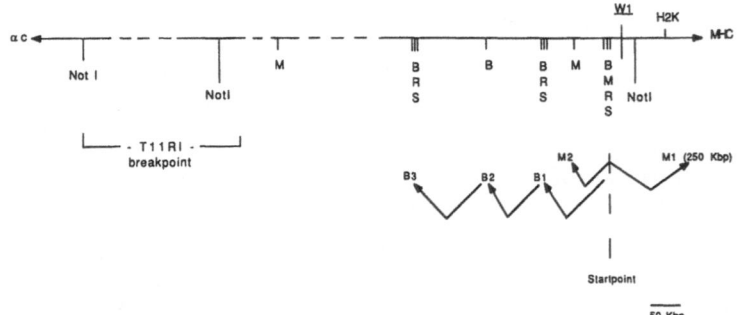

Figure 3. A restriction map extending proximally from the w1 probe toward *Crya-1*, including data from probes derived from jumping. B1,B2, and B3 are jumping clones selected from a BssH II library; M1 and M2 were isolated from a library constructed with MluI.

Mapping the distance between the flanking markers and the site of translocation

T11RI arose spontaneously on a C3Hx101 F1 hybrid, and has since been continously backcrossed with C3H. It is therefore possible, when comparing maps of DNA from mice of these wild type strains to that of T11RI, to relate restriction fragment length polymorphisms (RFLPs) detected by a flanking probe to the DNA rearrangement caused by translocation. Since we have found that the C3H and 101 strains give identical restriction maps for rare-cutting enzyme sites in this region (L. Stubbs, unpublished) , we will show only the comparison between DNA of C3H and T11RI mice. Neither flanking probe detects polymorphic fragments between mutant and wild type DNA after complete digestion with any enzymes tested (figure 2), including Not I. This suggests that the translocation breakpoint is at least 1.5 Mbp from the w1 probe, although it should be noted that our resolution of fragments of this size is not good enough to detect a polymorphism of several hundred kbp in either direction.

We next examined DNA samples cut partially by Not I, in order to yield larger fragments that might possibly cross the site of translocation. Since the Not I site lying just distal of w1 is so well cut, and since Not I fragments extending further distal into the MHC are relatively short, it was possible to orientate a partial fragment of approximately 2.5 Mbp detected by the w1 probe in wild type DNA as extending in the proximal direction (Figure 2). A fragment of comparable size is not detected in T11RI DNA after the same partial digest with Not I. In fact, no obvious partially cut fragment is detected with the w1 probe in T11RI DNA. Such a results suggests that the next well-cut Not I site brought in by translocation is either very close or very far from the end of the Not I band including w1: in the first case, the differences between the sizes of the complete and partially cut fragments would be too small to be detected, while a very large band >6 Mbp) would not enter our gel under these running conditions. Further experiments will favor one of the two alternative explanations, but data thus far do suggest that the T11RI translocation has occurred within the Not I band neighboring that containing w1, and within a distance of 1.5 to 2.5 Mbp from that probe. No RFLPs are detected by the Crya-1 probe between DNA from the translocation mutant and wild type mice, and so the distance from this marker to the site of translocation cannot be determined.

Closing the Gap between w1 and the Site of Translocation

A distance such as that predicted between w1 and the T11RI translocation breakpoint can only be bridged with innovations in even the most recent technologies. We are moving toward that goal by a series of jumps between neighboring rare-cutting enzyme sites within the region proximal to w1. Attempts to retrieve a jumping clone containing the endpoints of the 1.5 kb Not

I fragment have not yet been successful; most progress has been made so far with libraries constructed with the enzymes Mlu I and BSSH II (fig. 3), covering a total distance of 400 kb thus far. At present it is quite possible, given the appropriate spacing of useful restriction sites, to jump at least 450 kbp at a single step (T. Pohl and A. Poustka, unpublished) ; methods to increase the potential sizes of steps spanned by jumping clones are currently being explored. The cloning of fragments exicised from low-melting agarose gels (Michelis et al, 1986) , although more difficult for a single step, is a complementing strategy which can also be applied to longer DNA fragments. We are now in the process of applying all of these techniques to the region surrounding the T11RI translocation.

Jumping as a Means of Finding Genes

Recently, Bird (1986) has described sequences near the 5' end of many mammalian genes, which are highly enriched for undermethylated CpG doublets. Recognition sequences for the rare-cutting enzymes used in the construction of jumping libraries contain one or more CpGs, and are therefore often found clustered these CpG-rich "islands". This fact makes it likely that sequential jumps will quite frequently lead us directly to into the vicinity of neighboring genes within a genomic segment. Our data thus far supports the notion that jumping with libraries constructed with rare-cutting enzymes biases our movement into close proximity of transcribed sequences; jumping startpoints and endpoints, are often highly conserved in a variety of species, and frequently detect specific RNA species when applied as a probe to Northern blots containing RNA from selected mouse tissues (L. Stubbs, unpublished). These "islands" within the w1-*Crya-1* interval and their associated transcripts are of great interest, since they may be related to certain genetic loci which have been mapped to this region. Of particular interest is the gene corresponding to*tw5* , one of the t -complex embryonic lethal mutations , which is closely linked to, and thought to lie just proximal to, the H2K gene (Shin et al, 1984). For this reason, as we proceed toward the T11RI translocation breakpoint, and thus toward *Sl*, we are carefully analyzing all sequences lying close to our jumping endpoints for possible evidence of transcriptional activity.

CONCLUSION   AND SUMMARY

Toward the goal of the isolation and analysis of the functions of the mouse *Steel* locus, we have initiated a strategy using chromosome jumping and related techniques to move toward the gene from closely linked flanking markers. Since no cloned markers lie very near to *Sl* in wild type chromosome 10, we have used mice carrying a (10;17) translocation to bring the gene into close linkage with markers on chromosome 17. From the closest of the identified flanking markers, we have derived a series of probes closer and closer to the translocation breakpoint, with the eventual goal of jumping across the breakpoint into *Sl*. The fact that our libraries bias our movement directly into adjacent HTF islands may be helpful in the eventual identification of *Sl* coding sequences. Since TIIRI translocation is itself a *Sl* allele, it is likely that the breakpoint lies close to or within the gene. Therefore it is possible that our first jump over the breakpoint, with libraries constructed from T11RI DNA, will lead us directly into the *Steel* locus. If not, it is likely that we will be close enough to the gene to use the extensive collection of induced and spontaneous *Sl* mutations to guide us to the gene.

Acknowledgement
We thank Gene Rinchik for suggestions and helpful discussions on the Oak Ridge *Steel* mutations. L.S. was supported by an NIH postdoctoral fellowship.

REFERENCES

Bennett,D. (1956). Developmental analysis of a mutation with pleiotropic effects in the mouse. J. Morphol.. 98:199-234.

Bird, A. (1986). CpG-rich islands and the function of DNA methylation. Nature 331:209-213.

Cacheiro, M.L.A, and L.B. Russell (1975). Evidence that linkage group IV as well as linkage of the mouse are in chromosome 10. Genet. Res. Camb. 25: 193-195.

Herrmann, B. G.,.Bucan, M., Mains, P.E., Frischauf, A.M., Silver, L.M., and Lehrach, H. (1986). Genetic Analysis of the proximal portion of the mouse t-complex: evidence for a second inversion in t-haplotypes. Cell 44:469-476.

King, C., Shinoharo, T., and Piatogorsky, J. (1982). Alpha-crystallin messenger RNA: more non-coding than coding sequences. Science 215:985-987.

Mayer, T.C. (1973). Site of gene action in steel mice: analysis of the pigment defect by mesoderm-ectoderm recombinations. J. Exp. Zool. 184:345-352.

McCulloch, E.A., Siminovitch, L., Till, J.E., Russell, E.S., and Bernstein, S.E. (1965). The cellular basis of the genetically determined hemopoietic defect in anemic mice of the genotypeSl/Sld. Blood 26: 399-410.

Michiels, F., Burmeister, M. and Lehrach, H. (1986). Derivation of clones close to met by preparative field inversion gel electrophoresis. Science 236:1305-1307.

Poustka, A., and Lehrach, H. (1986). Jumping libraries and linking libraries: the next generationof molecular tools in mammalian genetics. TIGS 2:174-179.

Sarvella, P.A., and L.B. Russell. (1956). Steel, a new dominant gene in the house mouse. J. Hered. 47: 123-128.

Shin, H., Bennett, D., and Artzt, K. (1984). Gene Mapping within the T/t complex of Mouse. IV The inverted MHC is intermingled with several t-lethal genes. Cell 39: 573-578.

Skow, L.C., and Donner, M.E. (1985). The locus encoding A-crystallin is closely linked to H2-K on mouse chromosome 17. Genetics 11:723-732.

Steinmetz, M., Minard, K., Horvath, S., McNicholas, J., Srelinger, J., Wake, C., Long, E., Mach, B., and Hood, L. (1982). A molecular map of the immune response region from the major histocompatibility complex of the mouse. Nature 300: 35-42.

Weiss, E.H., Golden, L., Fahrner, K., Mellor, A., Devlin, J., Bullman, H., Tiddens, H. , Bud, H., and Flavell, R. (1984). Nature 310:650-655.

II. Complex Loci Involved in the Regulation of Developmental and Immunological Processes

Probing Mouse Origins with Random DNA Probes

J. Klein[1,2], V. Vincek[1], M. Kasahara[2], and F. Figueroa

Reading in chapter 17 of the mouse DNA chronicle

Until not so long ago, many villages and towns used to have their
own chroniclers who took it upon themselves to record for posterity
those events which they believed to be the most important in the
life of the community. They were, of course, no professionals; they
were farmers, bakers, shoemakers, or pursued whatever occupation
happened to be in their family tradition, and none of them were
particularly literate. The chronicles they kept were therefore a
mixture of trivia, as well as a source of important information
about the events that had molded the population.

The DNA of a species is much like a village chronicle. It, too, has
a touch of immediacy about it because it has recorded both inconse-
quential and notable events. The mouse DNA has 20 chapters, alto-
gether comprising some 1.1×10^8 letters. It makes fascinating as
well as challenging reading, and our ambition has been to read the
first half of Chapter 17 which records the events on the proximal
part of chromosome 17. Why this particular part? Because it records
the origin of one of the most enthralling group of genes -- the t
complex. We have not come very far as yet, mainly because we still
have the problem of distinguishing the trivia from the important
events, but what we have learnt thus far sheds light not only on the
t complex but also on the origin of the mouse species.

Random and Nonrandom DNA Probes

The problem we faced after having resolved to read Chapter 17 was
how to find it and how to obtain copies of the pages we wanted to
read. We could use the genes already isolated from the chromosome
17 as probes, and this we did (Figueroa et al. 1985; Bukara et al.
1985; Golubić et al. 1985). These probes, however, are limited in
number and cover only a very short segment of chromosome 17; we were
therefore anxious to find other ways of reading in the chronicle.
One such way has been pioneered by Lehrach and his associates (Fox
et al. 1985; Roehme et al. 1984), who isolated chromosome 17 under
the dissecting microscope and cloned parts of it in a plasmid. We
have used these probes (Figueroa et al. 1987a), too, but even they
are limited to only small bits of chromosome 17 and the need for a
broader access to the chromosome remained. To satisfy this need we
have embarked on a random cloning of chromosome 17.

The cloning has been made possible by the existence of a hybrid cell
line that carries Chinese hamster chromosomes and a single pair of
mouse chromosomes (Smiley et al. 1987). The pair is a metacentric
chromosome which combines chromosomes 17 and 18, as well as bits of
chromatin from unspecified origin (Richards et al. 1985). The idea
was to make a genomic library from DNA isolated from this cell line,
screen the library with mouse repetitive sequences that do not
hybridize with hamster DNA and hence identify mouse clones, and then
find clones derived from mouse chromosome 17 (Kasahara et al. 1987a,
1987b, Fig. 1). This last step could be accomplished with the help
of another cell line, JS17, produced in our laboratory (Szymura et

[1]Max-Planck-Institut für Biologie, Abteilung Immungenetik,
 Corrensstrasse 42, D-7400 Tübingen, F.R.G
[2]Department of Microbiology and Immunology, University of
 Miami School of Medicine, Miami, Florida 33101, U.S.A

Current Topics in Microbiology and Immunology, Vol. 137
© Springer-Verlag Berlin · Heidelberg 1988

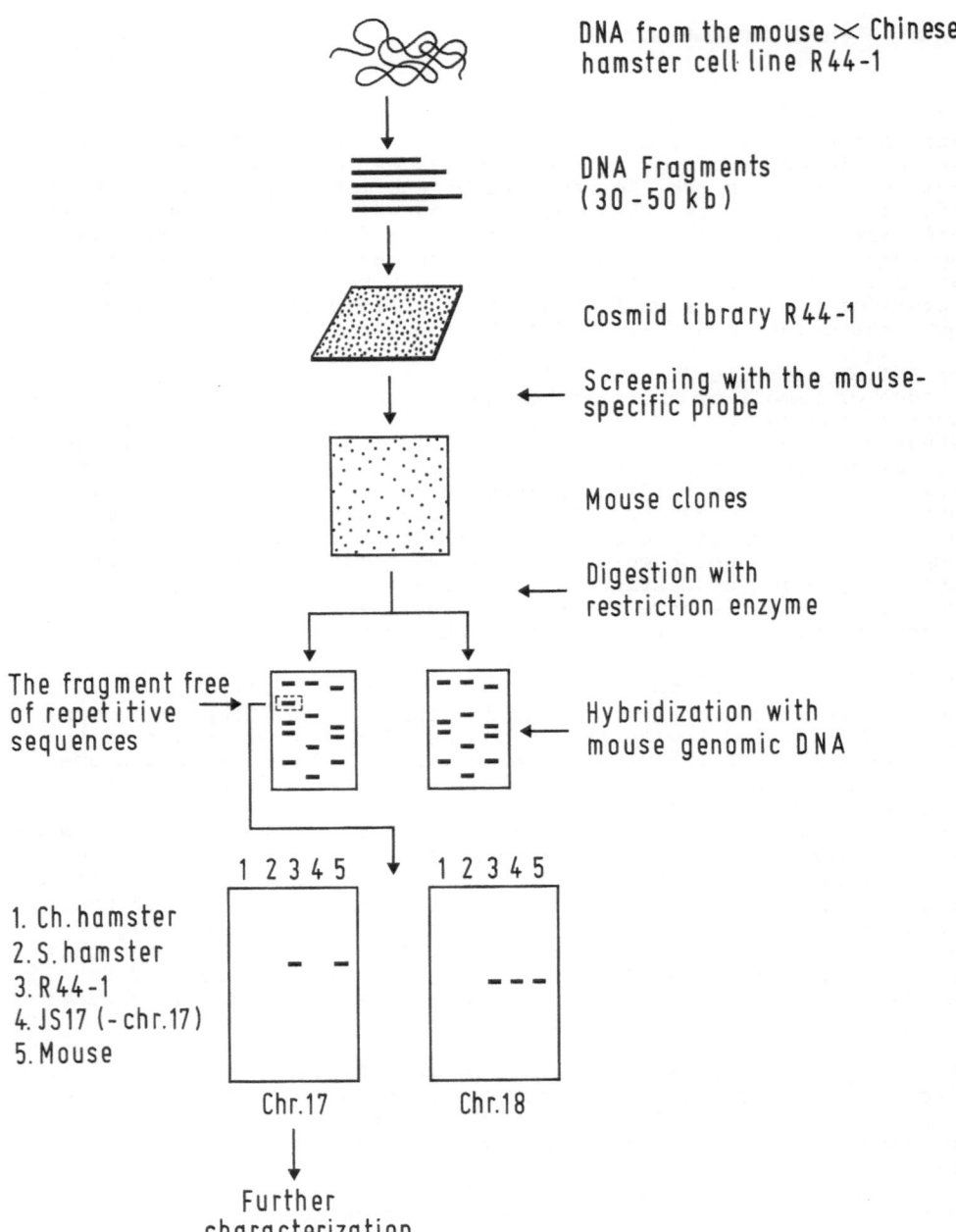

DNA from the mouse × Chinese hamster cell line R44-1

DNA Fragments (30-50 kb)

Cosmid library R44-1

Screening with the mouse-specific probe

Mouse clones

Digestion with restriction enzyme

The fragment free of repetitive sequences

Hybridization with mouse genomic DNA

1 2 3 4 5   1 2 3 4 5

1. Ch. hamster
2. S. hamster
3. R44-1
4. JS17 (-chr.17)
5. Mouse

Chr. 17   Chr. 18

Further characterization

Fig. 1. Experimental design used to isolate chromosome 17 specific sequences. Clones were identified by their positive hybridization with mouse and R44-1 derived DNA and their lack of hybridization with DNA derived from the JS17 cell line. These two mouse x hamster cell lines differ in that the former does and the latter does not carry the mouse chromosome 17.

al. 1981). This hybrid cell line contains Syrian hamster chromosomes
and all mouse chromosomes except number 17. Any DNA clone hybridizing with total mouse DNA but not with the DNA isolated from the
JS17 line should derive from mouse chromosome 17. The position of
the DNA on chromosome 17 can then be determined by testing a set of
recombinants involving different segments of this chromosome.

The random cloning approach has the potential for providing two
kinds of DNA probes -- probes for genes and probes for unique,
noncoding sequences. The genes can be detected by screening RNA or
cDNA libraries obtained from different mouse tissues. The unique
noncoding sequences can be detected by hybridization with total
mouse DNA. The main problem with this approach is the abundancy of
repetitive DNA in the mammalian genome. For a molecular biologist,
repetitive DNA may be an interesting material to study, but for a
geneticist it is a curse he has not yet learnt to avoid. Repetitive
DNA is found all over the clones and even in the cDNA. Its over-re-
presentation in the genome means that genes and other unique sequences are masked by thick bands or smears formed by this junk
material on both Southern and Northern blots. There are various ways
in which to deal with it but no foolproof way of avoiding it alto-
gether. The method we use is to compete out the repetitive DNA with
genomic mouse DNA and thus reveal the unique sequences, which then
could be used as probes. Using this method we have thus far been
able to isolate one new gene (Kasahara et al. 1987a, b) and two non-
coding probes (Kasahara et al. 1987b; Figueroa et al. 1987b) mapping
to chromosome 17. It will be the latter that we shall concentrate on
in this communication.

Polymorphism of D17Tu1 and D17Tu2 Probes

The two noncoding probes, designated D17Tu1 and D17Tu2 and abbre-
viated here to Tu1 and Tu2, are located on the opposite borders of
the segment that we are interested in (Fig. 2). The Tu1 element is
located near the centromere of the acrocentric chromosome 17,
whereas the Tu2 element maps into the S region of the H-2 complex
(in fact, the cosmid clone from which the Tu2 probe was isolated
carries the C4 gene). These two elements are therefore not very
useful for probing the t complex, but they have provided interesting
information about the mouse populations.

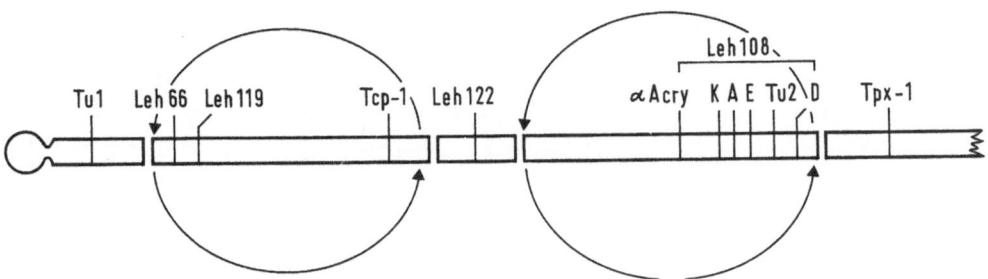

Fig. 2. Genetical map of the proximal part of the mouse chromosome
17. Tu1 and Tu2 refer to the D17Tu1 and D17Tu2 markers as described
in the text. The Leh numbers refer to the markers described in
Roehme et al. (1984); αAcry corresponds to the α-crystalline gene;
K, A, E, and D are Mhc loci and Tpx-1 is a gene described by Kasahara et al. (1987a, b).

58

Both elements are polymorphic in the laboratory and the wild mouse
(Figueroa et al. 1987b, Fig. 3 and 4). The polymorphism of the Tu2
element correlates well with the H-2 polymorphism in the sense
that all strains having a particular H-2 haplotype carry the same
form of the Tu2 element. This finding is not surprising considering
the location of the element within the H-2 complex. Since, however,
the same form of Tu2 is always shared by several H-2 haplotypes, it
is possible to group these H-2 haplotypes into higher-order categories presumably reflecting their evolutionary relationships.
Using this probe, as well as other markers and the sequences of the
H-2 loci themselves, it should therefore be possible to construct an
evolutionary tree not only of H-2 genes, but also H-2 haplotypes.
This tree would tell us a great deal about the origin of H-2 and
also of the mouse populations.

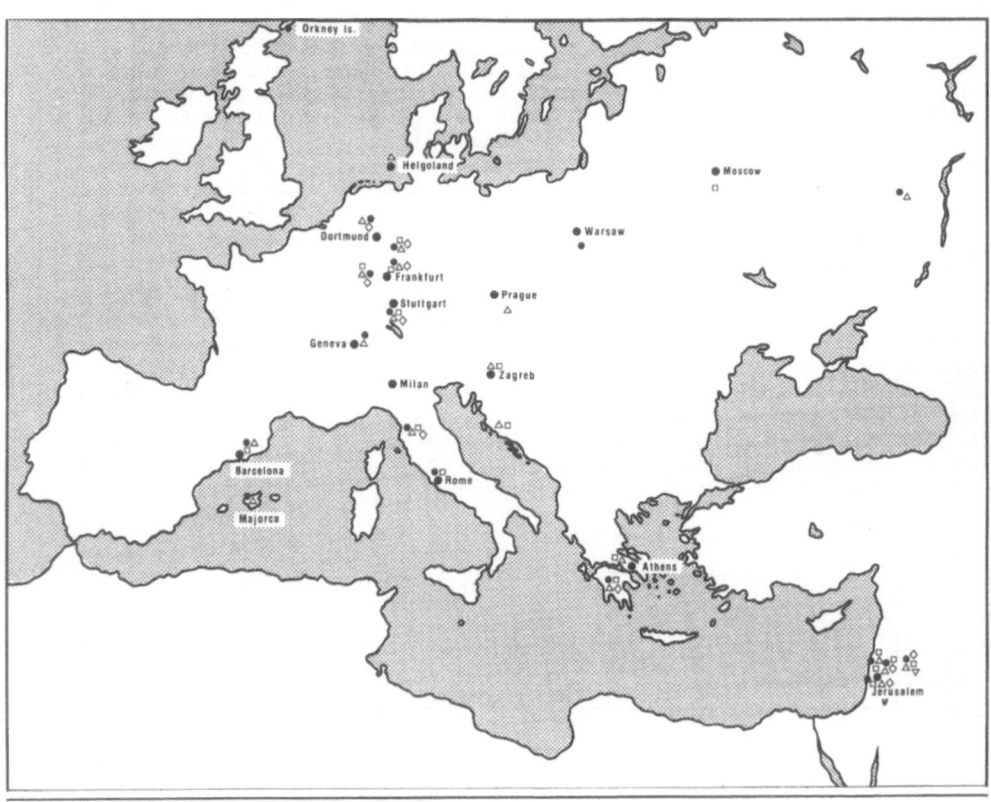

Fig. 3. Geographical distribution of the RFLP patterns defined by
hybridization with the D17Tu2 probe. The different patterns are
represented by different symbols.

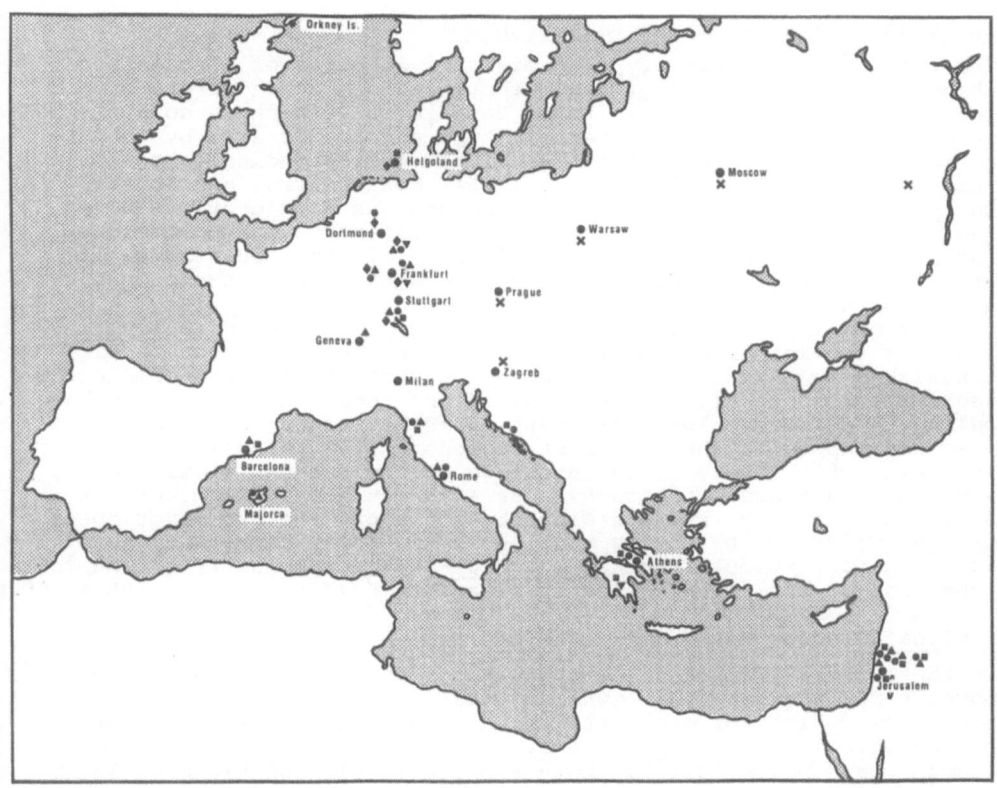

Fig. 4. Geographical distribution of the RFLP patterns defined
by hybridization with the D17Tu1 probe. The different patterns
are represented by different symbols.

The polymorphism of the Tu1 element does not, and this fact is not
surprising, correlate with the H-2 polymorphism. By studying the
distribution of this polymorphism, we could make two interesting
observations. First, the polymorphisms present in the laboratory
mouse are absent in European wild mice and vice versa. Second, while
the populations of Mus domesticus show high Tu1 polymorphism, the
populations of Mus musculus are monomorphic (with the restriction
endonucleases that we used). The former observation suggests that
European wild mice have not contributed in a significant way to the
derivation of the laboratory mouse. The second observation has
important implications for the origin of the mouse populations.
However, before we discuss these implications, we shall mention two
other observations of a similar nature.

Chromosomal and t-complex Polymorphisms

The standard mouse karyotype consists of 20 pairs of acrocentric chromosomes. About half of the European wild mice, however, have less than 40 chromosomes in their somatic cells because some of the chromosomes are of the metacentric type and are derived by Robertsonian fusions of the centromeres of the corresponding acrocentric chromosomes (reviewed in Winking 1986). Most Central and South European populations belonging to the species M. domesticus have individuals with at least one pair of metacentric chromosomes but the number is as high as 11 pairs in some of the populations. In striking contrast to this situation, no metacentric chromosomes have as yet been discovered in mice of the species Mus musculus. Another similar difference between M. domesticus and M. musculus concerns the lethal genes of the t complex. The genes can be distinguished by a genetic complementation test: genes that complement each other and permit the survival of the "homozygotes" presumably belong to different loci. At least 16 lethal genes have been identified and mapped to the different regions of the t complex (reviewed in Klein 1986). The various lethal genes are present in wild mice, sometimes in frequencies as high as 40%, but here again there is a striking asymmetry in their distribution among the two major species of Mus: wild mice belonging to M. domesticus may carry any one of 16 lethal genes, whereas when M. musculus individuals carry a t haplotype, one of the lethal genes is always t^{w73} (Klein et al. 1984).

Implications for the Origin of Mice

In these three examples, the populations of M. domesticus are polymorphic for a given trait, whereas the populations of M. musculus are monomorphic. For other traits, however, both populations are polymorphic. The K, D, A_β, and E_β loci of the H-2 complex, for example, are polymorphic in both species (Klein and Figueroa 1981; Figueroa and Klein, unpublished data). How can this situation be explained?

The two species are geographically clearly separated: M. domesticus occupies western Europe, the Americas, and Australia, whereas M. musculus is distributed in eastern Europe and northern Asia. In Europe the species meet in a narrow hybrid zone that runs across the Jutland peninsula, then across Holstein, south to the Elbe, and then roughly follows the line Dessau-Nürnberg-Regensburg-München-Salzburg (Zimmermann 1958; Reichstein 1978). It is believed that the distribution in Europe was attained some 5,000 to 8,000 years ago, after the retreat of the last glacials and spreading of farming from the Middle East. This belief is based on the supposition that no mice could have survived in central and northern Europe during the glacial periods, and on the lack of any mouse remains at European archeological sites dated before the spreading of agriculture. It is further believed that mice colonized Europe on the heels of man and with the spreading of farming. It is inconceivable that the two species separated after their emigration from the Middle East 8,000 years ago, first, because molecular data indicate their age to be more than one million years, and second, because it is difficult to think of a mechanism that would isolate them along their present border, where there is no unsurmountable physical barrier. One must assume, therefore, that the two species were separated long before the introduction of agriculture and that they moved into Europe in two separate waves. The present-day border between M. domesticus and M. musculus in Europe represents the area where the two waves met. It is commonly assumed that the two waves originated in the "fertile

crescent", but we consider this assumption extremely improbable.
What barrier would have kept the two species apart in the Middle
East and why is this region now occupied only by M. domesticus? What
happened to M. musculus in the Middle East if it used to exit there
and why is there no trace of it now? Why is M. musculus so homogeneous in certain traits and M. domesticus heterogeneous? These and
other questions cannot be answered by the hypothesis which postulates
the origin of both species from the Middle East.

To reconcile the available data, we propose an alternative explanation of how mice reached Europe (Klein et al. 1987). We postulate
that house mice originated from an ancestral stock that lived in the
area of present-day Pakistan, where the murids seem to have originated. Some two million years ago, changes in the climatic conditions
made the Iranean plateau traversable for mice, and a group of them
crossed it to reach the steppes of Central Asia, only to become
separated from the main stock when the plateau became impassable
again. An alternative possibility -- that the mice reached Central
Asia by migrating into India and then north along the coast -- seems
less likely to us since the Himalayas send out high crests that run
almost all the way into the ocean over a broad area of the South-east
Asian coast. The two populations then existed either independently
or transiently associated with man in both regions, but isolated
from each other and thus they evolved into two different species,
the population in present-day Pakistan into M. domesticus and the
population in present-day China into M. musculus. During the neo-
lithic revolution, the association with man began to assume a
tighter form and occurred independently in the two major agricultural
centers: in the near East (the mice spread from Pakistan to the
fertile crescent either before the introduction of farming or after
farming diffused into Pakistan and India) and in China. As farming
began to spread into Europe, so did the mice: M. domesticus from the
near East and M. musculus from China. There was, however, a basic
difference in the way this spreading took place. For the most part,
M. domesticus hitched a ride on ships sailing along the Mediterranean
coast and began to colonize the shores of Greece, Yugoslavia, Italy,
France, Spain, Portugal, Holland, Denmark, and Great Britain. Only
later did it begin to move inland. The colonization occurred in
spurts and erratically because of the dependence on ships. Small
colonies became established at different places along the coast,
isolated from one another and from the parental population. A
considerable mixing of the populations occurred when the colonies
spread out and began contacting neighboring colonies and when the
ships brought new immigrants into the region. When the mice began to
move inland, they spread primarily along the main northsouth trading
routes. Again, they spread erratically, first establishing isolated
colonies that frequently went through population bottlenecks and
were continually replenished with new immigrants. This mode of
dispersal favored mixing of populations and thus laid the founda-
tions for the great genetic heterogeneity observed today in M.
domesticus.

M. musculus spread to Europe in an entirely different manner. The
migration took place on a single great wave that progressed from
China across the Asiatic part of the Soviet Union and into Eastern
Europe. The wave moved westward without losing contact with the
parental population, exchanging genes with this population for a
long time. This mode of colonization, therefore, involved less
intermixing of populations and hence tended to keep the populations
more homogeneous.

Why did the advance of M. musculus stop at the present border with
M. domesticus? Most likely because of the climatic conditions. The
border between the two species coincides almost exactly with the
are of transition from the oceanic to the continental climate, and
is also the border for several other closely related species of
animals and plants. As M. musculus still shows a tendency to
live outdoors for part of the year (Tupikova 1947), it may, in the
northern zones, be more dependent on climatic conditions than M.
domesticus.

And that is what we believe the few passages we have been able to
read in Chapter 17 of the Mouse Chronicle tell us.

ACKNOWLEDGMENTS

This work was supported in part by grant no. IMB 1 R01 AI23667 from
the National Institutes of Health, Bethesda, Maryland. We thank Ms.
Lynne Yakes for editorial assistance.

REFERENCES

Bukara M, Vincek V, Figueroa F, Klein J (1985) How polymorphic are
    class II loci of the mouse H-2 complex? Immunogenetics 21: 569-
    579
Figueroa F, Golubić M, Nizetić D, Klein J (1985) Evolution of
    mouse major histocompatibility complex genes borne by t chromo-
    somes. Proc Natl Acad Sci USA 82: 2819-2823
Figueroa F, Neufeld E, Ritte U, Klein J (1987a) t-Specific DNA poly-
    morphisms among wild mice from Israel and Spain. Genetics (sub-
    mitted)
Figueroa F, Kasahara M, Tichy H, Neufeld E, Ritte U, Klein J
    (1987b) Polymorphism of unique noncoding DNA sequences in
    wild and laboratory mice. Genetics (in press)
Fox HS, Martin GR, Lyon MF, Herrmann B, Frischauf, AM, Lehrach H,
    Silver LM (1985) Molecular probes define different regions
    of the t complex. Cell 40: 63-69
Golubić M, Figueroa F, Tosi M, Klein J (1985) Restriction fragment
    length polymorphism of C4 genes in mice with t chromosomes.
    Immunogenetics 21: 247-256
Kasahara M, Figueroa F, Klein J (1987a) Molecular cloning of a
    testis-specific gene from mouse chromosome 17. Transpl Proc
    19: 815-816
Kasahara M, Figueroa F, Klein J (1987b) Random cloning of genes
    from mouse chromosome 17. Proc Natl Acad Sci USA 84: 3325-3328.
Klein J (1986) Natural History of the Major Histocompatibility
    Complex. Wiley, New York
Klein J, Figueroa F (1981) Polymorphism of the mouse H-2 loci.
    Immunol Rev 60: 23-57
Klein J, Sipos P, Figueroa F (1984) Polymorphism of t-complex
    genes in European wild mice. Gent Res Camb 44: 39-46
Klein J, Tichy H, Figueroa F (1987) On the Origin of mice. Ann
    Univ Chile. (in press)
Reichstein H (1978) Mus musculus Linnaeus, 1758 Hausmaus. In:
    Niethammer J, Krapp F (ed) Handbuch der Säugetiere Europas,
    vol. 1/5 Akademische Verlagsgesellschaft, Wiesbaden, pp 421-451
Richards JE, Pravtcheva DD, Day C, Ruddle FH, Jones PP (1985)
    Murine invariant chain gene: Chromosomal assignment and segre-
    gation in recombinant inbred strains. Immunogenetics 22: 193-
    199
Roehme D, Fox H, Herrmann B, Frischauf AM, Edstrom JE, Mains P,

Silver LM, Lehrach H (1984) Molecular clones of the mouse t complex derived from microdissected metaphase chromosomes. Cell 36: 783-788

Smiley JR, Steege DA, Juricek DK, Summers WP, Ruddle FH (1978) A Herpes Simplex virus 1 intergration site in the mouse genome defined by somatic cell genetic analysis. Cell 15: 455-468

Szymura JM, Wabl MR, Klein J (1981) Mouse mitochondrial superoxide dismutase locus is on chromosome 17. Immunogenetics 14: 231-240

Tichy H, Vucak I (1987) Chromosomal polymorphism in the house mouse (Mus domesticus) of Greece and Yugoslavia. Chromosoma 95: 31-36

Tupikova NV (1947) Ecology of the house mouse in the central part of the USSR In: Fauna: ekologia gryzunov 2: 5-67 (in Russian)

Winking H (1986) Some aspects of Robertsonian karyotype variation in European wild mice. Curr Top Microbiol Immunol 127: 68-74

Zimmermann K (1950) Zur Kenntnis der mitteleuropäischen Hausmäuse. Zool Jb 78: 301-322

Mouse t Haplotypes: A Tale of Tails and a Misunderstood Selfish Chromosome

L.M. Silver

INTRODUCTION

The mouse t haplotype system has aroused the curiosity of numerous biologists over the last half century. It has been used as a model system to probe questions in fields as diversified as embryonic development, spermatogenesis, meiotic recombination, chromosome organization and evolution, population biology and selfish genes (see Silver, 1985, Frischauf, 1985 and Klein, 1986 for original references and more detailed reviews of the background material presented here). Until the last decade, the t system appeared to be unnaturally complex and enigmatic, even to the few workers brave enough to study it. But with the advent of molecular biology, the secrets of the t haplotype have been exposed, and a unified understanding of what-were-once unrelated properties has been attained. Although t haplotypes have lost their original sex appeal as enigmatic entities, they have gained status as a prototypical system for the study of both the genetic control of differentiative events, and general aspects of genomic organization and evolution.

HISTORICAL PERSPECTIVES AND MISPERCEPTIONS

Mouse t haplotypes were first discovered by a quirk of fate in the Parisian laboratory of Dobrovoloskaia-Zavadskaia in 1932. Fate had to play a hand in this discovery because mice that carry t haplotypes (both t/t homozygotes and t/+ heterozygotes) are indistinguishable to the eye from "wild-type" mice, and the eye was the major piece of equipment used by geneticists in 1932. The fateful turn of events that brought t haplotypes to light began with the appearance of a spontaneous mutation at the T locus (later shown to be on mouse chromosome 17) that caused a shortening of tail length in T/+ heterozygotes. To keep her stock of T-mutant mice going, Dobrovoloskaia-Zavadskaia was forced to collect wild mice for use as mating partners. t haplotypes are present in up to 20% of mice in wild populations, and consequently Dobrovoloskaia-Zavadskaia unknowingly set up matings between T-carrying animals and t-carrying animals. Now, although t haplotypes are invisible when they are in genomic isolation, they are uncovered by their ability to enhance the tail shortening effect of T mutations, such that doubly heterozygous T/t animals have no tail at all.

Since the T mutation and t haplotypes were originally discovered because of their effects on tail length, their names are based on

Department of Molecular Biology
Princeton University
Princeton, NJ 08544

Current Topics in Microbiology and Immunology, Vol. 137
© Springer-Verlag Berlin · Heidelberg 1988

this property (t stands for tail). Early genetic experiments
(carried out mostly by L. C. Dunn and his colleagues) brought out
several additional features of this system. First, no recombination
was observed between T and t. From this result, it appeared that the
spontaneous T mutation and the wild-derived t haplotype were
alleles at a single genetic locus. (The t haplotype was originally
called a t mutation or a t allele.) Second, when tailless T/t
animals were mated to each other, only tailless T/t offspring were
born. Neither T/T nor t/t animals were born because both T and
t acted as recessive lethal mutations. Later, through the capture
and breeding of additional wild mice from around the world, it
became clear that different wild-derived t haplotypes could carry
non-complementing lethal mutations such that t^1/t^2 animals were
viable.

Further experiments by Dunn's group led to the discovery of two
unrelated, bizarre phenotypes expressed by all wild-derived t
haplotypes - transmission ratio distortion (TRD) and recombination
suppression. TRD refers to the inheritance of the t-carrying
chromosome from a heterozygous +/t male by 95% or more of his
offspring (rather than the expected 50%). Recombination suppression
occurs along the region of chromosome 17 extending from the T locus
distally to the major histocompatibility complex (MHC) in both males
and females heterozygous for a t haplotype - the observed frequency
of crossing over along this region is reduced from the expected
15% to 0.1%. Finally, with the discovery that viable t^1/t^2
males were sterile, a complete picture of the phenotypes expressed by
t haplotypes was in place. The problem was that no one could
understand how the various parts of the picture - tail
length effects, lethality, transmission ratio distortion,
recombination suppression and sterility - all fit together.

Although fate allowed for the early discovery of t haplotypes,
fate was also responsible for a series of long-lived misperceptions
concerning the true nature of these genetic entities. The first
misperception was that t haplotypes were "recessive" mutations at a
single locus - the T locus - which could also be mutated to
produce dominant T mutations. The seemingly-unrelated phenotypes
expressed by t haplotypes were considered to be the pleiotropic
effects of a single mutant allele. The second misperception was
that the effects of t haplotypes on embryogenesis were the "primary
t effects". (In retrospect, it would appear that this
misperception came about because the embryonic effects [both
taillessness and lethality] were the first of the various t
phenotypes to be discovered.) With the accumulation of data
demonstrating the action of different lethal t mutations at
different points during embryogenesis, it was suggested that the "T
locus" could be the master regulatory gene which controlled
early developmental decisions. How else could different alleles at
the same locus affect such an array of developmental stages?

MOUSE t HAPLOTYPES ARE DEFINED BY STRUCTURE RATHER THAN FUNCTION.

Although Lyon (1960) was the first to suggest that the single
locus model of t haplotypes was incorrect, this work went largely
unnoticed in the field until over a decade later. We now know
that all t haplotypes are closely related, structurally-variant
forms of a portion of mouse chromosome 17 that includes the "simple"

T locus, as well as the entire MHC, and extends over 20-30,000 kb. Within this structurally- variant region are all of the normally-functioning genes found on the wild-type form of this chromosome with the exception of a small number of independent mutant loci that mediate the characteristic t effects. The length of the t haplotype is defined by the region of chromosome held together as a single genetic entity from generation to generation by recombination suppression. Lethal mutations associated with different complementing t haplotypes are unrelated to each other and map to different positions along the length of t haplotypes (none are true alleles of the T locus), but because of recombination suppression, they do not usually recombine with mutations at the T locus.

With this new understanding of structure-function relationships in t haplotypes, the hypothesis of the T locus as a master regulatory gene in control of development fell apart. In fact, as discussed later, it now seems clear that the lethal mutations are a peripheral characteristic associated with some t haplotypes, while transmission ratio distortion and recombination suppression are the primary features necessary for their continued existence in wild populations of mice.

MOLECULAR PROBES PROVIDE TOOLS FOR DISSECTION OF t HAPLOTYPES

As a genetic entity extending over 20,000 kb of DNA, the mouse t haplotype presented a unique problem for molecular analysis. The various genetic components of the t haplotype were not well characterized and could not provide a handle for molecular forays. Instead, a novel approach (at that time) was used to obtain molecular clones from the t haplotype (Frischauf, 1985). This approach, called "microcloning", involved the direct micro-dissection of the t haplotype region of chromosome 17 with the use of a micropipet operated under a microscope. Several hundred chromosomal fragments could be dissected from a metaphase plate and placed together in a micro-droplet where they were de-proteinized, cut with a restriction enzyme and ligated to arms of a lambda-derived cloning vector. In this way, it was possible to obtain a large number of molecular markers distributed randomly along the length of t haplotypes. With the subsequent explosion in the general cloning and mapping of genes in mice, additional t haplotype markers have been defined. The accumulated molecular probes have been used to great success in exposing the secrets of the t haplotype which are described in the next section.

WHAT IS A t HAPLOTYPE?

1. All are derived from a single ancestor.

All t haplotypes present in mice around the world today are descendents of a single ancestral chromosome which had evolved apart from the wild-type form of mouse chromosome 17. The separate evolution of these two forms of chromosome 17 (which reside in the same nucleus) was dependent on the generation of several (from two to four) large non-overlapping inversions which distinguish the t haplotype from its wild-type counterpart. These inversions provide an explanation for the recombination properties characteristic of t haplotypes.

2. Selective mechanisms must act in favor of their existence.

But why did t haplotypes come into existence in the first place and why are they present at such a high frequency in wild mice? The answer must be that selective forces acted in favor of the formation of these variant genetic elements. Natural selection is usually viewed in the context of increased reproductive fitness of individual animals. However, none of the phenotypes expressed by t haplotypes would appear to be beneficial in any way to the t-carrying mice. On the contrary, lethality and sterility are both serious detriments to reproductive fitness. It has been suggested that lethal t haplotypes increase the chances of heterozygosity at the MHC [matings between two +/t heterozygotes with lethal mutations will produce primarily heterozygous offspring] and that MHC heterozygosity increases fitness. This suggestion is not valid for two reasons: first, even in the absence of t haplotypes, nearly 100% of wild mice are heterozygous at the MHC, and second, t haplotypes in some populations of mice do not carry lethal mutations and are still present at high frequencies. Therefore, selection must operate at a level other than the whole animal.

The obvious solution to this apparent paradox is that selection has operated at the level of the chromosome itself - the t form of mouse chromosome 17 has evolved the ability to propagate itself at the expense of its wild-type counterpart. In anthropomorphic terms, the t haplotype is a selfish chromosome [actually its a selfish subchromosomal region]. It is in this context that all of the varied phenotypes expressed by t haplotypes come together in a unified manner.

3. Evolution as a selfish chromosome.

The evolution of t haplotypes can now be envisaged as follows. First, by chance, mutations occurred at a number of testes-expressed genes in the proximal portion of chromosome 17. Second, when by chance these mutations were brought together onto a single chromosome through normal events of recombination, they interacted to increase the probability of their own transmission by depressing the fertilizing ability of sperm that carried their wild-type counterpart. A group of linked alleles acting in this manner would have an obvious selective advantage relative to a wild-type chromosome, and as such, this mutant allele group would be able to reproduce itself (within the context of mice of course) in large numbers. Once significant numbers of the allele group were in existence, subsequent mutations would allow divergence to occur between them. Those allele groups which evolved a relatively higher level of transmission ratio distortion would have a selective advantage over other allele groups.

In the form just described, the allele groups could never attain a transmission ratio of greater than 85%. This is because the individual genes involved in TRD are spread out over a genetic distance of 15 cM which means that approximately 15% of the time, recombination would occur between various members of the group. Only those chromosomes that carried a complete set of alleles express TRD at the maximal level. Therefore, recombination would destroy the selective advantage held by an allele group. An allele group able to suppress recombination between its members would clearly be at a great advantage relative to all other allele groups. This was accomplished by the accumulation of several non-overlapping inversions which served to lock together the allele group such that it was now transmitted essentially as a single genetic entity.

With the accumulation of inversions, the allele group would now be recognizable as a t haplotype, and all of the DNA included in the inverted regions would be free to evolve apart from the wild-type form of the chromosome. A comprehensive phylogenetic analysis indicates that this event occurred at least 2 to 4 million years ago (Mike Hammer and LM Silver, unpublished data). With TRD and recombination suppression alone, one would expect the t haplotype to be so successful that it should ultimately displace the wild-type form of chromosome 17 entirely. It is interesting to note that if this had happened, all evidence for the existence of the original variant allele group would have vanished, since the variant group would now be considered to be wild-type. What prevented this scenario from playing itself out?

The answer is that an unavoidable consequence of the genes involved in TRD is that males homozygous for t haplotypes are sterile (Lyon, 1986). Therefore, the t haplotype can never become fixed in a population of mice. From the viewpoint of the t haplotype, it is even worse, because sterile t/t males will compete for females and resources with +/t heterozygotes, without providing for the further propagation of the variant chromosome. Alas, the t haplotype has one more trick up its sleeve. By picking up a spontaneous recessive lethal mutation anywhere along the length of the inverted regions, all potentially sterile t/t males will die in utero. Contrary to what would be considered common sense, in the t haplotype system, selection favors lethal mutations.

All naturally-occurring t haplotypes are virtually identical in all expressed phenotypes with the exception of lethality. Of the naturally- derived t haplotypes analyzed to date, approximately 20% do not carry lethal mutations, whereas the others are associated with one or more of
sixteen independent, complementing, lethal mutations (Klein, 1986). The simplest explanation of the existing situation is that t haplotypes began to diverge apart from a highly evolved, common ancestor that possessed all of the properties characteristic of t haplotypes save one - lethality. Only when t haplotypes reached significant frequencies in individual populations (such that homozygous males became frequent) would selective pressure favor the addition of a lethal mutation. This phase of the evolution of t haplotypes is clearly still in progress since some populations remain devoid of lethal mutations. Selective pressure to accumulate lethal mutations provides an explanation for the observation that they are the most polymorphic genetic feature of t haplotypes.

4. A tale of tails.

The only property of t haplotypes left unexplained by the selfish chromosome model is (as fate would have it) the first property discovered and the one responsible for its name. Why do t haplotypes enhance the effect of mutations at the T locus to cause taillessness? It is difficult to explain the rationale for a phenotype that will rarely be expressed in wild mouse populations. The only explanation is an ad hoc one - without taillessness, it is possible that no one would ever have discovered this remarkable little piece of chromosome that has kept so many of us entertained for so many years.

ACKNOWLEDGMENTS

I thank my one year old daughter Rebecca Eve for bringing historical matter on the t haplotype to my attention, and I thank Susan Silver for keeping Rebecca away from my computer long enough to write this paper. The author's work was supported by a grant from the NIH (HD16092).

REFERENCES

Frischauf AM (1985) The T/t complex of the mouse. Trends in Genetics 1:100-103

Klein J (1986) Natural History of the major histocompatibility complex. pp. 683-705. Wiley and Sons, New York.

Lyon MF (1960) Effect of X-rays on the mutation of t-alleles in the mouse.Heredity 14:247-257

Lyon MF (1986) Male sterility of the mouse t-complex is due to homozygosity of the distorter genes. Cell 44:357-363

Silver LM (1985) Mouse t haplotypes. Ann. Rev. Genet. 19:179-208

Contrasting Patterns of Evolution in the Proximal and Distal Regions of the Mouse *t* Complex

M. A. Erhart, S. J. Phillips, and J. H. Nadeau

INTRODUCTION

One of the most perplexing but fascinating segments of the mouse genome is the t complex, a 12-15 cM region of Chromosome 17. A number of alternative allelic combinations called t haplotypes characterize this segment. Wild-derived t haplotypes affect a wide variety of biological properties including embryogenesis, male fertility, male transmission ratio, meiotic recombination, and tail length (Silver 1985). Since the discovery of t haplotypes 55 years ago (Dobrovoloskaia-Zavadskaia and Kobozieff 1932), many investigators have tried to account for this diverse array of attributes. It is evident that t haplotypes carry mutant alleles at loci such as tct (t complex tail) that interacts with the dominant mutation T (brachyury) to produce tailless offspring, tcr (t complex responder) and tcd-1 through tcd-4 (t complex distorter) that interact to distort transmission ratio in t/+ males (Lyon 1984, 1987; Silver and Remis 1987), tcs-1 through tcs-3 (t complex sterility) that cause male sterility (Lyon 1986, 1987), and recessive lethal mutations that map to 16 different loci and that affect different stages of embryonic development (Bennett 1975; Klein et al., 1984).

As a result of a combination of classical and molecular genetic approaches, the genetic organization of t haplotypes has begun to emerge. Artzt et al. (1982), Pla and Condamine (1984) and Herrmann et al. (1986) showed that at least two non-overlapping chromosomal inversions are associated with the t complex. These inversions encompass a large portion of the t complex and suppress recombination 50-100 fold between t-bearing and wild-type chromosomes (Forejt 1972; Lyon et al., 1979). An important consequence of recombination suppression is a "locking together" of mutant alleles in the t complex. Included among these alleles are those causing segregation distortion and sterility in males as well as variant alleles of "neutral" loci, i.e., loci not involved in the function of the t complex (such as H-2), that serve as markers for studying the organization and evolution of t haplotypes.

Despite the barrier to recombination, partial t haplotypes have been identified among offspring of crosses between wild-type and t-bearing individuals. There is evidence that partial t haplotypes can arise in natural mouse populations (Silver et al., 1987). In this chapter, we examine the structure of these exceptional recombinant haplotypes and discuss hypotheses concerning the origin of partial t haplotypes. We also describe how neutral marker loci within the t complex can be used to study recombination between t-bearing and wild-type chromosomes in natural populations. It is apparent from these data that the nature of recombination within the proximal inversion is fundamentally different from that occurring in the distal inversion. This has resulted in contrasting patterns of linkage disequilibrium in the two regions and suggests that different kinds of chromosome rearrangements occur in the proximal and distal portions of the t complex.

FORMATION AND CHARACTERIZATION OF PARTIAL t HAPLOTYPES

The composition of partial t haplotypes that arise in laboratory mice is intriguing in that most appear to result from an unequal exchange between a complete t haplotype and a wild-type version of Chromosome 17. As a result of

The Jackson Laboratory
Bar Harbor, ME 04609

unequal crossing-over within an inverted region, these partial t haplotypes have either expanded or contracted their total length when compared to parental chromosomes (Herrmann et al., 1986; Sarvetnick et al., 1986). Recently, Lehrach and his colleagues (Herrmann et al., 1987) and Silver and his colleagues (Schimenti et al., 1987) described the way in which repeated DNA sequences may have been involved in the recombination events that gave rise to these partial t haplotypes. Specifically, they showed that the partial t haplotypes t^{ae5} and t^{h45} arose by recombination involving a segment of DNA containing the Chromosome 17-specific elements D17Leh66 and D17Leh119, both of which map to the proximal region of the t complex. In addition, the vast majority of partial t haplotypes arising in the laboratory have resulted from recombination either within the proximal inversion or between the proximal and distal inversions (Klein and Hammerberg 1977). The only examples of partial t haplotypes that arose in laboratory mice with recombination breakpoints in the distal inversion are the members of the t^9 complementation group, t^{w18}, t^4, and t^{ks1} (Bucan et al., 1987). There is no evidence for the involvement of repetitive DNA elements in the formation of these distal partial t haplotypes.

Naturally occurring partial t haplotypes may have escaped detection because of a bias in the way t haplotypes are identified (Klein 1979). A cross between a normal tailed wild mouse (+/?) and a mouse carrying the brachyury mutation (T/+) should yield tailless offspring (T/t) because of the t complex tail-interaction component (tct) present in complete t haplotypes and in many proximal partial t haplotypes. Mice lacking the tct segment of the t complex are undetectable even though they might retain a significant portion of the t complex. With molecular probes now available for the t complex (Rohme et al., 1983), the discovery of RFLPs between t haplotypes and wild-type chromosomes (Silver 1982; Shin et al., 1982; Fox et al., 1984; Skow et al., 1987; Nadeau and Phillips 1987), and the presence of biochemical (Silver et al., 1983; Nadeau 1986) and serological (Hammerberg and Klein, 1975; Hammerberg et al., 1976) variants unique to the t complex, a wild mouse can be screened for any portion of the t complex. This has provided an unbiased and efficient way of identifying partial t haplotypes.

CONTRASTING LEVELS OF VARIATION IN THE PROXIMAL AND DISTAL REGIONS

The numerous markers for the t complex could prove very useful in elucidating the evolutionary history of t haplotypes. Although polymorphisms have been documented between t haplotypes and wild-type chromosomes, however, very little variation has been detected among different t haplotypes (Silver et al., 1987). This is believed to be the result of both the recent origin of the t complex (Silver et al., 1987) and recombination suppression between t haplotypes and wild-type chromosomes, which creates strong linkage disequilibrium. In the proximal inversion, for example, the DNA markers D17Leh48, D17Leh66, D17Rp17 and the polypeptide marker Tcp-1 are each represented by indistinguishable forms among t haplotypes. By contrast, loci in the distal inversion do not exhibit complete linkage disequilibrium among t haplotypes. Pim-1 (Nadeau and Phillips 1987), Crya-1 (Skow et al., 1987), and H-2 (Dembic et al., 1984, 1985) are all examples of genes that vary among t haplotypes. To date, the only locus in the distal inversion that does not vary among t haplotypes is the allozyme glyoxalase-1 (Glo-1; Nadeau, 1986). The difference in variability must reflect different modes of evolution between the two inversions.

EVIDENCE FOR SEGMENTAL EXCHANGE IN THE DISTAL REGION

Three separate surveys suggest that recombination between wild-type and t haplotypes in the distal inversion accounts for the contrasting patterns of variation between the proximal and distal regions. The three surveys involved the alpha-crystallin (Crya-1) locus (Skow et al., 1987), the Pim-1 locus (Nadeau and Phillips 1987), and the MHC Class I locus E_α (Dembic et al., 1984, 1985). Each of these loci has an allele that is associated either exclusively or predominantly with t haplotypes (called t-specific alleles). The order of these three loci on wild-type chromosomes is believed to be: centromere - Pim-1 - Crya-1 - E_α (Nadeau and Phillips 1987). Because all three loci map within the distal inversion, their order in t haplotypes is reversed with respect to the centromere.

The data from these surveys show that not all t haplotypes have the t-specific alleles at the Crya-1, Pim-1, and E_α loci, and that there is no linkage disequilibrium among alleles at these loci in the t haplotypes examined. Skow et al. (1987) identified three different alpha-crystallin alleles (Crya-1^a, Crya-1^b, and Crya-1^t) among laboratory mice. The majority of t-bearing mice have an allele (Crya-1^t) which is found only in t haplotypes (Table 1). A few t haplotypes, however, contain an allele (Crya-1^a) which is prevalent in inbred mice, and one t haplotype (t^{w121}) has another allele (Crya-1^b) also found among standard inbred strains. Nadeau and Phillips (1987) have similarly categorized t haplotypes with respect to Pim-1 alleles. As with alpha-crystallin, the Pim-1 locus has an allele (Pim-1^t) that is found only among t haplotypes. Strikingly, only three of the ten t haplotypes examined have this allele. The majority of t haplotypes have an allele (Pim-1^b) which is widespread in laboratory strains of mice. Finally, the MHC Class I locus E_α has a null allele whose molecular defect is a 627 bp deletion spanning the promoter region and the signal peptide exon. This E^0 deletion is found in many t haplotypes (Dembic et al., 1984, 1985) as well as in several inbred strains. The fact that the three markers Crya-1^a, Pim-1^b, and E^0 are not found in all t haplotypes suggests that the widespread occurrence of the three markers is not simply due to common ancestry among t haplotypes, but that they have been spread by segmental exchange (either gene conversion or double crossing-over) between t haplotypes and their wild-type homologues. Whether these alleles arose on wild-type or t-bearing chromosomes is uncertain, and consequently, the direction of spread for each is unknown.

Strong linkage disequilibrium among alleles at the Crya-1, Pim-1, and E_α loci in t haplotypes is expected because these loci lie within an inversion, and thus would be associated with one another, reflecting a history of presumed genetic isolation by recombination suppression (Nadeau 1983, Silver et al., 1987). Contrary to expectation, however, there is no concordance between alleles at the Crya-1, Pim-1, and E_α loci among t haplotypes (table 1). The t-specific allele of one locus is often associated with the wild-type allele of another locus, suggesting that the distal region of t haplotypes has experienced segmental exchanges with wild-type homologues.

To examine the variability of loci throughout the t complex and to document more fully the apparent segmental recombination in the distal region, we have begun a survey of wild mice (M. musculus and M. domesticus) from Europe (M.A. Erhart, S.J. Phillips, F. Bonhomme, F. Figueroa, G. Gaechelin, J. Klein, E. Wakeland, and J.H. Nadeau, in preparation). Using molecular probes for the structural loci Pim-1 and Crya-1, anonymous loci D17Leh48, D17Leh54, and D17Leh66, and the alpha-globin pseudogene Hba-4ps, chromosomes were scored as having the wild-type or t-type RFLP at each of the six loci. This was done by using one or two restriction enzymes that distinguish variant markers at each locus. The chromosomes can be placed in

Table 1. Distribution of E_α, Crya-1, and Pim-1 alleles in t-haplotypes.

t-haplotype	tcl	E_α [a]	Crya-1	Pim-1
t^0	0	−	a	t
t^6	0	+	a	t
t^{w32}	12	−	t	t
t^{w1}	w1	+	t	b
t^{12}	w1	.	t	b
t^{w12}	w1	+	a	b
t^{w71}	w1	+	t	b
t^{w75}	w1,w5	−	t	b
t^{w2}	w2	.	t	.
t^{w8}	w2	−	t	b
t^{w73}	w73	.	t	.
t^{LUB-1}	Lub-1	.	a	.
t^{w120}	.	.	a	.
t^{w121}	.	.	b	.

[a] Scored by presence (+) or absence (−) of the E molecule on the cell surface.

Sources of data are as follows: E. Wakeland, personal communication (for E_α); Skow et al., 1987 (for Crya-1); Nadeau and Phillips 1987 (for Pim-1).

The symbols a, b, and t denote which allelic form of either Crya-1 or Pim-1 is present in each haplotype.

Dots denote data not available.

one of three categories: wild-type (+) at every locus, t-type (t) at every locus, or mosaic with (+) at some loci and (t) at others. Members of this third class are most interesting because they may represent naturally occurring partial t haplotypes.

Of nearly 100 wild-derived chromosomes examined, less than 5% possessed the t-specific RFLP at all six loci. This percentage is significantly smaller than the 10 to 40% estimate of t haplotype frequency in natural populations (Bennett 1975). There were, however, numerous examples of mosaic haplotypes containing a mixture of wild-type and t-specific RFLPs. These mosaic haplotypes can be sub-divided into different classes, depending on the specific distribution of t-specific RFLPs on the chromosome. One particular class may represent chromosomes with only the proximal inversion because its members possess t-specific markers only in the proximal region. Another class is characterized by t-specific RFLPs at a single locus, whereas wild-type alleles are present at the remaining loci. The majority of these examples exhibit t-specific alleles at either the Hba-4ps or the D17Leh54 locus, both of which probably lie in the region between the inversions (H. Lehrach, personal communication; J.H. Nadeau and M.-B. Tchetgen, unpublished). A third class of wild-derived chromosomes with t-specific markers at four or five out of six loci surveyed were found. In these instances, a wild-type RFLP of either Pim-1 or Crya-1 (or both) is present in a putative t haplotype.

The mosaic patterns observed suggest that segmental exchange and not single crossovers are the predominant means of recombination between t haplotypes and their wild-type homologues in the region distal to the proximal inversion. Segmental recombination can result from either double crossover or gene conversion. Our population survey would seem to suggest that non-reciprocal gene conversion is the primary mechanism of recombination. For instance, there are several examples of the wild-type allele $Pim-1^b$ in t haplotypes, but no examples of the reciprocal product $Pim-1^t$ in a normal chromosome (M.A. Erhart, S.J. Phillips, F. Bonhomme, F. Figueroa, G. Gaechelin, J. Klein, E. Wakeland, and J.H. Nadeau, in preparation). This implies a unidirectional transfer from wild-type chromosomes to t haplotypes. The outcomes of double crossing-over and gene conversion are difficult to distinguish, because one can only be certain of the nature of the process by examining all the products of a given meiosis. The situation is complicated by the fact that "hitch-hiking" of a wild-type allele on a t haplotype invariably increases the frequency of the wild-type allele in mouse populations. Conversely, the t-specific allele in a wild-type chromosome would usually suffer the fate of most mutations, i.e. it would be lost by random drift. It is noteworthy that both gene conversion (Chovnick 1973) and double crossing over (Levine 1956) occur at appreciable frequencies in inversion heterozygotes in Drosophila.

SUMMARY

Comparison of the proximal and distal regions of the t complex reveals a number of contrasting features. First, the number of partial t haplotypes arising in laboratory mice with breakpoints in or near the proximal inversion greatly outnumber those with breakpoints in the distal inversion. Of all the partial t haplotypes characterized to date, only the six members of the t^9 complementation group (Bucan et al., 1987) arose by recombination in the distal inversion. Second, the level of disequilibrium among loci in the proximal inversion is very high in all t haplotypes that have been examined, whereas it is low for loci in the distal inversion. This suggests that distally recombinant chromosomes may have gone undetected because of the size and nature of the region involved in the exchange. With the discovery of polymorphic markers in the distal inversion, the identification of these small segments has been made possible. Interestingly, evidence of segmental exchange has not been observed in the proximal inversion. Thus, although unequal single crossovers leading to partial t haplotypes occur readily in the proximal inversion, segmental exchange has taken place only between the two inversions or within the distal inversion. One could argue that the number of tcr, tcd, and tcs loci is higher in the proximal inversion, making segmental exchanges there unfavorable in terms of t haplotype propagation. Alternatively, segmental recombination in the distal region may be inherently higher perhaps due to DNA sequences that act as recombination "hot spots". Sequences of this nature have been discovered in the MHC region of both M.m. molossinus (Shiroishi et al., 1982) and M.m. castaneus (Steinmetz et al., 1986). However, a higher level of recombination in the distal region may be more apparent than real, owing to the fact that the distal inversion encompasses a larger region than the proximal inversion (6 cM compared to 4 cM). A third, and most intriguing possibility, is that the structure of the proximal and the distal inversions may be different. The distal region may be a simple, continuous inversion while the proximal region may consist of a number of smaller "inversions within an inversion" as suggested by recent analyses (Herrmann et al., 1987; Schimenti et al., 1987). This hypothesized difference in structure could have a profound effect on the type and frequency of recombination in each region.

AKNOWLEDGEMENTS

We thank Ward Wakeland for permission to use unpublished data, and Muriel Davisson
and Priscilla Tucker for critically reading a draft of the manuscript. This work
was supported by NSF grants PCM8215004 and DCB8610297. M.A.E. is supported by
institutional postdoctoral training grant HD07065-09 from the NIH. The contents of
this paper are solely the responsibility of The Jackson Laboratory and do not
necessarily represent the official views of the National Institutes of Health.

LITERATURE CITED

Artzt K, Shin H-S, Bennett D (1982) Gene mapping within the T/t-complex of
the mouse. II. Anomolous position of the H-2 complex in t haplotypes. Cell
28: 471-476

Bennett D (1975) The T-locus of the mouse. Cell 6: 441-454

Bucan M, Herrmann BG, Frischauf A-M, Bautch VL, Bode V, Silver LM, Martin GR,
Lehrach, H (1987) Deletion and duplication of DNA sequences is associated
with the embryonic lethal phenotype of the t^9 complementation group of the
mouse t complex. Genes and Devel 1:376-385

Chovnick A (1973) Gene conversion and transfer of genetic information within
the inverted region of inversion heterozygotes. Genetics 75:123-131

Dembic Z, Singer PA, Klein J (1984) E^0: a history of a mutation. EMBO J
3:1647-1654

Dembic Z, Ayane M, Klein J, Steinmetz M, Benoist CO, Mathis DJ (1985) Inbred
and wild mice carry identical deletions in their E_α MHC genes. EMBO J 4:127-
131

Dobrovoloskaia-Zavadskaia N, Kobozieff N (1932) Les souris anoures et la
queue filiforme qui se reproduisent entre elles sans disjunction. R Soc Biol
Paris 110:782-784

Forejt J (1972) Chiasmata and crossing-over in the male mouse (Mus musculus).
Suppression of recombination and chiasma frequencies in the ninth linkage
group. Folia Biol Praha 18:161-170

Fox H, Silver LM, Martin G (1984) An α globin pseudogene is located within
the mouse t complex. Immunogenetics 19:125-130

Hammerberg C, Klein J (1975) Linkage disequilibrium between H-2 and t-
complexes in chromosome 17 of the mouse. Nature 258:296-299

Hammerberg C, Klein J, Artzt K, Bennett D (1976) Histocompatability-2 system
in wild mice. II. H-2 haplotypes of t-bearing mice. Transplantation 21:199-
212

Herrmann B, Bucan M, Mains PE, Frischauf A-M, Silver LM, Lehrach H (1986)
Genetic analysis of the proximal portion of the mouse t-complex: evidence
for a second inversion within t haplotypes. Cell 44:469-476

Herrmann BG, Barlow DP, Lehrach H (1987) A large inverted duplication allows
homologous recombination between chromosomes heterozygous for the proximal t
complex inversion. Cell 48:813-825

Klein J (1979) Population genetics of the murine chromosome 17. Israel J Med
Sci 15:859-866

Klein J, Hammerberg C (1977) The control of differentiation by the T-complex.
Immunol Rev 33:70-104

Klein J, Sipos P, Figueroa F (1984) Polymorphism of t-complex genes in
European wild mice. Genet Res 44:39-46

Levine RP (1956) Crossing over and inversions in coadapted systems. Amer Nat
90:41-45

Lyon MF (1984) Transmission ratio distortion in mouse t-haplotypes is due to
multiple distorter genes acting on a responder locus. Cell 37:621-628

Lyon MF (1986) Male sterility of the mouse t-complex is due to homozygosity
of the distorter genes. Cell 44:357-363

Lyon MF (1987) Distorter genes of the mouse $\underline{t}$-complex impair fertility when heterozygous. Genet Res 49:57-60

Lyon MF, Evans EP, Jarvis SE, Sayers I (1979) t-Haplotypes of the mouse may involve a change in intercalary DNA. Nature 279:38-42

Nadeau JH (1983) Absence of detectable gametic disequilibrium between the t-complex and linked allozyme-encoding loci in house mice. Genet Res 42:323-333

Nadeau JH (1986) A glyoxalase-1 variant associated with the $\underline{t}$-complex in house mice. Genetics 113:91-99

Nadeau JH, Phillips SJ (1987) The putative oncogene Pim-1 in the mouse: its linkage and variation among $\underline{t}$ haplotypes. Genetics 117:533-541

Pla M, Condamine H (1984) Recombination between two mouse $\underline{t}$ haplotypes ($\underline{t}^{w12tf}$ and $\underline{t}^{Lub-1}$): Mapping of the H-2 complex relative to the centromere and tufted ($\overline{tf}$) locus. Immunogenetics 20:277-285

Rohme D, Fox H, Herrmann B, Frischauf A-M, Edstrom J-E, Mains P, Silver LM, Lehrach H (1983) Molecular clones of the mouse t complex derived from microdissected metaphase chromosomes. Cell 36:783-788

Sarvetnick N, Fox HS, Mann E, Mains PE, Elliott RW, Silver LM (1986) Nonhomologous pairing in mice heterozygous for a $\underline{t}$-haplotype can produce recombinant chromosomes with duplications and deletions. Genetics 113:723-734

Schimenti J, Vold L, Socolow D, Silver LM (1987) An unstable family of large DNA elements in the center of the mouse t complex. J Mol Biol 194:583-594

Shin H-S, Stavnezer J, Artzt K, Bennett D (1982) Genetic structure and origin of t haplotypes of mice analyzed with H-2 cDNA probes. Cell 29:969-976

Shiroishi T, Sagai T, Moriwaki K (1982) A new wild-derived H-2 haplotype enhancing K-IA recombination. Nature 300:370-372

Silver LM (1982) Genomic analysis of the H-2 complex region associated with mouse t haplotypes. Cell 29:961-968

Silver LM (1985) Mouse t haplotypes. Ann Rev Genet 19:179-208

Silver LM, Remis D (1987) Five of the nine genetically defined regions of mouse t haplotypes are involved in transmission ratio distortion. Genet Res 49:51-56

Silver LM, Hammer M, Fox H, Garrels J, Bucan M, Herrmann B, Frischauf A-M, Lehrach H, Winking H, Figueroa F, Klein J (1987) Molecular evidence for the rapid propagation of mouse $\underline{t}$ haplotypes from a single, recent, ancestral chromosome. Molec Biol Evol 4:473-482

Silver LM, Uman J, Danska J, Garrels JI (1983) A diversified set of testicular cell proteins specified by genes within the mouse $\underline{t}$ complex. Cell 35:35-45

Skow LC, Nadeau JH, Ahn JC, Shin H-S, Artzt K, Bennett D (1987) Polymorphism and linkage of the A-crystallin gene in $\underline{t}$-haplotypes of the mouse. Genetics 116:107-111

Steinmetz M, Stephan D, Fischer-Lindahl K (1986) Gene organization and recombinational hotspots in the murine major histocompatability complex. Cell 44:895-904

From Phenotype to Gene: Molecular Cloning in the *Brachyury* (*T*) Locus Region

B. G. Herrmann and H. Lehrach*

INTRODUCTION

The *t* complex of the mouse is located on the proximal half of chromosome 17 and spans approximately 1% of the genome (for Review see Frischauf 1985; Silver 1985). Wild mouse populations of the species Mus.m.musculus and M.m.domesticus carry two variant forms of this chromosomal region, designated wild type (+) and *t* haplotype (*t*). The *t* haplotype form has several very unusual properties. If a mouse is heterozygous for a *t* haplotype (+/*t*), meiotic recombination is strongly suppressed between the markers *T* and H-2 that are separated by 12cM. Therefore a *t* haplotype behaves as a genetic unit. In heterozygous (+/*t*) males the *t* chromosome has a selective advantage. Up to 99% of the offspring of such a male will inherit the *t* chromosome. Several factors have been shown to be responsible for this property of *t* haplotypes (Lyon 1984), but no biochemical explanation has been found so far.

Most *t* haplotypes that were isolated from wild mouse populations carry recessive embryonic lethality factors. 16 different factors have been identified (Klein et al. 1984) and a few of them have been mapped to specific subregions of the *t* haplotype (Artzt et al. 1982; Shin et al. 1984). Several *t* lethal factors affecting a variety of embryonic structures have been studied in more detail (Mc Laren 1976). In addition to these factors in the *t* haplotype a number of interesting gene loci have been mapped to the wild type form of the *t* complex. Among those are recessive lethals (*T*, *Ki*), a maternal effect gene (*Tme*)(Johnson 1975) and an autosomal sex determining factor (*Tas*) (Washburn and Eicher 1983). 12 new embryonic lethal factors have recently been generated in the wild type *t* complex by chemical mutagenesis (Shedlovsky et al. 1988).

There are therefore well over 30 different gene loci known in the *t* complex region which are defined by the phenotype of their mutant forms. The molecular isolation and analysis of these genetic disease loci would clearly provide important insights into embryonic development, sex determination and spermatogenesis of mammals. We have therefore decided to undertake a detailed analysis of the *t* complex in order to isolate some of these factors.

In particular we have focussed our attention on the molecular cloning of the *Brachyury* (*T*) locus gene. The *T* mutation affects the organization of the body axis of the mouse. Heterozygotes are usually short tailed. Homozygotes die at about 8-10 days of gestation. They lack the notochord and are deficient in somite formation. Larger parts of the posterior region including hind limb buds are missing in *T/T* embryos (Grüneberg 1958).

How Can a Genetic Disease Locus Be Cloned ?

The molecular cloning of a genetic disease gene requires the chromosomal localization of the trait and DNA probes from the genome fragment encoding the gene. These probes can be used as tools to clone the entire region of the gene. The cloned region can then be screened for coding sequences by various ways. Finally the identity of the cloned gene with the genetic disease locus must be established, e.g. by complementation of the mutant phenotype by providing the wild type gene product.

The major constraints of this approach to gene cloning is the size of the genome, the accuracy of localization of the trait and the degree of selectivity of cloning of specific regions. For instance the giant polytene chromosomes in Drosophila allow the precise localization of genetic traits to specific bands of only a few hundred kb or less in size; such bands can be selectively cloned by microdissection which allows direct entry to the gene locus (Scalenghe et al. 1981). The major step for cloning in Drosophila is therefore the precise localization of the trait to a chromosomal band by genetic means.

The large size of mammalian genomes allows at present only the isolation of random DNA fragments from chromosomal regions of minimally a few thousand kb. Laborious linkage analyses have to be carried out to obtain the positions of these fragments on the chromosome and with respect to the genetic trait. Once markers in the vicinity of the gene have been identified, pulsed field gel analysis

Laboratory of Molecular Embryology, National Institute for Medical Research, The Ridgeway, Mill Hill, London NW7 1AA
* Imperial Cancer Research Fund Laboratories, P.O. Box No.123, Lincoln's Inn Fields, London WC2A 3PX

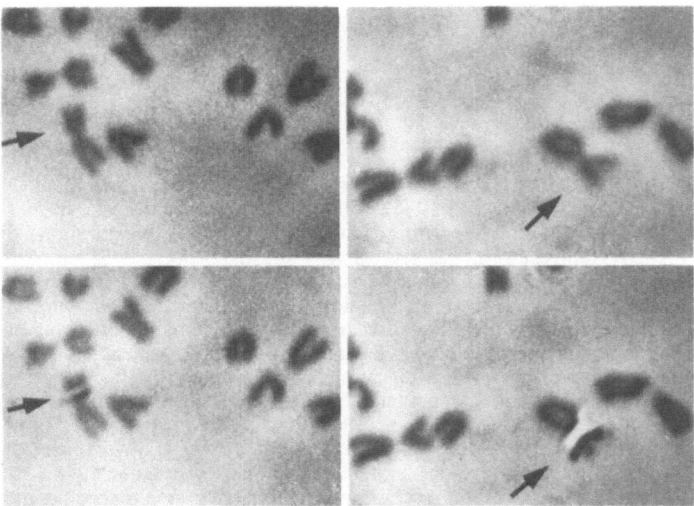

Fig. 1. Mouse metaphase chromosomes before (upper panel) and after (lower panel) microdissection of a proximal fragment of chromosome 17 (arrows). The two examples represent extremes of the range of excised fragments. The Fig. is reprinted, with permission (© Cell Press), from Röhme et al. (1984).

(Schwartz and Cantor 1984; Barlow and Lehrach 1987) can be used to obtain a physical map of the relevant region. Chromosome walking and novel jumping techniques (Poustka and Lehrach 1986) can then be applied to clone the region containing the gene of interest. We would like to stress that the genetic definition of this region is the crucial step in this approach of gene cloning, since the "assay" for the gene is to look for coding sequences on the DNA cloned. The more precisely the gene region is defined, the less sequences have to be assayed to identify the "right" gene. This constraint may be overcome once a functional assay for the presence of the "right" gene becomes available.

RESULTS AND DISCUSSION

Genetic Analysis of the *t* Complex with Molecular Probes

We have made use of the microcloning technique to obtain random DNA markers from the *t* complex. Pieces of minimally several thousand kb in size can be dissected from spread mammalian metaphase chromosomes using fine glass needles. Figure 1 demonstrates the size range of fragments that are usually cut from the chromosomes. In a typical experiment several hundred chromosomal fragments are cut out, collected and processed in nanoliter droplets. The restricted DNA is cloned into a lambda insertion vector.

We have obtained a large number of random DNA fragments from the proximal part of chromosome 17 using this technique (Röhme et al. 1984). Low copy number fragments were selected and investigated for their ability to recognize polymorphic restriction fragments in genomic DNA of strains used for genetic mapping. Polymorphic markers were then localized to chromosomal subregions of the *t* haplotype using a panel of overlapping partial *t* haplotypes (analogous to intra H-2 recombinant haplotypes) (Fox et al. 1985), and to subregions of the wild type chromosome using recombinant inbred strains (BXD lines) and partial *t* haplotypes.

Several important findings resulted from this analysis. We showed that the proximal region of the *t* complex is inverted in *t* haplotypes with respect to the wild type. This inversion is independent from the earlier detected inversion in the distal region of the *t* complex (Artzt et al.1982). From these results one of the phenomena associated with the mouse *t* complex, the strong suppression of meiotic recombination between *t* and wild type chromosomes could be explained (Herrmann et al. 1986). Furthermore we were

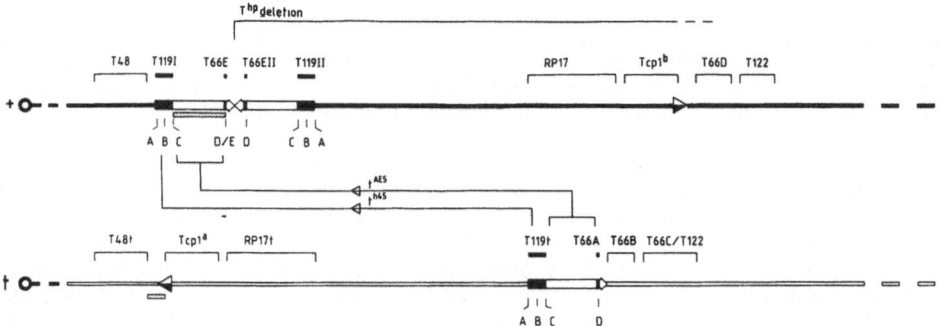

Fig. 2. Schematic representation of the genetic fine structure of the proximal region of the wild type (+) and t haplotype (t) form of mouse chromosome 17. Dashed lines indicate an undefined distance. Black bars above the chromosomes represent cloned regions. The thin lines and arrowheads between the t and + chromosome indicate the joining of chromosome parts in the recombination events producing t^{h45} and t^{AE5}. Brackets represent intervals. DNA loci are shown above the maps and the probes defining the markers and cloned regions are shown beneath. The Fig. is reprinted, with permission (© Cell Press), from Herrmann et al. (1987).

able to explain on a molecular level how chromosomes can recombine across an inversion. This phenomenon has already been described in Drosophila in the 1930s by Sturtevant and Beadle(1936). Nonhomologous recombination was generally assumed to be the mechanism allowing such crossover events. We could show that recombination between the t haplotype and the wild type chromosome across the proximal inversion is in fact homologous and is mediated by an element of 650kb that is present in the same orientation in both forms of the chromosome (see Fig. 2). The wild type chromosome contains an inverted duplication of this element. The chromosomes resulting from such recombination events contain a duplication of 3-5cM (6-10 x 10^3kb) (Herrmann et al. 1987). These duplication chromosomes have provided important additional information about the position of the T gene (see below).

Positioning of the T Locus Region with Respect to Molecular Markers

The location of the T gene has been determined by several sets of data. The comparison of data on the genetic linkage of T to tf and the MHC, derived from classical breeding analyses, with data on linkage of cloned DNA markers to the MHC, derived by RI strain mapping, showed that the markers T48, T119I and T66E are located in the vicinity of the T locus. To establish the genetic linkage and position of these markers with respect to the T mutation we then carried out a classical genetic mapping cross involving the T mutation as a marker. The centromere (marked by a Robertsonian translocation and assayed in metaphase chromosome spreads) and the recessive hair loss mutation tf were used as flanking markers. 380 offspring were scored for recombination in the interval centromere -T, 808 offspring were scored for recombination within the interval T-tf. None of the recombinant chromosomes had separated any of the markers of the inverted duplication shown in Fig. 2 from the T mutation. The marker T48, however, could be localized proximal to T (Herrmann and Lehrach, manuscript in preparation). On this level of analysis the T mutation can not be positioned more accurately with respect to the cloned markers.

A more precise localization was achieved by the analysis of the deletion chromosome T^{hp}. This chromosome contains an allele of the T mutation due to the deletion of a large region of the chromosome (Johnson 1975). We were able to place the proximal deletion breakpoint between the markers T66E and T66EII (see Fig. 2). Therefore the markers T119I and T66E could be excluded from being adjacent to the T mutation, leaving the other half of the inverted duplication and more distal parts of the chromosome defining the region containing the T gene.

The analysis of a particular partial t haplotype, t^{Tu3}, allowed an even more precise positioning of T. This chromosome complements the T mutation. Animals of the genotype T/t^{Tu3} are phenotypically normal. We were able to show that this chromosome arose by a homologous recombination event across the proximal t complex inversion, similar to the events generating the duplication chromosomes t^{h45} and t^{AE5} shown on Fig. 2. Therefore this chromosome contains a large duplication including the normal T gene. It thus possesses two doses of the normal gene (Herrmann, Bode and Lehrach, manuscript in preparation). These data allowed us to position the T gene proximal to the recombination breakpoint of t^{Tu3} in the t haplotype, and (since the crossover event was homologous) distal to the corresponding point in the wild type chromosome. This point is located in the cloned region T119II (see Fig. 2). In addition the two duplication chromosomes shown on Fig. 2 fail to complement the T mutation because they contain the mutant gene in the distal part of the duplication and therefore possess only a single dose of the normal gene.

Molecular Cloning of a Gene from the T Locus Region

Using several systems of genetic mapping we were therefore able to define the proximal border of the region containing the T gene. We had reached the present limit of accuracy of defining this border. The distal border of the relevant region could not be defined with the markers available at the time. However, we have obtained data showing that the cloned region T119II is in linkage disequilibrium with the T mutation suggesting that it is very close to the T gene. This finding encouraged us to screen the cloned T119II region (distal to the t^{Tu3} breakpoint) for the presence of coding sequences. Our approach was to look for DNA fragments detecting homologous sequences in other vertebrates such as man, monkey, dog, chicken and xenopus. We found a fragment that detected a band in genomic chicken DNA upon hybridization. This probe was then used to screen a mouse embryo cDNA library (Fahrner et al. 1987). We isolated several cDNA clones originating from a gene located in the T119 regions. This gene is presently being investigated (Herrmann, Labeit, Carr, Hogan and Lehrach, manuscript in preparation). Although the isolated gene is located in the region genetically defined to contain the T gene, it appears at present unlikely to be identical with the T gene, since this gene is duplicated in the wild type chromosome. An inactivation of one copy would still leave an intact gene copy. Homozygous lethality of T/T embryos would thus be hard to explain, especially since t haplotypes have only one copy and are homozygous normal. There is a slight possibility that the one copy in the wild type chromosome is inactivated. However, we have not found any evidence for that possibility.

CONCLUSION

We have described a genetic and molecular approach to the cloning of genetic disease loci in mammalian genomes. We have genetically analyzed the mouse t complex using molecular probes as markers. This and similar analyses will provide the basis for the molecular cloning of factors of the t complex involved in mouse embryogenesis, spermatogenesis and sex determination. In particular we have focussed our attention on the cloning of the T gene involved in the formation of the embryonic body axis. We have genetically defined the T locus region and isolated a gene. We are therefore optimistic that this approach of cloning specific genes from the t complex will be successful.

ACKNOWLEDGMENTS

We thank D.P. Barlow for critical comments on the manuscript. B.G.H. was supported by an EMBO fellowship.

REFERENCES

Artzt K, Shin HS, Bennett D (1982). Gene mapping within the T/t complex of the mouse. II. Anomalous position of the H-2 complex in t haplotypes. Cell 28: 471-476.

Barlow DP, Lehrach H (1987) Genetics by gel electrophoresis: the impact of pulsed field gel electrophoresis on mammalian genetics. Trends in Genetics 3: 167-171

Fahrner K, Hogan BLM, Flavell RA (1987) Transcription of H-2 and Qa genes in embryonic and adult mice. EMBO J 6: 1265-1271

Fox HS, Martin GR, Lyon MF, Herrmann BG, Frischauf AM, Lehrach H, Silver LM (1985). Molecular probes define different regions of the mouse t complex. Cell 40: 63-69.

Frischauf AM (1985). The T/t complex of the mouse. Trends in Genetics 1: 100-103.

Grüneberg H (1958) Genetical studies on the skeleton of the mouse XXIII: The development of Brachyury and Anury. J Embryol Exp Morphol 6: 424-443

Herrmann BG, Bucan M, Mains PE, Frischauf AM, Silver LM, Lehrach H (1986). Genetic analysis of the proximal portion of the mouse t complex: evidence for a second inversion within t haplotypes. Cell 44: 469-476.

Herrmann BG, Barlow DP, Lehrach H (1987) A Large Inverted Duplication Allows Homologous Recombination between Chromosomes Heterozygous for the Proximal t Complex Inversion. Cell 48: 813-825

Johnson DR (1975). Further observations on the hairpin-tail (T^{hp}) mutation in the mouse. Genet. Res. Camb. 24: 207-213.

Klein J, Sipos P, Figueroa F (1984). Polymorphism of t-complex genes in European wild mice. Genet. Res. Camb. 44: 39-46.

Lyon MF (1984). Transmission ratio distortion in mouse t-haplotypes is due to multiple distorter genes acting on a responder locus. Cell 37: 621-628.

Mc Laren A (1976) Genetics of the early mouse embryo. Ann Rev Genet 10: 361-388

Poustka A, Lehrach H (1986) Jumping libraries and linking libraries: the next generation of molecular tools in mammalian genetics. Trends in Genetics 2:174-179

Röhme D, Fox HS, Herrmann BG, Frischauf AM, Edström JE, Mains P, Silver LM, Lehrach H (1984) Molecular clones of the mouse t complex derived from microdissected metaphase chromosomes. Cell 36: 783-788

Scalenghe F, Turco E, Edström JE, Pirrotta V, Melli M (1981) Microdissection and cloning of DNA from a specific region of Drosophila melanogaster polytene chromosomes. Chromosoma 82: 205-216

Schwartz DC, Cantor CR (1984). Separation of yeast chromosome-sized DNAs by pulsed field gradient gel electrophoresis. Cell 37: 67-75.

Shedlovsky, A., King TR, Dove WF (1988) Saturation germline mutagenesis of the murine t-region: coisogenic mutations amenable to high resolution mapping, including a lethal allele of the *quaking* locus. Proc Natl Acad Sci USA, in press

Shin HS, Bennett D, Artzt, K (1984) Gene mapping within the T/t complex of the mouse.IV. The inverted MHC is inter-mingled with several t-lethal genes. Cell 39: 573-578

Silver LM (1985). Mouse t haplotypes. Ann. Rev. Genet. 19: 179-208.

Sturtevant AH, Beadle, GW (1936). The relations of inversions in the X chromosome of Drosophila melanogaster to crossing over and disjunction. Genetics 21: 554-604.

Washburn LL, Eicher E (1983) Sex reversal in XY mice caused by dominant mutation on chromosome 17. Nature 303: 338-340

Murine Hox Genes – A Multigene Family

M. Fibi, M. Kessel, and P. Gruss

INTRODUCTION

The embryonal development of higher organisms is conducted by a network of many different structural and regulatory gene functions whose complexity is yet poorly understood. Some genetic elements identified as being involved in specifying segment identity of the fruit fly *Drosophila melanogaster* are the homeotic genes (Ouweneel 1976). Several homeotic genes of *Drosophila* belonging to either the engrailed gene complex (EN-C; Garcia-Bellido and Santamaria 1972) or the antennapedia and bithorax complex (ANT-C/BX-C; Regulski et al. 1985) contain a 180 bp conserved region, the "homeo box", coding for a protein domain of the helix-turn-helix type (McGinnis et al. 1984a, b; Scott and Weiner 1984). This type of DNA-binding domain was first detected in procaryotes. Interestingly, the two yeast mating-type proteins MAT a-1 and MAT α2 (Shepherd et al. 1984; Laughon and Scott 1984) show significant similarities to the consensus homeodomain sequence. MAT α2 is a transcriptional repressor (Wilson and Hershkowitz 1984; Hartig et al. 1986). It was therefore hypothesized that the *Drosophila* homeodomain proteins might also have regulatory functions, e.g., by interacting directly or indirectly in trans with their own promoter regions or those of other genes (Desplan et al. 1985).

Using *Drosophila* probes several homeo box-containing genes could also be identified in the mouse. Because of their high degree of homology (<90% amino acid level) these mouse genes are suggested to possess functions of similar importance for embryonal development of the mouse as the insect genes have for the development of the fly.

Up to today morphological mutations could not be shown by restriction mapping to be connected with mutational defects of Hox genes. Therefore, the investigation of functional traits of murine homeodomain proteins is based on expressional analyses of wild-type animals.

Since the development of the mouse leads from a single cell, the zygote, to an organism with many different tissues and organs, there must be a sufficiency of specific gene functions to direct morphogenesis. On the other hand, for primitive eucaryotes such as yeast one would expect only specific functional requirements for generation of a limited number of distinct cellular phenotypes (Hershkowitz and Oshima 1981; Sprague et al. 1983; Hershkowitz 1986) where mating type genes with the helix-turn-helix motif are involved (Laughon and Scott 1984). If the homeo box-containing genes of higher organisms are evolutionarily derived from helix-turn-helix type genes like the yeast MAT genes, the requirement for more gene functions must have been met by mechanisms such as tandem duplication and moderate alteration of existing genetic information generating new morphogenetic functions. In the following evidence is provided from the mouse Hox genes and the human Hox genes that such mechanisms did occur during evolution to generate a multigene family directing correct pattern formation in higher animals.

ANTENNAPEDIA-LIKE GENES OF THE MOUSE (HOX) ARE ARRANGED IN CLUSTERS AND LOCATED ON DIFFERENT CHROMOSOMES

So far 20 Hox genes have been mapped on the murine genome (Martin et al. 1987) and from five murine Hox genes cDNA sequences are described (Krumlauf et al. 1987; Odenwald et al. 1987; Kessel et al. 1987a; Meijlink et al. 1987; Baron et al. 1987; Fibi et al. 1987).

Department of Molecular Cell Biology, Max Planck Institute of Biophysical Chemistry, Am Fassberg, D-3400 Göttingen

Table 1. Murine Hox genes - overview of those detected so far

Chromosome	Locus	Genes and antp homologies of the homeodomain with the Antennapedia domain						Reference
6	Hox 1	1.1 82%	1.2 81%	1.3 74%	1.4 73%	1.5 72%	1.6 64%	1, 2
11	˙Hox 2	2.5	2.4	2.3 97%	2.2 90%	2.1 90%	2.6 ?	3
15	Hox 3	3.2	3.1 79%					4, 5
12	Hox 4	4.1 72%						6

The different murine Hox loci on the different chromosomes are listed and the percentage of homology of the respective homeo box regions to antennapedia is indicated. The references are: 1 = Colberg-Poley et al. 1985; 2 = Duboule et al. 1986; 3 = Ruddle et al. 1985; 4 = Breier et al. 1986; 5 = Awgulewitsch et al. 198?; 6 = Lonai et al. 1987

The murine Hox genes are arranged in clusters of up to seven genes in one locus and each locus is located on a different chromosome (Table 1). It seems likely that more Hox genes will be detected. A sequence comparison of the homeo boxes in the murine Hox 1 cluster with the prototype Antennapedia homeo box of *Drosophila* reveals that the similarity decreases stepwise in the direction of transcription. Thus, the Hox 1.1 box is very similar to the Antennapedia box while the Hox 1.6 box only shows a loose relationship. This suggests the 5' gene of the Hox 1 cluster is an ancestral gene from times of the phylogenetic division of insects and animals and the genes following in the 3' direction are the duplicated derivatives generated in later times of evolution. Although there are no cognate gene clusters in the fly and the mouse genome based on linkage to the same genes, they can be delineated by comparison of the mouse and the human genome (Bucan et al. 1986; Rabin et al. 1986), indicating that the clustered genes must have existed before the phylogenetic division of mouse and man.

HOX GENES EXPRESS A VARIABLE AND A CONSTANT REGION

Comparing homeodomain proteins encoded in the Hox 1 cluster, strong homologies exist only in the homeo box (region E, Fig. 1) and in a short hexapeptide (region c, a sequence at the 3' end of exon 1 (Fig. 1; for detailed information on Hox protein domains see Kessel et al. 1987b)). Besides these generally conserved domains there are variable regions in Hox proteins in the N-terminal half and at the carboxy terminus (regions A, B, D, and F). However, between homologous proteins from different species and proteins otherwise related (see below) the regions at the N-terminus (A) between the hexapeptide and the box (D) and at the carboxy terminus (F) may also be conserved. Region B, however, seems not to be conserved and varies also between related proteins. Assuming a

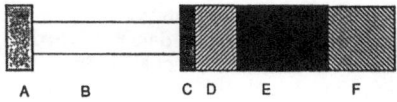

Fig. 1. Hox protein regions

certain function of a Hox protein being different from that of another Hox protein, the variable region B becomes a candidate. The high degree of conservation in the homeodomain indicates a more general function common to all proteins with a helix-turn-helix motif containing the homeodomain recognition helix. If the homeodomain provides the sites for DNA binding (Laughon and Scott 1984; Desplan et al. 1985) and for oligomerization with homologous molecules the variable regions might be responsible for the binding of further specific factors. If variable regions provide evolutionary advantages, organisms develop mechanisms to raise the variability to use a basic function (Ig genes). Simeone and co-workers (A. Simeone, D. Acampora, M. D'Esperito, M. Pannese, and E. Boncinelli, manuscript submitted) recently showed that for human Hox 3 genes there exist different transcripts generated by differential splicing. Since also for other Hox genes of other chromosomes more than one transcript of different size exists differential splicing or differential promoter usage seems to be a common mechanism (Odenwald et al. 1987; Krumlauf et al. 1987; Fibi et al. 1987) that might increase the variability of Hox genes..

DIFFERENT SETS OF HOX GENES WERE GENERATED DURING EVOLUTION BY CLUSTER DUPLICATION

If the protein coding sequences of some Hox genes of different chromosomes are compared, there are extended homologies in region C and E and additional homologies in the N-terminal variable region of exon 1 (region A) and the splice region (region D, Fig. 1), which are not detected in genes of one cluster. Since this is the case not only for one gene of a cluster but rather for a set of genes, namely Hox 1.1, Hox 1.2, Hox 1.3 on chromosome 6 and Hox 2.3, Hox 2.2, and Hox 2.1 on chromosome 11 (Fig. 2), it seems likely that a part of the Hox 1 cluster on chromosome 6 has been duplicated and segregated to chromosome 11, generating a part of the Hox 2 cluster. Furthermore, Hox 1.5 has its most homologous counter gene Hox 4.1 on chromosome 12, suggesting a further duplication event. This seems also to be the case for the pair Hox 2.4 on chromosome 11 (Lonai et al. 1987) and Hox 3.1 on chromosome 15 (Awgulewitsch et al. 1986; Breier et al. 1986).

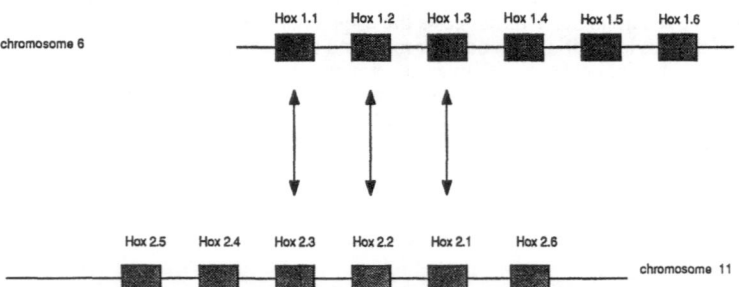

Fig. 2. Duplication of the Hox gene cluster

HOX GENES ARE SPATIALLY EXPRESSED IN EMBRYO AND ADULT MICE

Although the structural features of Hox genes are straightforward to delineate, it is much more complicated to interpret the *in situ* expression data of the murine Hox genes and even more complicated to come to a conclusion about gene function. Since appropriate analogs of the *Drosophila* mutants are not available to study the mouse homeo box genes, the information has to be drawn from the spatial expression pattern of the genes during the time course of embryonal development and adult life. In Table 2 we give an overview of Northern expression data published so far from different laboratories (Awgulewitsch et al. 1986; Baron et al. 1987; Breier et al. 1986; Colberg-Poley et al. 1985; Duboule et al. 1986; Fibi et al. 1986; Kessel et al. 1987a; Krumlauf et al. 1987; Meijlink et al. 1987; Odenwald et al. 1987; Ruddle et al. 1985). Obviously there are murine Hox genes which are highly expressed in many adult tissues, e.g., Hox 1.3, and others expressed at low levels in a limited number of tissues such as Hox 2.1, Hox 2.3, Hox 1.1, and Hox 3.1. Most strikingly, however, genes also exist that are expressed only in one specific tissue as in the case of Hox 1.4 in testis and Hox 1.6 in intestine. Another interesting result comes from the comparison of the very similar genes Hox 1.3 and Hox 2.1. Although both genes are expressed in spinal cord only Hox 1.3 is expressed in liver and testis. Furthermore, it becomes evident from the data that there are genes only expressed in one organ, such as Hox 1.3 in adult liver and Hox 2.1 in adult lung, and there are tissues in which a combination of Hox genes seems to be expressed simultaneously. Thus, Hox genes could be involved in the specific maintenance of adult tissue functions and this could be accomplished either by the expression of one Hox gene or by a combination of different Hox genes. In embryonal tissue all known Hox genes are expressed and there seems to be a peak of expression on day 12. However, the data are preliminary and in the near future a large amount of data will have to be collected and compared to gain greater insight into the Hox gene expression pattern and to delineate the basic mechanisms of Hox gene function during embryonal development and adult life of the mouse.

Table 2. Hox gene expression in different tissues of adult mice detected by Northern and *in situ* hybridization analysis

	Hox 1.3	Hox 2.1	Hox 2.3	Hox 1.1	Hox 3.1	Hox 1.6	Hox 1.4
Liver	++	-	-	-	-	-	-
Kidney	++	(+)	++	++	(+)	-	-
Ovary	++	n.d.	-	-	n.d.	n.d.	-
Testis	++	-	++	++	n.d.	-	++
Spinal cord	+++	++	++	n.d.	++	n.d.	n.d.
Brain	++	n.d.	-	n.d.	-	-	-
Lung	n.d.	+++	-	n.d.	n.d.	-	-
Spleen	n.d.	-	-	-	-	-	
Heart	n.d.	-	-	n.d.	n.d.	-	-
Intestine	n.d.	-	-	n.d.	n.d.	+	n.d.

n.d. = not done

REFERENCES

Awgulewitsch A, Utset MF, Hart CP, McGinnis W, Ruddle FH (1986) Spatial restriction in expression of a mouse homoeo box locus within the central nervous system. Nature 320:328-335

Baron A, Featherstone MS, Hill RE, Hall A, Galliot B, Duboule D (1987) Hox 1.6: A mouse homeo box containing gene member of the Hox-1 complex. EMBO J 6:2977-2986

Boncinelli E, Simeone A, LaVolpe A, Faiella A, Fidanza V, Acampora D, Scotto L (1985) Human cDNA clones containing homeo box sequences. Cold Spring Harbor Symp Quant Biol 50:301-306

Breier G, Bucan M, Francke U, Colberg-Poley AM, Gruss P (1986) Sequential expression of murine homeo box genes during F9 EC cell differentiation. EMBO J 5:2209-2215

Bucan M, Yang-Feng T, Colberg-Poley AM, Wolgemuth DJ, Guenet J-L, Francke U, Lehrach H (1986) Genetic and cytogenetic localisation of the homeo box containing genes on mouse chromosome 6 and human chromosome 7. EMBO J 5:2899-3905

Colberg-Poley AM, Voss SD, Chowdhury K, Stewart CL, Wagner E, Gruss P (1985) Clustered homeo boxes are differentially expressed during murine development. Cell 43:39-45

Desplan C, Theis J, O'Farrell PH (1985) The *Drosophila* developmental gene, *engrailed*, encodes a sequence-specific DNA binding activity. Nature 318:630-635

Duboule D, Baron A, Mähl P, Galliot B (1986) A new homeo-box is present in overlapping cosmid clones which define the mouse *HOX*-1 locus. EMBO J 5:1973-1980

Fibi M, Zink B, Kessel M, Colberg-Poley AM, Labeit S, Lehrach H, Gruss P (1987) Coding sequence and expression of the homeo box gene Hox 1.3. Development, in press

Garcia-Bellido A, Santamaria P (1972) Developmental analysis of the wing disc in the mutant engrailed or Drosophila melanogaster. Genetics 72:87-104

Hartig A, Holly J, Saar G, MacKay VL (1986) Multiple regulation of STE-2, a mating-type specific gene of Saccharomyces cerevisiae. Mol Cell Biol 6:2106-2114

Hershkowitz I, Oshima Y (1981) Control of cell type in Saccharomyces cerevisiae: Mating type and mating-type interconversion. In: Strathern JH, Jones EW, Broach JR (eds) The molecular biology of the yeast Saccharomyces: Life cycle and inheritance. Cold Spring Harbor Laboratory, New York, p 181

Hershkowitz I (1986) Specialized cell types in yeast: Their use in addressing problems in cell biology. In: Hides J (ed) Yeast cell biology. Alan R. Liss, New York, p 625

Kessel M, Schulze F, Fibi M, Gruss P (1987a) Primary structure and nuclear localization of a murine homeodomain protein. Proc Natl Acad Sci USA 84:5306-5310

Kessel M, Fibi M, Gruss P (1987b) Organization of homeodomain proteins. In: Sato GH, Harris SE (eds) Cellular factors in development and differentiation - embryos, teratocarciomas and differentiated tissues. Alan Liss, New York, in press

Krumlauf R, Holland PWH, McVey JH, Hogan BLM (1987) Developmental and spatial patterns of expression of the mouse homeo box gene Hox 2.1. Development 99:603-617

Laughon A, Scott MP (1984) Sequence of a Drosophila segmentation gene: Protein structure homology with DNA binding proteins. Nature 310:25-31

Lonai P, Arman E, Czosnek H, Ruddle FH, Blatt C (1987) New murine homeoboxes - structure chromosomal assignment and differential expression in the embryo and in adult erythropoiesis. DNA, in press

Martin GR (1986) Nomenclature for homeo box-containing genes. Nature 325:21-22

McGinnis W, Garber RL, Wirz J, Kuroiwa A, Gehring WJ (1984a) A homologous protein coding sequence in Drosophila homeotic genes and its conservation in other metazoans. Cell 37:403-408

McGinnis W, Levine MS, Hafen E, Kuroiwa A, Gehring WJ (1984b) A conserved DNA sequence in homeotic genes of the Drosophila Antennapedia and bithorax complex. Nature 308:428-433

Meijlink F, de Laaf R, Verrijzer P, Destrée O, Kroezen V, Hilkens J, Deschamps J (1987) A mouse homeo box containing gene on chromosome 11: Sequence and tissue-specific expression. Nucl Acids Res 15:6773-6786

Odenwald WF, Taylor CF, Palmer-Hill FJ, Friedrich Jr V, Tani M, Lazzarini RA (1987) Expression of a homeo domain protein in non-contact-inhibited cultured cells and postmitotic neurons. Genes & Development 1:482-496

Ouweneel WJ (1976) Developmental genetics of homeosis. Adv Genet 18:179-248

Rabin M, Ferguson-Smith A, Hart CP, Ruddle F (1986) Cognate homeo box loci mapped on homologous human and mouse chromosomes. Proc Natl Acad Sci USA 83:9103-9108

Regulski M, Harding K, Kostriken R, Karch F, Levine M, McGinnis W (1985) Homeo box genes of the Antennapedia and bithorax complexes of Drosophila. Cell 43:71-80

Ruddle F, Hart C, Awgulewitsch A, Fainsod A, Utset M, Dalton D, Kerk N, Rabin M, Ferguson-Smith A, Fienberg A, McGinnis W (1985) Mammalian homeo box genes. Cold Spring Harbor Symp Quant Biol 50:277-284

Scott MP, Weiner AJ (1984) Structural relationships among genes that control development: Sequence homology between Antennapedia, Ultrabithorax and fushi tarazu loci of Drosophila. Proc Natl Acad Sci USA 81:4115-4119

Shepherd JCW, McGinnis W, Carrasco AE, De Robertis EM, Gehring WJ (1984) Fly and frog homeo domains show homologies with yeast mating type regulatory proteins. Nature 310:70-71

Sprague Jr GF, Blair LC, Thornes J (1983) Cell interactions and regulation of cell type in the yeast Saccharomyces cerevisiae. Ann Rev Microbiol 37:623-660

Wilson KL, Hershkowitz I (1986) Sequences upstream of the STE6 gene required for its expression and regulation by the mating type locus in Saccharomyces cerevisiae. Proc Natl Acad Sci USA 83:2536-2540

Expression of the Homeobox Genes Hox 2.1 and 2.6 During Mouse Development

A. Graham, P. W. H. Holland[2], A. Lumsden[3], R. Krumlauf, and B. L. M. Hogan[1]

INTRODUCTION

The homeobox is a conserved DNA sequence of about 183 nucleotides identified within a number of Drosophila genes which regulate certain aspects of early development. The homeobox sequence encodes a 61 amino acid homeodomain containing a helix-turn-helix motif which is probably involved in DNA binding. Drosophila genes containing a homeobox include some segmentation genes which are involved in generating a metameric pattern, and many homeotic genes (Gehring 1987). Homeotic genes have roles in establishing segment identity, which involves the specification of positional values along the anteroposterior body axis - a process which must occur in the embryos of all bilateral animals, not only those with a segmented body plan. It is therefore significant that several Drosophila homeobox-containing genes are expressed in patterns which suggest roles in positional specification independent of the process of segmentation (Doyle 1986; Hoey et al., 1986; Akam 1987; Gehring 1987).

About 20 homeobox-containing genes have been identified in Drosophila (Akam 1987; Gehring 1987). Most of the homeotic genes which are involved in the specification of segment identity or positional value are organised into two clusters, the Antennapaedia and bithorax complexes. Homeobox sequences have also been identified in a wide range of segmented and non-segmented animals besides insects, including molluscs, annelids, echinoderms and vertebrates (McGinnis 1985; Holland and Hogan 1986).

In the mouse, more than 20 homeobox-containing genes have so far been identified (Colberg-Poley et al., 1987). Several of these genes are organised in two clusters, known as Hox 1 and Hox 2, on chromosomes 6 and 11 respectively. At present the Hox 1 cluster contains 7 characterised genes and the Hox 2 cluster contains 6 (Colberg-Poley et al., 1987; Rubin et al., 1987). It seems likely that the genes within these clusters have evolved via duplication and divergence of an ancestral gene (or part of a gene). Sequence analysis and restriction enzyme mapping of the Hox 1 and Hox 2 clusters have allowed some insight into the possible genealogy of these duplication events.

The distances (in kilobase pairs) between the homeoboxes of four neighbouring genes within the Hox 1 cluster (Hox 1.1, 1.2, 1.3 and 1.4) are very similar to the distances between the homeoboxes of four genes within the Hox 2 cluster (Hox 2.3, 2.2, 2.1 and 2.6). Thus, there may have been a relatively recent duplication of an ancestral cluster containing at least four genes, which gave

[1]To whom correspondence should be addressed at Dept. Cell Biology, Vanderbilt University Medical School, Nashville, Tennessee 37232, U.S.A.

Laboratory of Molecular Embryology, National Institute for Medical Research, Mill Hill, London NW7 1AA, U.K., and [2]Department of Anatomy, Guy's Hospital Medical School, London SE1 9RT, U.k. [3]Present address: Department of Zoology, University of Oxford, South Parks Road, Oxford OX1 3PS, U.K.

Hox 1 Locus Chromosome 6

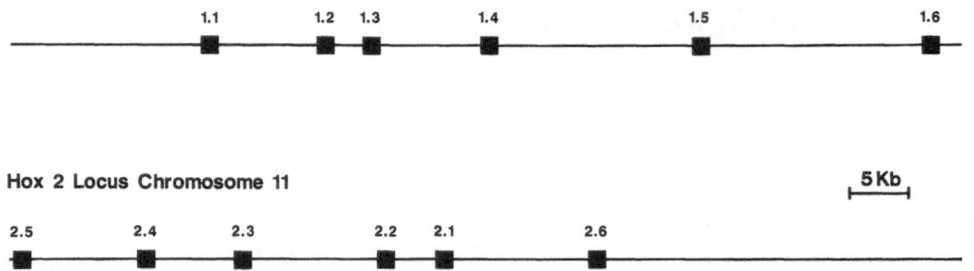

Fig. 1. Genomic organization of the Hox 1 and Hox 2 clusters. For details, see text.

rise to part of the Hox 1 and Hox 2 clusters. The other genes may be accounted for by later rearrangement and duplication events. This hypothesis is consistent with evidence from comparisons of Hox 1 and Hox 2 homeobox sequences, which reveal high degrees of sequence identity between Hox 1.1 and 2.3 (82% nucleotide identity, 93% amino acid identity) (Kessel et al., 1987; Meijlink et al., 1987), between Hox 1.3 and 2.1 (84% nucleotide, 100% amino acid) (Krumlauf et al., 1987; Odenwald et al., 1987), and between Hox 1.4 and 2.6 (82% nucleotide, 90% amino acid) (Duboule et al., 1986, and data not shown). Where more extensive sequence is available for comparison, high degrees of identity are also observed between the N-terminal regions of the coding sequences of these gene pairs (e.g. Hox 1.3 versus 2.1 (Krumlauf et al., 1987; Odenwald et al., 1987) and Hox 1.1 versus 2.3 (Kessel et al., 1987; Meijlink et al., 1987)). These additional domains of identity are consistent with the suggestion that duplication of an ancestral gene cluster has contributed to the evolution of the Hox 1 and Hox 2 clusters. However, the high degree of conservation in gene organization may also reflect functional constraints on the spacing and structure of mouse homeobox-containing genes, perhaps related to transcription, RNA processing and protein functions. Such constraints could lead to convergent evolution, such that precise evolutionary history may be obscured.

EMBRYONIC EXPRESSION OF HOX 2.1 AND HOX 2.6

Hox 2.1 and Hox 2.6 are 13kb apart at the 3' end of the Hox 2 cluster, which maps at the distal end of mouse chromosome 11, near the Dlb-1 locus (Jackson et al., 1985; Holland and Hogan 1987). As discussed above, sequence analysis indicates that the genes may be more closely related to Hox 1.3 and Hox 1.4 respectively, than they are to each other. It was therefore of interest to compare the patterns of Hox 2.1 and 2.6 expression in the embryo. This was achieved using in situ hybridization with ^{35}S-labelled single-stranded RNA probes (Holland and Hogan 1987). With both genes, expression is detected in regions of the central nervous system (CNS), peripheral nervous system (PNS), and in the mesodermal component of several visceral organs.

Expression in the CNS and PNS

Within the CNS at 12.5 days post coitum, Hox 2.1 expression is detected in a single continuous domain, with a sharp anterior boundary in the hindbrain, just posterior to the otic vesicle. This limit does not seem to correlate with any visible change in cell phenotype, and corresponds to about the level of the first occipital somite. There is no clear posterior boundary, and expression in the spinal cord extends at least to the level of the thirtieth somite. At 13.5 to 15.5d p.c., the region of expression in the CNS becomes more restricted, and extends posteriorly only to the level of the seventh somite (Holland and Hogan 1987).

Expression of Hox 2.1 is also detected in specific ganglia of the PNS which are derived from the neural crest. At 12.5d p.c. high levels of Hox 2.1 are seen in all dorsal root ganglia and in ganglia of the myenteric plexus, but only in one cranial ganglion, situated in the post-otic region, dorsal to the anterior oesophagus. We have previously suggested that this is the inferior (or nodose) ganglion of the Xth (or vagus) nerve (Holland and Hogan 1987).

We have now examined this expression in more detail, using specific antibodies against neurofilament proteins to identify the expressing structures. Immuno-staining of whole and partially dissected mouse embryos with antineurofilament anti-bodies reveals the positions of the cranial nerves and ganglia. This approach indicated that the inferior ganglia of the IXth and Xth cranial nerves are very closely apposed at 12.5d p.c., and lie in the position of the paired structure expressing Hox 2.1 RNA (Fig. 2).

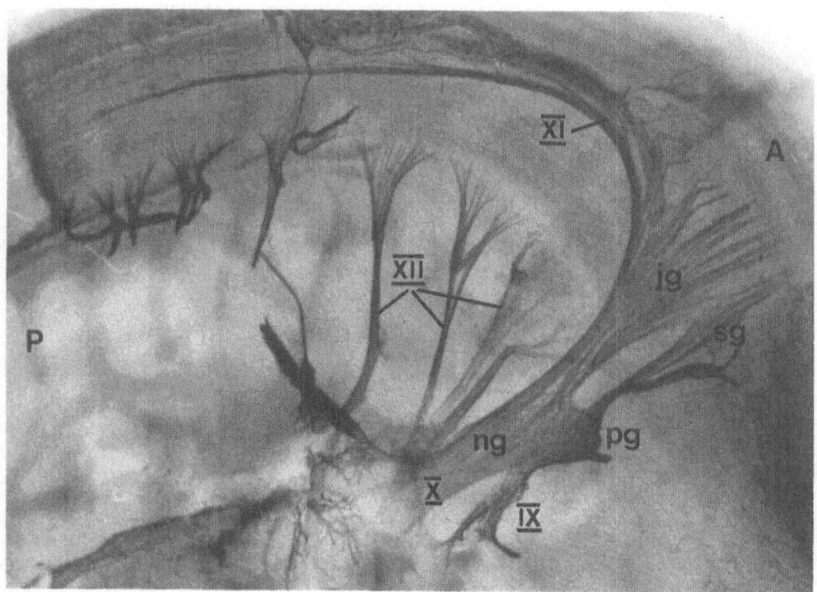

Fig. 2. Distribution of neurofilament in whole mouse embryos (12.5d p.c.) revealed by immunocytochemistry. Embryos were fixed in 4% paraformaldehyde in PBS (16 hr, 4°C), rinsed in PBS and incubated in PBS, 0.3% Triton X-100 (PBST buffer)

containing 0.09% hydrogen peroxide (24 hr, 4°C). After washing in PBST (4 x 2 hr, 4°C), specimens were incubated in serum containing the anti-155kD neurofilament monoclonal antibody, 2H3, and 0.3% Triton X-100 (4 days, 4°C). Embryos were washed in PBST, 1% goat serum (3 x 2 hr, 4°C) and incubated in peroxidase conjugated goat anti-mouse IgG (Pharmacia) diluted 1:100 in PBST, 1% goat serum (20 hr, 4°C), incubated in 0.1M Tris-HCl (pH 7.2) (30 min, 4°C), pretreated with 0.05% (w/v) diaminobenzidene (DAB) in 0.1M Tris-HCl (pH 7.2) (3 hr, 4°C in the dark), and then transferred to fresh Tris-HCl, DAB containing 0.018% hydrogen peroxide. The reaction was allowed to develop in the dark for 3 to 10 min and stopped in PBS. Abbreviations: IX, X, XI, XII, cranial nerves. A = anterior, P = posterior. sg, pg, superior and inferior (petrosal) ganglia of the IXth cranial nerve. jg, ng, superior (jugular) and inferior (nodose) ganglia of the Xth cranial nerve

To ascertain if the hybridizing structure corresponds to one (or both) of these cranial ganglia, adjacent face-to-face parasagittal sections were taken from a 12.5d p.c. embryo. One section was stained with an anti-neurofilament antibody (Fig. 3a,c), and the other hybridized with Hox 2.1 antisense probe (Fig. 3b,d,e). This revealed that cells within the hybridizing structure express neurofilament protein, and that associated with the structure are several major nerve tracts. This strengthens the suggestion that the hybridizing structure is a ganglion. Figure 3c,d,e also clearly shows that the intensely hybridizing ganglion is the larger, and the more posterior of the two closely associated ganglia. Within this ganglion, hybridization is not seen in the nerve tracts, but is localized to the region containing nerve cell bodies and accessory cells. The smaller ganglion (which does not hybridize to Hox 2.1 antisense probe) is associated with a major nerve leading caudally and ventrally (Fig. 3). Comparison with whole embryos stained with an anti-neurofilament antibody indicates that the inferior ganglion of the IXth nerve is associated with a nerve tract in this position, leading to the third branchial arch. This suggests that the smaller (non-hybridizing) ganglion is the inferior ganglion of the IXth cranial nerve. The relative position, and nerve associations of the larger, more posterior, ganglion indicate that it is the inferior (or nodose) ganglion of the Xth cranial nerve.

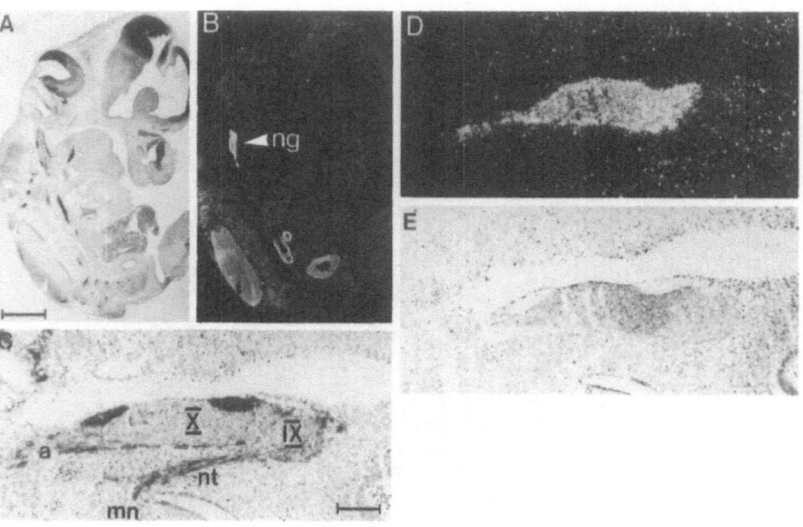

Fig. 3. Neurofilament distribution and Hox 2.1 expression visualised in sections of a 12.5d p.c. embryo. Embryos were fixed and frozen sections prepared as

described (Hogan et al., 1986). One of a pair of adjacent sections (A,C) was stained with an anti 200-155kD neurofilament antibody, RT97 (Wood and Anderton 1981). After fixation, slides were incubated in PBS, 0.1% Triton X-100 (10 min, 20°C), washed in PBS, and endogenous peroxidase blocked in 0.3% hydrogen peroxide in methanol (30 min, 20°C). Slides were washed in PBS, blocked with 10% rabbit serum in PBS (45 min, 20°C) and incubated in ^{1}/250 dilution of RT97 in PBS (20 hr, 4°C). Slides were washed in PBS, treated with ^{1}/100 biotinylated sheep anti-mouse Ig (Amersham) (1 hr, 20°C), washed and overlayed with ^{1}/200 streptavidin-peroxidase conjugate (Amersham) (1hr, 20°C). Peroxidase was detected utilizing DAB as a substrate (Hume and Gordon 1983), followed by silver enhancement using a kit supplied by Amersham International. The other section of each pair was hybridized with an antisense probe for Hox 2.1 RNA (probe 2, Krumlauf et al., 1987) as previously described (Holland and Hogan 1987), and exposed for 5 days. A, low magnification, neurofilament staining. Scale bar 1mm. B, adjacent section to A, distribution of Hox 2.1 RNA. Dark ground illumination. Note hybridization to lung, stomach, spinal cord and nodose ganglion (ng). Scale as for A. C, higher magnification of the occipital region in A, showing the inferior ganglia of the IXth and Xth cranial nerves. a = accessory nerve, nt = nerve tract, mn = mandible. Scale bar 150µm. D and E, higher magnification of occipital region in B. D, dark ground; E, bright field. Scale as for C.

Thus, comparison of Figures 2 and 3 indicates that Hox 2.1 RNA is expressed in the nodose ganglion, but not in the inferior ganglion of the IXth cranial nerve. At least in the chick, the nodose ganglion has a mixed origin, with the neurones being predominantly of placodal origin, and the neuroglia of neural crest origin (Le Douarin 1982). Hence, this expression may be comparable with that seen in the neural crest-derived dorsal root ganglia and myenteric plexus.

The embryonic expression of Hox 2.6 in the CNS and PNS is very similar to that described for Hox 2.1, except that the ganglia of the myenteric plexus may be negative.

Expression in the mesoderm

Both in situ hybridization and Northern analysis show that Hox 2.6 and Hox 2.1 are expressed in a subset of mesodermal cells. These include nephrotome derivatives, lung and stomach mesoderm and, for Hox 2.6 only, the longitudinal muscle of the gut. We have never seen expression of either gene in mesodermal cells of the heart, somite derivatives or limb, or in cells of endodermal origin.

DISCUSSION

Both Hox 2.1 and Hox 2.6 are clearly expressed in a specific anteroposterior domain of the CNS. In addition, since the dorsal root ganglia, myenteric plexus (at least for Hox 2.1) and nodose ganglion receive neural crest contributions from posterior to the first somite (Narayanan and Narayanan 1980; Le Douarin 1982), we would suggest that a similar anteroposterior restriction is imposed upon expression in the PNS.

Expression of Hox 2.1 and 2.6 in cells of mesodermal origin is not uniform, but appears to be restricted to a subset of derivatives from the medial lateral plate and intermediate mesoderm derived from a domain extending posterior to the occipital region (Holland and Hogan 1987; Graham et al., in preparation). The heart, for example, originates from a region anterior of this point and it does not express either of these genes. However, anteroposterior position alone cannot account for the observed patterns of mesodermal expression. Hox 2.1 and Hox 2.6

are not expressed in somite derivatives or in the limbs, both of which arise posterior of the occipital region. Thus, while position appears to be an element in determining expression, it cannot be viewed in a simple anteroposterior restriction. More detailed analysis must await accurate mapping of the embryonic origin of the mesodermal components of organs such as the stomach and lungs (see Holland and Hogan 1987 for discussion).

This description of the embryonic expression patterns of Hox 2.1 and 2.6 has parallels with the expression of some Drosophila homeobox-containing genes, in particular those which have been implicated in the control of anteroposterior positional specification independent of the process of segmentation (Hoey et al., 1986; Akam 1987; Gehring 1987).

In conclusion, the homeobox-containing genes of the mouse seem to have duplicated and diversified via a complex pathway. Tight clustering of these genes may reflect their evolutionary history, but also seems to have functional implications. For example, Hox 2.1 and 2.6 are in close proximity and seem to be expressed in very similar patterns in the embryo. These patterns of expression are themselves of great interest, since they are consistent with mouse homeobox-containing genes playing a role in specifying positional values along the anteroposterior axis of the embryo.

ACKNOWLEDGEMENTS

We thank M. Snow for valuable discussion, V. Harrison and J. Lorimer for assistance, and Lydia Pearson for preparing the manuscript.

REFERENCES

Akam M (1987) The molecular basis for metameric prepattern in the Drosophila embryo. Development 101:1-22
Colberg-Poley AM, Voss SD, Gruss P (1987) Homeobox genes of the mouse. Oxford Surveys in Eukaryotic Genes 4, Oxford University Press, Oxford, in press
Doyle, HJ, Harding K, Hdey T, Levine M (1986) Transcripts encoded by a homeobox gene are restricted to dorsal tissue of Drosophila embryos. Nature 323:76-79
Duboule D, Baron A, Mahl P, Galliot B (1986) A new homeobox is present in overlapping cosmid clones which define the mouse Hox 1 locus. EMBO J 5:1973-1980
Gehring WJ (1987) Homeoboxes in the study of development. Science 236:1245-1252
Hoey T, Doyle HJ, Harding K, Weeden C, Levine M (1986) Homeobox gene expression in anterior and posterior region of the Drosophila embryo. Proc Natl Acad Sci USA 83:4809-4813
Hogan BLM, Costantini F, Lacy E (1986) Manipulating the mouse embryo: a laboratory manual. Cold Spring Harbor Laboratory, Cold Spring Harbor, New York
Holland PWH, Hogan BLM (1986) Phylogenetic distribution of Antennapedia like homeoboxes. Nature 321:251-253
Holland PWH, Hogan BLM (1987) Spatially restricted patterns of expression of the mouse homeobox-containing gene, Hox 2.1, during mouse embryogenesis. Development (in press)
Hume DA, Gordon S (1983) Mononuclear phagocyte system of the mouse defined by immunohistochemical localisation of antigen F4/80. J Exp Med 157:501-531
Jackson IJ, Schofield, P, Hogan BLM (1985) A mouse homeobox gene is expressed during embryogenesis and in adult kidney. Nature 317:745-748
Kessel M, Schulze F, Fibi M, Gruss P (1987) Primary structure and nuclear localisation of a murine homeodomain protein. Proc Natl Acad Sci USA 84:5306-5310

Krumlauf R, Holland PWH, McVey JH, Hogan BLM (1987) Developmental and spatial patterns of expression of the mouse homeobox gene, Hox 2.1. Development 99: 603-617

Le Douarin N (1982) The Neural Crest. Cambridge University Press

McGinnis W (1985) Homeobox sequences of the Antennapedia class are conserved only in higher animal genomes. Cold Spring Harbor Symp Quant Biol 50:263-270

Meijlink CF, De Laaf R, Verrijzer P, Destree O, Kroezen V, Hilkens J, Deschamps J (1987) A mouse homeobox-containing gene on chromosome 11: sequence and tissue-specific expression. Nucl Acid Res 15:6773-6786

Narayanan CH, Narayanan Y (1980) Neural crest and placodal contributions in the development of the glossopharyngeal-vagal complex in the chick. The Anatomical Record 196:71-82

Odenwald WF, Taylor CF, Palmer-Hill FJ, Friedrich V, Tani M, Lazzarini RA (1987) Expression of a homeodomain protein in noncontact-inhibited cultured cells and post mitotic neurons. Genes and Development 1:482-496

Rubin MR, King W, Toth LE, Sawzuk IS, Levine MS, D'Eustachio P, Chi Nguyen-Huu M (1987) Murine Hox 1.7 homeobox gene: cloning, chromosomal location and expression. Mol Cell Biol 7:3836-3841

Wood JN, Anderton BH (1981) Monoclonal antibodies to mammalian neurofilaments. Bioscience Reports 1:263-268

Studies of V(D)J Recombination with Extrachromosomal Substrates

M. R. Lieber, J. E. Hesse, K. Mizuuchi, and M. Gellert

INTRODUCTION

We have developed a series of new substrates to study the mechanism and regulation of lymphoid V(D)J recombination. The substrates remain extrachromosomal and are recovered and analyzed for recombination within one to two days after transfection into murine cells. Extrachromosomal substrates have several advantages over substrates that integrate into the genome. Because integrating substrates incorporate into the genome at different sites in each host cell, recombination may be variably influenced by different chromosomal contexts, thereby introducing an uncontrolled parameter into comparisons between different host lines or substrates. Also, a considerable length of time is required to establish cells with integrated exogenous DNA, and drug selection or cellular subcloning steps are necessary to isolate the recombinant clones. Quantitative studies are thus difficult or in many cases impossible.

The family of substrates that we have described recently (Hesse et al., 1987) allows an assay that is sensitive and rapid; a frequency of rearrangement can easily be measured, so that experiments that vary the host cells or the recombination substrates can be meaningfully compared (Lieber et al., 1987). We have thus begun to study the way in which the level of V(D)J recombination activity and its sites of action are regulated, as well as some aspects of the reaction mechanism. The following sections briefly describe the experimental system and our results on the distribution of the recombination activity among cell lines representative of various tissues and developmental stages. Details can be found in two recent papers (Hesse et al., 1987; Lieber et al., 1987).

DESCRIPTION OF THE ASSAY

The strategy used to measure levels of recombination activity employs a plasmid, pJH200 (Fig. 1), which contains the heptamer/nonamer joining signals as well as genes conferring antibiotic resistance. This substrate DNA is transfected into the eukaryotic cells to be tested, recovered 48 hrs later, and introduced into E. coli by transformation (Fig. 2). All plasmid DNA confers ampicillin resistance (Amp^r). Because recombination excises a transcription stop signal upstream of the cat gene in pJH200, recombinant molecules also confer chloramphenicol resistance (Cam^r). Thus, the ratio of doubly resistant (Amp^{r}Cam^r) colonies to Amp^r colonies reflects the fraction of DNA which is rearranged at the heptamer/nonamer joining signals. HgiAl restriction analysis of plasmids recovered from doubly resistant colonies confirmed that a precise signal junction (heptamer to heptamer fusion) was formed in the large majority of recombinants (Hesse et al., 1987). Some exceptions to this rule will be discussed in a later paper.

Several useful features of this assay deserve mention:
1)   It is quite sensitive. In cell lines where plasmid transfection is efficient, recombination can easily be detected down to a level of 0.1% or less.

Laboratory of Molecular Biology, NIDDK, NIH, Bethesda, MD 20892

2) In some cell lines the recombination frequency is quite high, in excess of 20%.

3) Recombination is seen only among DNA molecules which have replicated in the eukaryotic cells. Although the mechanism is not yet understood, this requirement is very useful in comparing recombination frequencies between different cell lines, because it allows one to ignore DNA molecules which are merely adsorbed to the cells.

V(D)J Recombination in the Lymphoid Lineage

We have used this assay to ask some questions about the regulation of the recombination activity. Is the activity really present only in lymphoid cells? Is the activity merely switched on and then off during B lymphoid

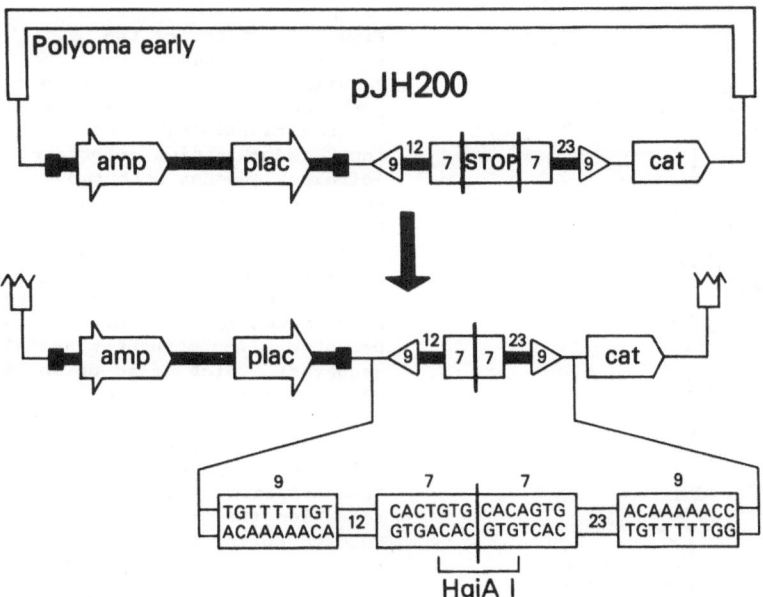

Figure 1. Outline of Recombination Reaction
Plasmid pJH200 contains two heptamer/nonamer immunoglobulin joining signal sequences flanking a prokaryotic transcription terminator (labelled "stop"). The signals in turn are flanked by the E. coli plac promoter on one side and the gene for chloramphenicol acetyl transferase (CAT) on the other. The terminator prevents expression of the cat gene when the plasmid is in E coli. After V(D)J rcombination in lymphoid cells (lower part of Figure), the terminator has been deleted, allowing cat expression in E. coli, and the joining signals have been fused, heptamer to heptamer. The signal joint contains a novel HgiA1 restriction site.
Plasmid pJH200 is identical to pJH201 previously described (Hesse et al., 1987), except that pJH200 lacks the kappa transcription enhancer.

differentiation, or is its level also modulated? And to what extent is the activity present in cell lines which are no longer rearranging their endogenous V, D, and J loci? After measuring recombination in more than thirty mouse cell lines, we have arrived at a fairly coherent picture (Lieber et al., 1987; Figs. 3 and 4).

First of all, no activity was found outside the hematopoietic lineage. Cell lines we tested included neural, embryonic liver, epithelial, fibroblast, and smooth muscle. Recombination was found at a low level in a myelo-monocyte precursor cell line (see Fig. 4). Thus the activity persists beyond the branching of the myelo-monocytic lineage from the lymphoid lineage. Activity was not found in later granulocytic or monocytic cells.

Second, there are major changes in the level of recombination activity during B lymphoid development. Results from the 24 cell lines surveyed in this pathway are summarized in Fig. 3. Activity is low in pro-GMB cell lines, but then increases greatly in pro-B cells. The two cell lines representing this

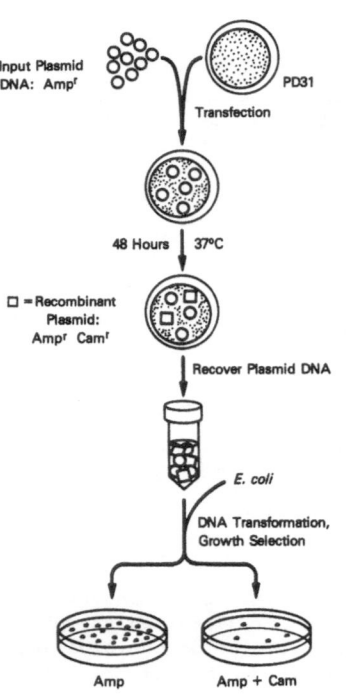

Figure 2 Outline of the Recombination Assay.

Plasmid DNA is introduced into eukaryotic cells by the DEAE-dextran transfection method. This input recombination substrate (circles) encodes both Amp resistance and Cam resistance, but transcription of the latter gene in an E. coli host would be blocked by the presence of the prokaryotic transcription terminator located between the cat gene and the lac promoter. Recombinant plasmids (squares), which arise during the 48 hr residence in the eukaryotic cells, have deleted or relocated the terminator and have thereby restored the potential for transcription of the cat gene (no selection for Cam resistance is imposed during this period). Plasmid DNA is recovered from the transfected cells and introduced into E. coli by transformation. Aliquots of each transformation mix are dispensed to two types of solid growth media, one containing Amp and one containing Amp and Cam. Only recombinant plasmids can give rise to Amp^r Cam^r transformants.

Plasmid DNA is isolated from Amp^r Cam^r transformants and structurally characterized. A frequency of recombination is given by the ratio of the number of Amp^r Cam^r transformants to the number of Amp^r transformants after correction for dilution.

latter stage (BASC6 and NFS70) had the highest recombination frequencies found. From there on, the level of activity declines progressively, with pre-B cells at the stage of heavy chain rearrangement generally higher than those that are rearranging their light chains, with mature B cell lines showing even lower or zero activity, and with no activity detectable at the later immunoblast and plasma cell stages. The one exception to this apparent progression is the λ-rearranging line ABC-1, which has much higher activity than any κ-rearranging line. However, in the light of a recent suggestion that some λ-rearranging cells form a distinct B-lymphoid sub-lineage, this may not be a real exception.

Recombination was also found in pre-T cell lines, but not in a mature T cell line, indicating that the activity may also be developmentally regulated in the T-cell lineage.

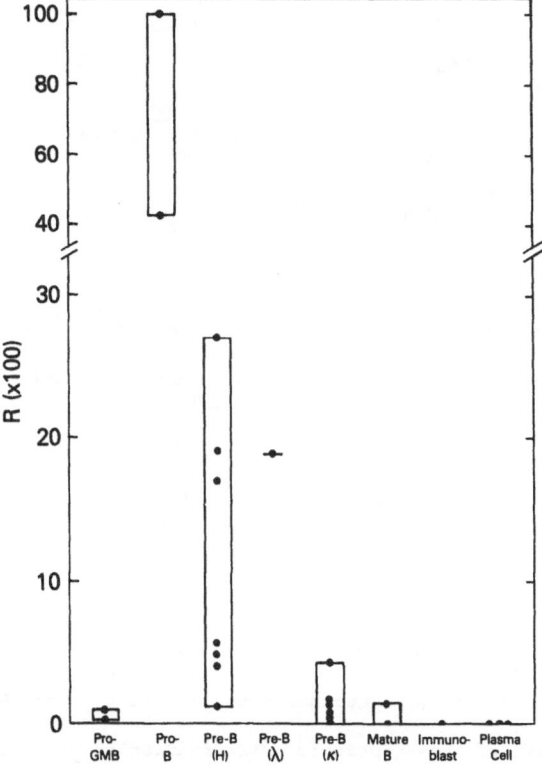

Figure 3. Recombination Frequency in Cell lines of the B Lineage.

Recombination frequencies (R) are plotted as a function of the developmental stage of the cell lines; each point represents one cell line. The boxes enclose the range of R in that category of cells. For each stage, the current or most recent locus of Ig recombination is indicated: H, heavy chain locus; λ, lambda locus; κ, kappa locus.

Third, it is clear from our results that extrachromosomal DNA can recombine in some cell lines that are no longer rearranging their endogenous Ig genes. We focused on the cell lines 38B7 (which has undergone nonproductive VDJ rearrangement on both heavy chain alleles and has exhausted the D segments), and 1-8 (which has a nonproductive VDJ rearrangement at one heavy chain allele and a DJ rearrangement on its other); both recombine our introduced substrate rather efficiently.

From these results, one can conclude that V(D)J recombination is controlled in at least two ways. The level of the activity is modulated during lymphoid development, and within a single cell, some substrate regions are available for recombination while others are blocked.

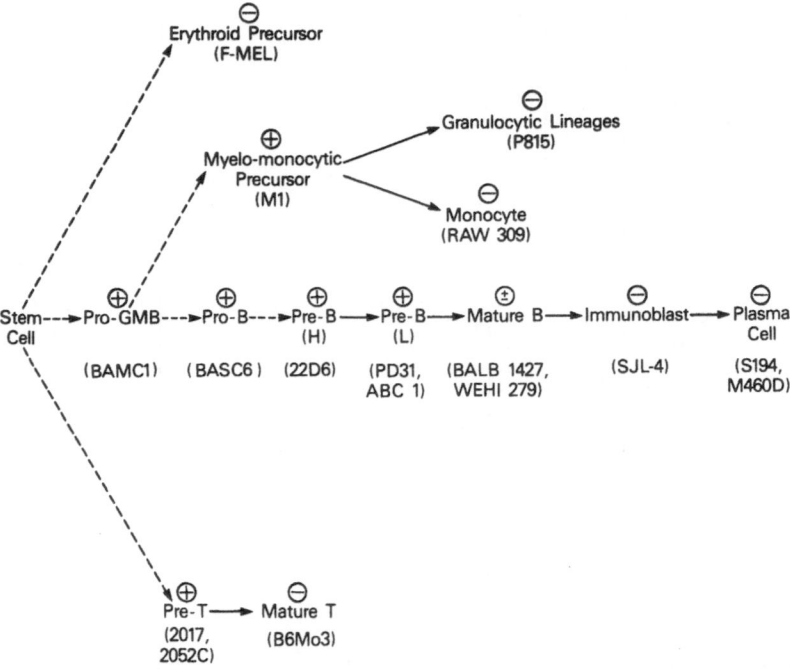

Figure 4.   Distribution of V(D)J Recombination Activity Among Hematopoietic
           Cell Types.
        The pathway of hematopoietic differentiation is summarized.   Known
lineage relationships are indicated by solid lines, more tenuous relationships by
dashed lines.   Specific cell lines representing each stage are named below it.   A
        circled (+) or (−) above the cell stage indicates the presence or absence
of detectable V(D)J recombination activity in the corresponding cell lines.

References:

Hesse JE, Lieber MR, Gellert M, Mizuuchi K (1987) Extrachromosomal Substrates in Pre-B Cells Undergo Inversion or Deletion at Immunoglobulin V-(D)-J Joining Signals. Cell 49: 775-783.

Lieber, MR, Hesse JE, Mizuuchi K, Gellert M (1987) Developmental Stage Specificity of the Lymphoid V(D)J Recombination Activity. Genes and Development 1: 751-761.

Transcription Factors in Terminally Differentiated B Cells

C.L. Peterson, B. Tsao, E. Kakkis, and K.L. Calame

INTRODUCTION

During B cell development differentiation is accompanied by the selective activation of some genes and the repression of other genes. We wish to identify and characterize transcription factors responsible for the activation and repression of gene expression.

Early in B cell development, an immunoglobulin heavy chain (IgH) gene is activated by rearrangment, positioning the promoter close to a transcriptional enhancer that is crucial for tissue-specific expression of IgH genes (Calame 1985). In vivo and in vitro studies show the IgH enhancer interacts with cellular proteins to activate transcription (Mercola et al 1985; Scholer and Gruss 1985). We report a functional analysis of protein binding sites within the IgH enhancer as well as the purification of two of these enhancer binding proteins.

The c-myc proto-oncogene is expressed in early proliferating B cells, but in plasma cells, c-myc expression is repressed (Kakkis et al 1987). Somatic cell hybrid studies suggest that the c-myc gene is controlled by a trans-dominant repressor in Human Burkitt lymphoma cells (Feo et al 1985). We have identified a protein (myc-PCF) which recognizes sequences in the c-myc promoter region and whose binding activity is restricted to plasmacytomas which do not express the normal unrearranged c-myc gene (Kakkis and Calame 1987). We report further characterization of myc-PCF and of a common upstream factor (myc-CUF1) binding nearby. The myc-PCF protein is a likely candidate for a developmental repressor of c-myc expression.

FUNCTIONAL ANALYSIS OF THE IGH ENHANCER

We have identified eight binding sites within the mouse immunoglobulin heavy chain enhancer which bind a minimum of six different proteins (Peterson and Calame 1987). We created deletions of each binding site by oligonucleotide-directed mutagenesis and cloned the mutated enhancers 3' to the chloramphenicol acetyltransferase (CAT) gene in the vector pA10CAT-2. Wild type and mutant enhancers were tested for enhancer function after transient transfection into plasmacytoma P3X63-Ag8 cells (Mercola et al. 1985), using a cotransfected B-galactosidase plasmid to normalize for transfection efficiency.

Deletion of site E, B, C1 or C2 from the 1 kb mouse IgH enhancer significantly reduces enhancer activity, demonstrating that each of these sites is important for enhancer function (Fig.1). Deletions of sites

Department of Biological Chemistry and The Molecular Biology Institute, University of California, Los Angeles, Los Angeles, CA. 90024

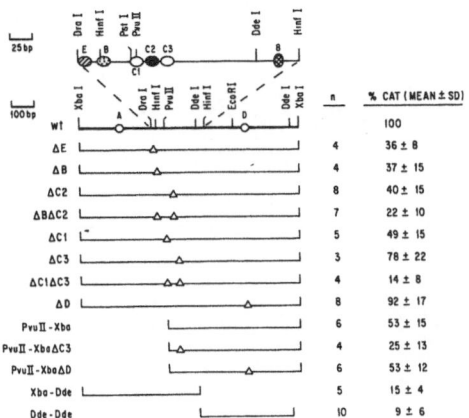

Fig.1 Functional analysis of protein binding sites on the IgH enhancer

C3 or D showed no significant diminution of enhancer activity. Simul taneous deletion of sites B and C2 reduced enhancer activity to a level similar to that observed with the individual deletion mutants. However, combining C1 and C3 deletions resulted in less activity than either individual mutant, suggesting both sites may be functionally important. Since no single site deletion completely abolished enhancer activity, and deletion of two binding sites was not always additive, there appears to be functional redundancy within the enhancer element, a conclusion also reached by others (Kadesch et al 1986; Lenardo et al 1987).

In addition to testing internal deletions of the IgH enhancer, we also examined several truncated enhancer fragments (Fig. 1). A 600 bp Pvu II-Xba I fragment, which contains sites C2, C3, octamer, and D, was 50% as active as the 1kb Xba I enhancer fragment. When the C3 and D sites were deleted from this fragment, no large decreases in enhancer activity were observed in comparison to the wild type Pvu II-Xba I fragment. Therefore, truncation of the 1 Kb Xba I enhancer did not reveal any importance for sites D and C3. We also divided the 1 Kb Xba I fragment into about two equal parts with Dde I. To our surprise, neither half contained much enhancer activity, even though the Xba I-Dde I enhancer fragment contained six of the eight identified protein binding sites. This result suggests that there might be interactions between proteins bound to sites on each half of the enhancer which may be important for enhancer function.

PURIFICATION AND CHARACTERIZATION OF IGH ENHANCER PROTEINS

We have reported the partial purification and characterization of proteins which bind to sites E, B, and C2 on the IgH enhancer (Peterson and Calame 1987). Proteins which bind to sites E and C2 were designated uEBP-E and uEBP-C2, respectively. We determined the

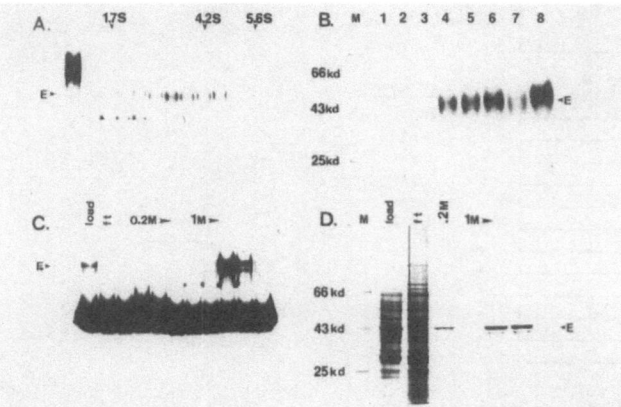

Figure 2. Characterization and purification of uEBP-E. (A) Glycerol gradient sedimentation analysis. Gradient fractions were assayed by gel retardation for uEBP-E. Lane 1 is the load. Arrows indicate positions of marker proteins cytochrome C, catalase, and E. coli Pol I. (B) UV crosslinking. Lane 1 contains probe without DNAse I, lane 2 contains probe treated with UV for 30 min. without protein, lane 3 contains a complete reaction mixture not treated with UV, lane 4, 5, 6, 7, and 8 contain complete reaction mixtures treated with UV for 5 min., 15 min., 30 min., and 30 min., respectively. The reaction in lane 7 also contained a 50-fold molar excess of the 1 kb Xba I fragment, and the reaction in lane 8 contained a 300-fold molar excess of salmon sperm DNA. (C).Affinity purification. Fractions were assayed by gel retardation. (D) Silver stained SDS PAGE of affinity purification. Samples were precipitated with 10% TCA, and each lane contained: load and ft 50 ul, .2M and 1M fractions 200 ul.

sedimentation coefficients for these proteins by glycerol gradient sedimentation. The results using proteins partially purified by FPLC Mono Q or Mono S chromatography (Peterson and Calame 1987) are shown in Fig. 2A for uEBP-E, and Fig. 3A for uEBP-C2. uEBP-E migrated with a sedimentation coefficient of 3.5 S, and uEBP-C2 migrated at 4.5 S. Assuming globular proteins with average partial specific volume and hydration, this corresponds to molecular weights of approximately 40,000 to 45,000 daltons for uEBP-E, and 62,000 to 67,000 daltons for uEBP-C2.

We have used a modified version of the UV crosslinking procedure of Chodish et al (1987) to further characterize the molecular weight of uEBP-E. A 60 bp Dra I-Pst I DNA fragment which contains site E was labelled by nick-translation and used in a binding reaction with partially purified uEBP-E. The binding reactions were exposed to UV light, treated with DNAase I, and electrophoresed on SDS PAGE. The results (Fig. 2B) show that after 5 minutes of UV treatment, one protein is crosslinked to the enhancer fragment (lane 4). The

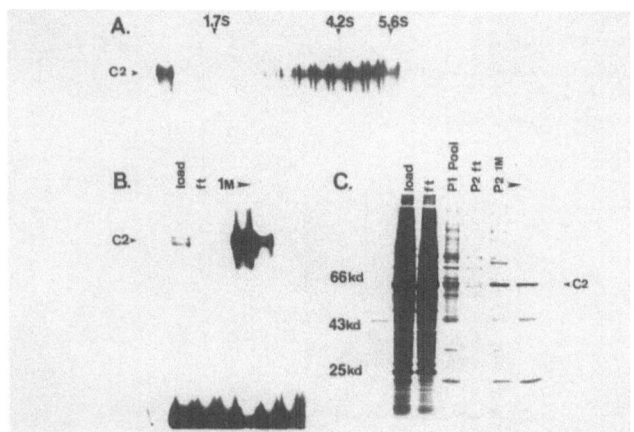

Figure 3. Characterization and purification of uEBP-C2. (A) Glycerol
gradient sedimentation analysis. (B) Affinity purification. (C) SDS
PAGE of affinity purification step. Lane labeled P1 represents the
pool of uEBP-C2 from the first pass on the affinity resin. P2 desig-
nates the second pass on the affinity resin. Refer to the figure 2
legend for details. Samples were treated as in Fig. 2, each lane contained 200 ul, except for the P1 load and ft which contained 100 ul.

crosslinking of this protein is due to sequence specific interactions,
since unlabelled enhancer DNA is able to compete for crosslinking
whereas salmon sperm DNA is unable to compete (compare lanes 7 and 8).
This crosslinked protein likely represents uEBP-E. Assuming that 10
bp of labelled DNA is bound to protein, the approximate molecular
weight for uEBP-E is 45,000 daltons, consistent with the size
predicted from glycerol gradient sedimentation analysis (Fig. 2A).

We then initiated further purification using oligonucleotide affinity
columns (Kadonaga and Tjian 1987) for sites E and C2. Nuclear extract
obtained from approximately 80 grams of plasmacytoma tumor tissue was
purified through the FPLC Mono Q step essentially as described previously, except that the heat step was omitted. Mono Q pools containing uEBP-E or uEBP-C2 were then chromatographed on 3 ml affinity
columns. The binding assay from an affinity chromatography step are
shown in Fig. 2C for uEBP-E, and Fig. 3B for uEBP-C2.

Both uEBP-E and uEBP-C2 are effectively purified by a factor greater
than 100-fold, with greater than 60% yields. A protein gel of fractions from the site E affinity column (Fig. 2D) shows that one protein
of 45,000 daltons is specifically retained. We believe this protein
to be uEBP-E since (i) it corresponds to the size predicted for uEBP-E
by glycerol gradient sedimentation and UV crosslinking, (ii) it specifically binds and elutes from site E affinity matrix, and (iii)
Scatchard analysis of uEBP-E binding activity from the column yields a
concentration of active protein very similar to the quantities of
45,000 dalton protein present in this fraction (C.P. in prep.).

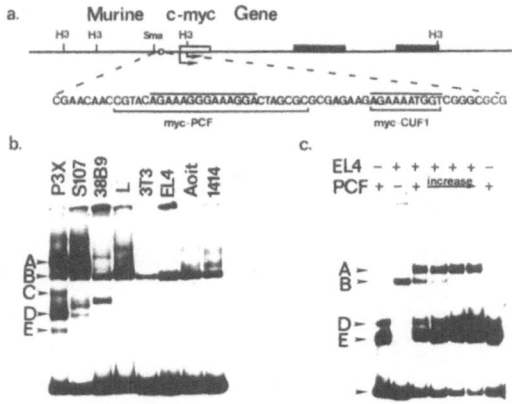

Figure 4. Analysis of myc-PCF distribution and binding. (A) Restriction map of the mouse c-myc gene. Exons are shown as boxes, and the
two start sites for transcription are indicated by arrows. The sequence of the myc-PCF and myc-CUF1 binding sites is expanded. The
binding site boundaries as determined by in vitro footprinting are indicated by brackets below the sequence, and regions of sequence
homology between the mouse and human c-myc genes are indicated above
the sequence by lines. (B) Distribution of myc-PCF and myc-CUF1 using
gel retardation. Complexes A,C,D,E are due to myc-PCF; complex B is
due to myc-CUF1. (C) Mixing experiments with myc-PCF and myc-CUF1.
"PCF" indicates the addition of oligo column-purified PCF and EL4 indicates the addition of crude EL4 nuclear extract.

When uEBP-C2, eluted from the first pass on the affinity column (Fig.
3C) and still containing multiple proteins, was chromatographed again
on the affinity matrix many contaminating proteins were removed and
the active fractions contain primarily three proteins of 65 kd, 43 kd,
and 20 kd. Based upon the predicted size of 62-67 kd for uEBP-C2, we
believe that the 65 kd protein represents intact uEBP-C2. Further
purification is necessary to determine whether the additional proteins
are proteolytic fragments of uEBP-C2 or proteins which copurify.

AN ANALYSIS OF MYC-PCF, A POTENTIAL REPRESSOR OF TRANSCRIPTION

We have identified a protein (myc-PCF) in plasmacytomas which binds to
sequences within the normal murine c-myc gene promoter and may be involved in repression of c-myc (Kakkis and Calame 1987). We previously
showed that gel shift complexes C,D and E were due to plasmacytoma-
specific binding at a single site by myc-PCF; complex B was due to
binding of another protein to a site 10 bp 3' to the myc-PCF site
(Kakkis and Calame 1987). We have investigated the distribution of
myc-PCF and of protein producing complex B in different cell lines and
tissues (Fig. 4). Oligonucleotide competition for myc-PCF binding was
used as a control to confirm the presence of myc-PCF (data not shown).

In combination with previous results (Kakkis and Calame 1987), we find that 4 plasmacytomas contain myc-PCF (P3X63-Ag and S107, complexes A, C, D, and E in Fig. 4b) while it is not found in 4 early B cell lines (38B9), 2 fibroblast lines (3T3, L), 2 T cell lines (EL4, AOIT), liver, spleen, kidney and brain (not shown). Cell line 1414 is a B cell line with an amplified c-myc gene, and it does contain a small amount of myc-PCF (complex A, Fig. 4b). Protein binding at the adjacent site (complex B) occurs in all tissues tested except brain (Fig. 4), thus we denote it myc-CUF1 (common upstream factor 1).

Myc-PCF and myc-CUF1 bind to sequences separated by only 10 bp of DNA and previous footprinting data suggested that the slowest migrating complex (complex A) was due to binding of both proteins. To confirm this, we tested whether addition of affinity purified myc-PCF, which does not form complex A (lane 1, Fig. 4c), to a T cell extract containing myc-CUF1 would generate complex A. The results in Fig. 4C show that as increasing amounts of myc-PCF are added, complex A is generated with the concomitant disappearance of complex B. These data suggest that myc-PCF and myc-CUF1 may bind cooperatively within the promoter of the c-myc gene, and lead us to postulate that this interaction may be important for the repressor function of myc-PCF.

CONCLUSION

Site-directed mutagenesis of the IgH enhancer has demonstrated that protein binding sites E, B, C1, and C2 are required for optimal enhancer function in vivo and suggests that protein-protein interactions are functionally important. Proteins binding to sites E and C2, uEBP-E and uEBP-C2, have been purified and characterized by sedimentation analysis. The availability of purified enhancer proteins will allow investigation into potential protein-protein interactions between enhancer factors. Repressors of transcription may also function through protein-protein interactions. We have presented preliminary evidence that a potential repressor of c-myc transcription, myc-PCF, interacts with an adjacent DNA binding protein, myc-CUF1. It seems probable that myc-CUF1 might be an activator of c-myc transcription, and that interaction with myc-PCF disrupts this activating function.

ACKNOWLEDGEMENTS

Supported by grants from USPHS #GM29361 and #CA38571 to K. C. and from the Life and Health Insurance Medical Research Fund to E. K..

REFERENCES

Calame K (1985) Mechanisms that regulate immunoglobulin gene expression. In: Paul WE (ed) Annual review of immunology, vol. 3. Annual Reviews Inc., CA., p 159
Chodosh LA, Carthew RW, Sharp PA (1986) A single polypeptide possesses the binding and transcription activities of the Adenovirus major late transcription factor. Mol. Cell. Biol. 6: 4723-4733
Feo S, ar-Rushdi A, Heubner K, Finan J, Nowell P, Clarkson B, Croce C (1985) Suppression of the normal mouse c-myc oncogene in human lymphoma cells Nature (London) 313:493-495.
Kadesch T, Zervos P, Ruezinsky D (1986) Functional analysis of the

murine IgH enhancer: evidence for negative control of cell-type specificity. Nucleic Acids Res. 14: 8209-8221

Kadonaga JT, Tjian R (1986) Affinity purification of sequence-specific DNA binding proteins. Proc. Natl. Acad. Sci. USA 83: 5889-5893

Kakkis E, Mercola M, Calame K (1987) Strong transcriptional activation of translocated c-myc genes occurs without a strong nearby enhancer or promoter. (manuscript submitted)

Kakkis E, Calame K (1987) A plasmacytoma-specific factor binds the c-myc promoter region. Proc. Natl. Acad. Sci. USA (in press)

Lenardo M, Pierce JW, Baltimore D (1987) Protein-binding sites in Ig gene enhancers determine transcriptional activity and inducibility. Science 236: 1573-1577

Peterson CL, Calame K (1987) Complex protein binding within the mouse immunoglobulin heavy chain enhancer. Mol. Cell. Biol. (in press)

Mercola M, Goverman J, Mirell C, Calame K (1985) Immunoglobulin heavy-chain enhancer requires one or more tissue-specific factors. Science 227: 266-270

Scholer HR, Gruss P (1985) Cell type-specific transcriptional enhancement in vitro requires the presence of trans-acting factors. EMBO J. 4: 3005-3013

Selective and Neutral Evolution in the Murine *Igh-V* Locus

A. Tutter[1,2] and R. Riblet[1]

INTRODUCTION

The Igh-V locus in the mouse is comprised of at least nine families of homologous genes encoding immunoglobulin heavy chain variable (Vh) regions (Brodeur and Riblet 1984; Dildrop 1984; Brodeur *et al*. 1985; Winter *et al*. 1985). These gene families are, for the most part, organized into discrete clusters with little interspersion; in addition, they are highly polymorphic. These features make this locus a good system for the study of the evolutionary mechanisms and constraints operative on a complex multi-gene system. Our studies show that both selective and neutral forces contribute to the evolution of the Igh-V locus; here, we focus on the evolution of Vh family size, or copy number, and Vh family divergence.

RESULTS AND DISCUSSION

Evolution of Vh Family Copy Number

A survey of the Igh-V locus in 72 inbred strains of mice, using blot hybridization techniques and probes specific for 8 of the 9 known Vh families, has shown that variation in the Igh-V locus characteristically involves the gain or loss of one or few cross-hybridizing bands from a single family (Tutter and Riblet, submitted). For example, Fig.1 demonstrates variation in the Vh3609P family. Changes were found in the four largest Vh families, and appear to have occurred at random. Tandemly repeated genes are subject to duplication and deletion through homologous, but unequal recombination (reviewed in Maeda and Smithies 1986), and it is likely that recombination between closely linked, homologous genes has generated the small changes in copy number observed. In contrast, coupled duplications involving members of different families have been observed in the human Vk and Vh regions (Pech *et al*. 1985; Kodaira *et al*. 1986). These patterns reflect the organizations of the different V region loci, the murine Vh gene families being predominantly clustered, while the human Vh and Vk families are extensively interspersed (reviewed in Brodeur 1987). We suggest that the clustered organization of the murine Vh families imposes constraints on not only the number of Vh genes, but also the number of Vh families that may be affected by a single unequal recombination event within this locus, as diagrammed in Fig. 2.

The examination and comparison of Vh family content in various *Mus* species (representing all four *Mus* subgenera), *Rattus* and *Peromyscus* has allowed us to infer

---

[1] Medical Biology Institute, La Jolla, CA 92037 and the
[2] University of Pennsylvania, Philadelphia, PA 19104

108

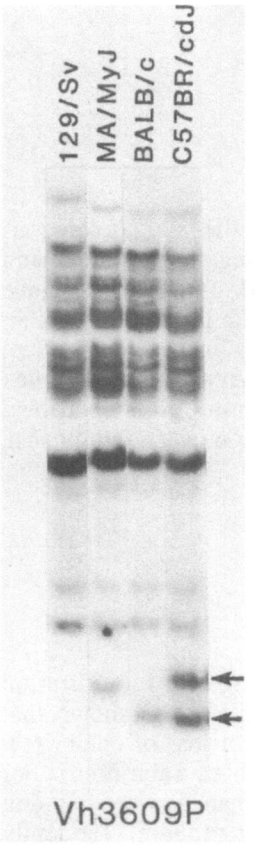

129/Sv MA/MyJ BALB/c C57BR/cdJ

Vh3609P

Fig. 1. Variation in the content of the Vh3609P family in inbred strains of mice. All other Vh families in these strains appear identical. The variable 1.5 and 1.7 kb bands are indicated with arrows. In this and in all Southern blots, EcoRI digested DNA was electrophoresed through 0.7% agarose gels, blotted onto nitrocellulose, and hybridized in the presence of 10% dextran sulphate, 0.1% SDS, and 10^6 cpm/ml labelled probe, with final wash at 0.2XSSC, 0.1% SDS at 65°C.

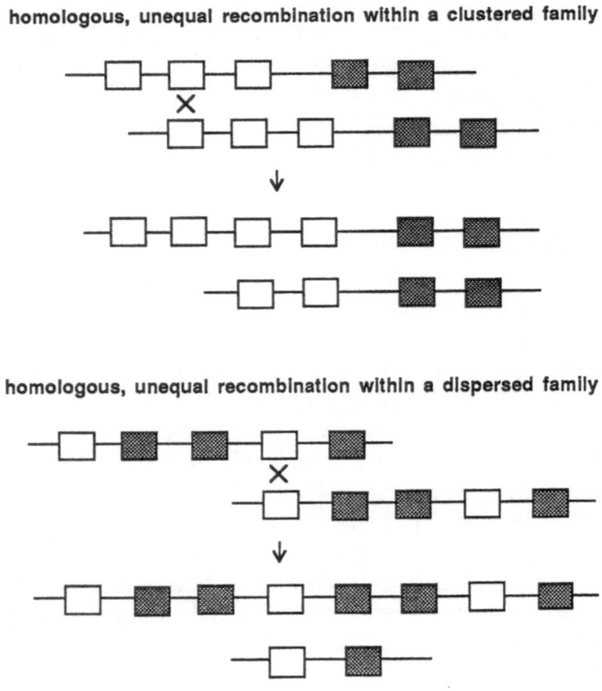

homologous, unequal recombination within a clustered family

homologous, unequal recombination within a dispersed family

Fig. 2. Influence of clustered versus dispersed organizations on the families affected by homologous, unequal recombination between members of the same family. Open and shaded boxes represent members of two different families. Unequal recombination within an interspersed family can result in copy number changes in several gene families.

the evolutionary history of individual Vh family copy number (Tutter and Riblet, submitted). By correlating the range of Vh family size seen in a given species with the phylogenetic distance of that species from *M. domesticus,* certain trends of Vh family copy number are made apparent. As shown in Fig. 3, the size of VhJ558 has gradually increased in the lineage leading to *M. domesticus,* while that of Vh7183 has decreased; on the other hand, VhQ52N appears to have remained relatively stable in size since the divergence of *Mus, Rattus* and *Peromyscus* from their common ancestor. Similar trends are also seen in other Vh families of *M. domesticus.* In addition, different

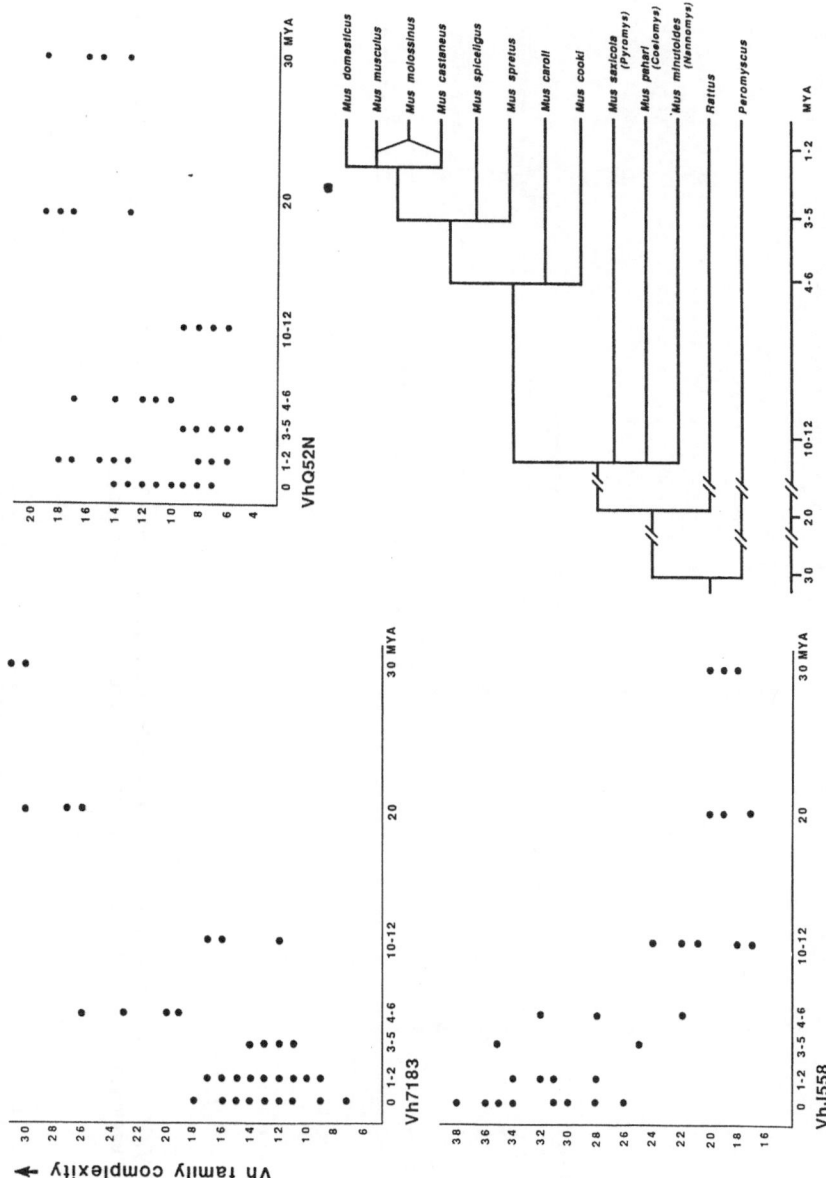

Fig. 3. Correlation of Vh family size range in *Mus* species, *Rattus* and *Peromyscus* with phylogenetic distance from *M. domesticus* (at 0 MYA), for three Vh families. Several polymorphic individuals were scored for each species indicated in the phylogenetic tree, lower right. Divergence times and phylogenetic relationships are taken from Brownell (1983), Ferris *et al.* (1983), Bonhomme *et al.* 1984, Sarich (1985), and E. Prager and V. Sarich, personal communication.

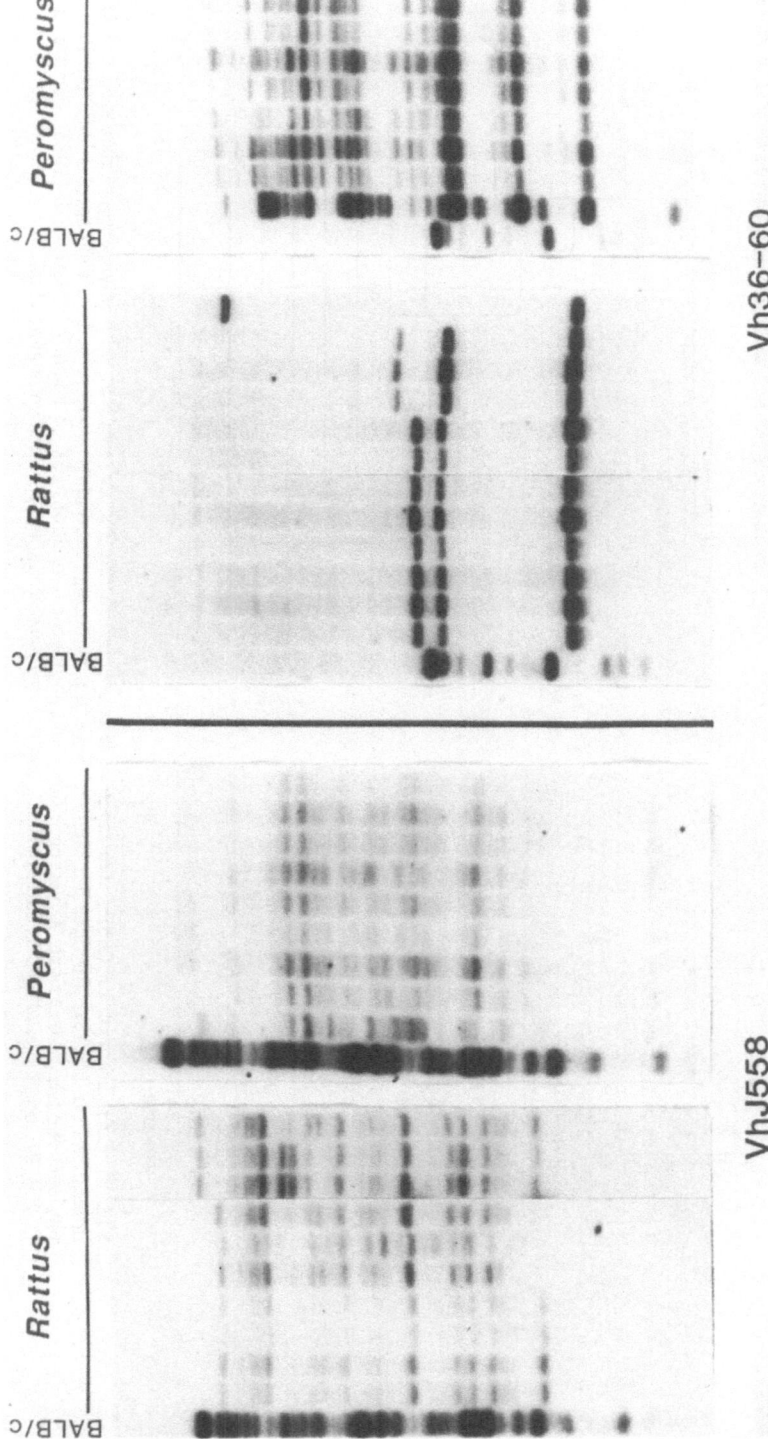

Fig. 4. The VhJ558 and Vh36-60 families in *Rattus norvegicus* and *Peromyscus maniculatus*. The VhJ558 family is contracted in both species, while the Vh36-60 family is contracted in *Rattus*, and expanded in *Peromyscus*, relative to *M. domesticus*.

families have expanded or contracted in various lineages. Figure 4 shows that the VhJ558 family is contracted in both *Rattus* and *Peromyscus*, relative to *Mus*; however, while the Vh36-60 family is similar in size in *Mus* and *Rattus*, this family is expanded in *Peromyscus*.

Several points can be made from these results. First, the gradual evolutionary trends observed are consistent with the notion of incremental variation in Vh gene copy number, as seen in inbred strains (Fig. 1). Large or frequent gene loss and gain would be expected to result in wider ranges of Vh family size within and between species, with little relationship to phylogenetic distance. Second, the fact that individual Vh families have experienced different trends of expansion or contraction in the *M. domesticus* lineage supports the notion that the clustered organization of the murine Igh-V locus generally precludes the coupled expansion and contraction of different families, allowing the copy number of different Vh families to evolve independently (Fig.2). Implicit in this argument is the supposition that all examined muroid Igh-V loci are similarly organized. Third, because different Vh families have expanded or contracted differently in separate lineages, we conclude that Vh family copy number variation is essentially stochastic. This apparently neutral evolution of individual Vh gene family size argues against any direct selection for the amplification of particularly large families in *M. domesticus*, or in other species.

Divergence and Selection of Vh Families

Kabat (1979) originally grouped murine N-terminal Vh protein sequences into five groups; subsequently, Vh genes were redivided into smaller groups, or families, on the basis of both cross-hybridization (Brodeur and Riblet 1984; Brodeur *et al.* 1985) and similarity of full length protein sequences (Dildrop 1984). We thought it reasonable that families that are more similar to each other than to other families might be related by common divergence from ancestral families, subsequent to the divergence of these ancestral families. A proposed Vh family divergence tree is presented in Fig. 5, in which we have grouped the nine known murine Vh families on the basis of nucleotide similarity into three groups (I, II, and III) which correspond roughly, but not entirely, with those of of Kabat (1987). The presence of sequences homologous to these three groups in both mouse and man (Rechavi *et al.* 1982, 1983; Takahashi *et al.* 1984; Kodaira *et al.* 1986) indicates that the divergence of these groups occurred prior to the mammalian radiation, 60-80 million years ago (MYA; Sarich 1985).

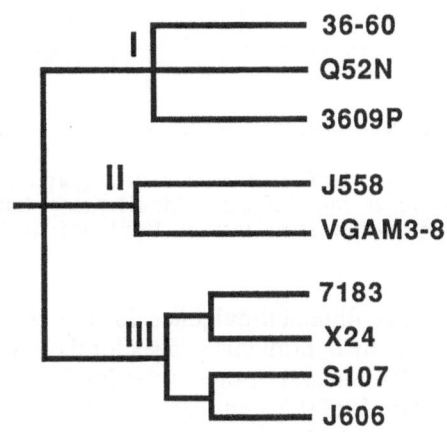

Fig. 5. Proposed divergence of murine Vh families, inferred from coding region nucleotide similarity. These families are divided into groups I, II, and III, which correspond roughly, but not entirely, to the grouping of Kabat (1987).

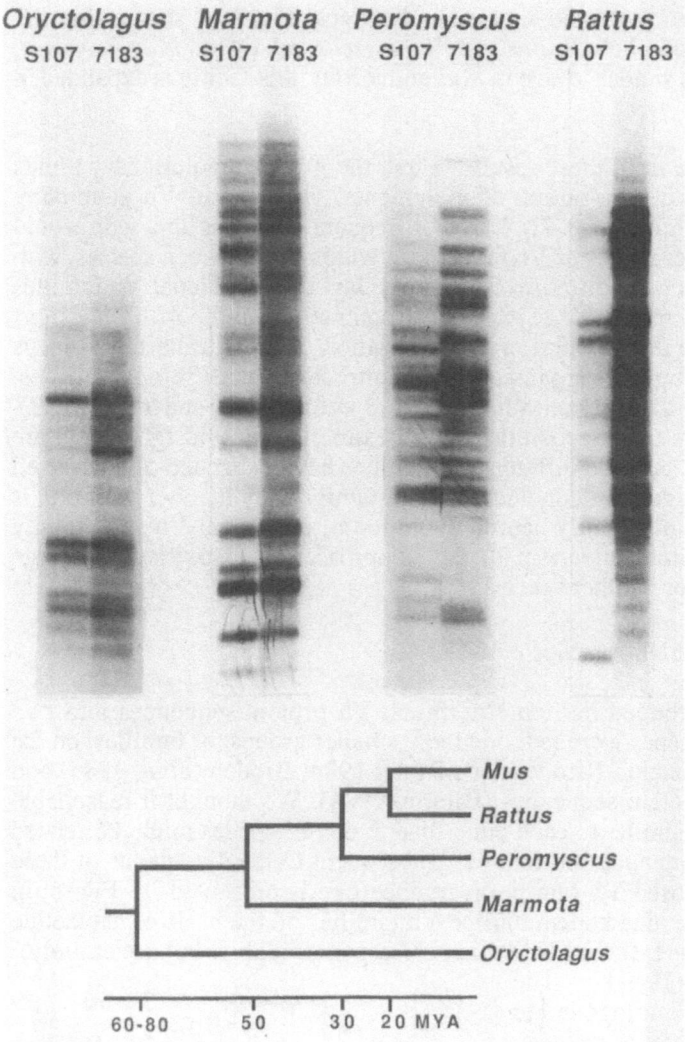

Fig. 6. The progressive divergence of the murine VhS107 and Vh7183 (group III) families in *Oryctolagus cuniculus* (rabbit), *Marmota monax* (woodchuck), *Peromyscus maniculatus* (deer mouse), and *Rattus norvegicus* (rat). References for divergence times are listed in the text. Other exposures reveal that only four bands crosshybridize in Rattus.

We have obtained evidence for the common ancestry of the four murine group III families by hybridizing probes for these families with progressively distant mammalian taxa (Tutter and Riblet, submitted). As shown in Fig. 6, probes for the group III families VhS107 and Vh7183 detect the same set of RFLPs in both *Oryctolagus* (rabbit) and *Marmota* (woodchuck), which diverged from *Mus* 60-80 and 50 MYA, respectively (Hafner 1984; Sarich 1985). In *Peromyscus* (deer mouse), which diverged from *Mus* 30 MYA (Brownell 1983; Sarich 1985), these probes detect overlapping sets

113

of bands, with most bands shared in common, and others detected uniquely. Only a few cross-hybridizing bands are seen in *Rattus*, which separated from *Mus* appx 20 MYA (Brownell 1983; Sarich 1985). In *Mus*, by the definition of Vh gene families (Brodeur and Riblet 1984), these two families have diverged such that no bands are detected in common. Taken together, these data indicate that the divergence of Vh7183 and VhS107 from a common, ancestral group III family began after the *Mus/Marmota* divergence 50 MYA, and was essentially complete before the *Mus/Rattus* divergence 20 MYA.

This analysis has been extended to the other group III families, and also to the group I families VhQ52N and Vh36-60, which all appear to have diverged subsequent to the *Marmota/Mus* divergence (not shown). However, hybridization of the VhQ52N and Vh36-60 murine families in *Marmota* is considerably weaker than that obtained with the group III families discussed above, and they fail entirely to crosshybridize with species more distantly related to *Mus* than *Marmota*, while another group I family, Vh3609P, and the group II family VhJ558 fail to detect crosshybridizing sequences in species more distant than *Peromyscus* (Tutter and Riblet, submitted). This differential conservation is illustrated by the hybridization analysis of *Marmota* DNA, using murine Vh family probes representing the three major groups (Fig. 7). As discussed above, these groups of Vh gene families diverged prior to the mammalian radiation, and thus the lack of high-stringency crosshybridization in certain species reflects either the divergence or loss of these sequences in these lineages. For example, sequencing of rabbit Vh genes indicates that all Vh genes are of group III, and that groups I and II have apparently been lost (Bernstein *et al.* 1983, 1984; Gallarda *et al.* 1985).

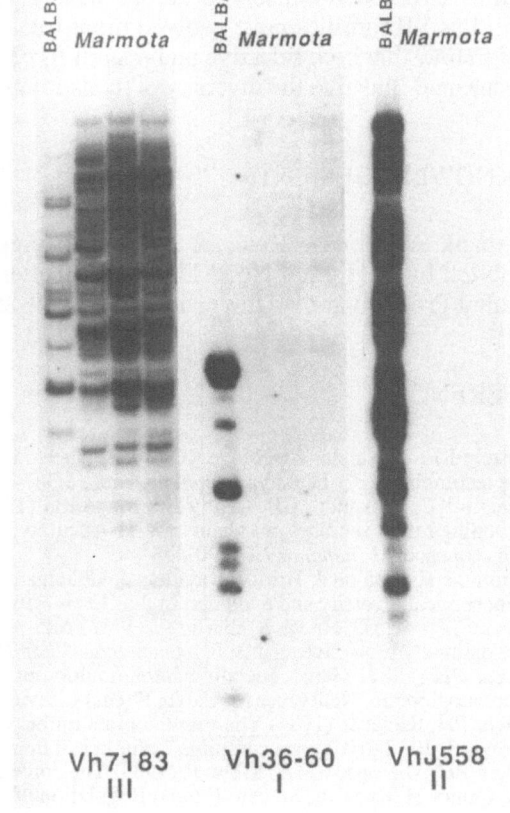

Fig. 7. Differential conservation of representative group I (Vh36-60), group II (VhJ558), and group III (Vh7183) families in *Marmota monax*. Blots were washed under stringent conditions. Note the overexposure of the BALB/c control lane in the Vh36-60 and VhJ558 blots.

Vh7183
III

Vh36-60
I

VhJ558
II

The conservation of group III sequences in species in which group I and/or group II sequences are lost or diverged has been consistently observed in different mammalian orders, and argues strongly for the selective preservation of these sequences. The conservation of group III sequences across Mammalia is underscored by the identification of group III sequences in such remote lineages as the crocodile and shark (Litman 1983, 1985). This suggests that group III sequences are in fact the modern descendants of the primordial Vh family. Unfortunately, there is no clear evidence for any specific selective advantage that group III sequences may confer. In the mouse, group III sequences encode binding specificities for a variety of bacterial capsid carbohydrate antigens (Brodeur and Riblet 1984), and confer protection against infection (Briles et al. 1982), but a similar role has not been documented in other mammals. The comparison of different Vh group homologues from different species should help to elucidate the particular structures that are conserved by selection.

SUMMARY

The evolution of Vh family copy number in the mouse is primarily stochastic, achieved through small, random duplication/deletion events usually restricted to a single family. The analysis of homologous Vh families in other species reveals that the group III Vh families have been conserved across widely separated mammalian lineages, while group I and II families have evolved more freely, and in one case, disappeared. These results show that both selective and neutral forces of evolution are operative in the Igh-V locus, and illustrate the diversity of constraints imposed on this multi-gene system.

ACKNOWLEDGEMENTS

We thank Annemarie Reid for helping to prepare the manuscript. This work was supported by NIH grant No. AI23548. A. Tutter is a trainee of the Medical Scientist Training Program at the University of Pennsylvania.

REFERENCES

Bernstein KE, Alexander CB, Mage RG (1983) Nucleotide sequence of a rabbit IgG heavy chain from the recombinant F-1 haplotype. *Immunogenet 18*:387-397

Bernstein KE, Alexander CB, Reddy EP, Mage RG (1984) Complete sequence of a cloned cDNA encoding rabbit secreted mu-chain of V-H-A2 allotype: comparisons with V-H-A1 and membrane mu sequences. *J Immunol 132*:490-495

Bonhomme F, Catalan J, Britton-Davidian J, Chapman VM, Moriwaki K, Nevo E, Thaler L (1984) Biochemical diversity and evolution in the Genus *Mus*. *Biochem Genet 22*:275-303

Briles DE, Forman C, Hudak S, Claflin JL (1982) Anti-phosporycholine antibodies of the T15 idiotype are optimally protective against *S. pneumoniae*. *J Exp Med 156*:1177-1187

Brodeur PH (1987) Genes encoding immunoglobulin variable regions. In: Molecular genetics of immunoglobulin. Neuberger M, Calabi F (eds) Elsevier Science Publishers, Amsterdam

Brodeur PH, Riblet R (1984) The immunoglobulin heavy chain variable region (Igh-V) locus in the mouse. I. 100 Igh-V genes comprise 7 families of homolgous genes. *Eur J Immunol 14*:922-930

Brodeur PH, Thompson MA, Riblet R (1984) The content and organization of mouse Igh-V families. In: Cantor H, Chess L, Sercarz E (eds) Regulation of immune system. Alan R Liss, New York, pp 445-453

Brownell E (1983) DNA/DNA hybridization studies of muroid rodents: symmetry and rates of molecular evolution. *Evolution 37*:1034-1051

Dildrop R (1984) A new classification of mouse Vh sequences. *Immunol Today 5*:85-87

Ferris SD, Sage RD, Prager EM, Ritte U, Wilson AC. 1983. Mitochondrial DNA evolution in mice. *Genetics 105*:681-721.

Gallarda JL, Gleason KS, Knight KL (1985) Organization of rabbit immunoglobulin genes. I. Structure and multiplicity of germ-line Vh genes. *J Immunol 135*:4222-4228

Hafner DJ (1983) Evolutionary Relationships of the Nearctic Sciuridae. In: Murie JO, Michener GR (eds) The biology of ground dwelling squirrels. Univ of Nebraska Press, Lincoln, pp 3-23

Kabat EA, Wu TT, Bilofsky H (1979) Sequences of immunoglobulin chains. NIH publication no. 80-2008

Kabat EA, Wu TT, Reid-Miller M, Perry HM, Gottesman KS (1987) Sequences of proteins of immunological interest (4th ed). NIH publication no. 165-462

Kodaira M, Kinashi T, Umemura I, Matsuda F, Noma T, Ono Y, Honjo T (1986) Organization and Evolution of variable region genes of the human immunoglobulin heavy chain. *J Mol Biol 190*:529-451

Litman GW, Berger L, Murphy K, Litman R, Hinds K, Jahn CL, Erickson BW (1983) Complete nucleotide sequence of an immunoglobulin Vh gene homologue from *Caiman*, a phylogenetically ancient reptile. *Nature (Lond) 303*:349-352

Litman GW, Berger L, Murphy K, Litman R, Hinds K, Erickson BW (1985) Immunoglobulin Vh gene structure and diversity in *Heterodontus*, a phylogenetically primitive shark. *Proc Natl Acad Sci USA 82*:2082-2086

Maeda N, Smithies O (1986) The evolution of multigene families: human haptoglobin genes. *Ann Rev Genet 20*:81-108

Pech M, Smola H, Pohlenz H-D, Straubinger B, Gerl R, Zachau HG (1985) A large section of the gene locus encoding human immunoglobulin variable regions of the kappa type is duplicated. *J Mol Biol 183*:291-299

Rechavi G, Bienz B, Ram D, Ben-Neriah Y, Cohen JB, Zakut R, Givol D (1982) Organization and evolution of immunoglobulin Vh gene subgroups. *Proc Natl Acad Sci USA 79*:4405-4409

Rechavi G, Ram D, Glazer L, Zakut R, Givol D (1983) Evolutionary aspects of immunoglobulin heavy chain variable region (Vh) gene subgroups. *Proc Natl Acad Sci USA 80*:855-859

Sarich VM (1985) Rodent macromolecular systematics. In: Lucket WP, Hartenberger J-L (eds) Evolutionary relationships among rodents: a multidisciplinary analysis, Plenum, New York, pp 423-452

Takahasi N, Noma T, Honjo T (1984) Rearranged immunoglobulin heavy chain variable region (Vh) pseudogene that deletes the second complementarity- determining region. *Proc Natl Acad Sci USA 81*:5194-5198

Winter E, Radbruch A, Krawinkel U (1985) Members of novel Vh families are found in VDJ regions of polyclonally activated B-lymphocytes. *EMBO J 4*:2861-2867

The Organization of the Immunoglobulin Kappa Locus in Mice

L. D'Hoostelaere[1,2], K. Huppi[1], B. Mock[1], C. Mallett[1], D. Gibson[3], J. Hilgers[4], and M. Potter[1]

The genetic locus that codes for the immunoglobulin kappa (Igκ) light chains in the mouse is located on chromosome 6 approximately 32 centimorgans from the centromere (Hengartner et al., 1978; Gibson et al., 1979; D'Hoostelaere et al., 1985). The number of germline sequences for variable kappa (Vκ) in inbred mice has been estimated to be from 90 to 320 (Cory et al., 1981; Briles and Carroll, 1981; Potter et al., 1982; Gibson, 1984; Nishi et al., 1985). Cory et al. (1981) made their estimates on the basis of 7 cDNA probes which detected non-overlapping sets of restriction endonuclease fragments (REFs). The sum of these sets of related Vκ genes are believed to correspond to a part but not all of the Vκ groups identified by partial or complete amino acid sequencing (Potter et al., 1982). Some of the sets are clusters of nearest neighbor exons, e.g. as with Vκ21 (Heinrich et al., 1984). Clustering must be demonstrated for each Vκ exon group since human Vκ groups have been found to be interspersed (Jaenichem et al., 1984; Peck et al., 1985). All of the Igκ genes are believed to be on chromosome 6 of the mouse; however, the organizational patterns have not been examined in great detail. We have selected a series of DNA probes for different kappa exons in combination with inbred recombinant inbred and congenic strains and backcross populations of mice to detect different allelic forms which could be used to examine diversity, and used to detect crossover events within Igk for a genetic map.

Identification of Different Vκ Exon groups

Using the N-terminal amino acid sequences from a large number of κ light chains Potter et al., (1982) has described 18 groups or families of V regions which have sequence similarities. This suggested that members of a group may be coded for by a single or small number of closely related exons. Members of different groups may be coded for by exons which would not have enough similarity to cross hybridize in Southern analysis.

In an attempt to determine if this assumption was correct, we selected DNA probes for Vκ exons from 12 of the different groups. We also used a probe which included the Jκ and Cκ exons, and a probe for a Vκ exon, which had not been included in the previous amino acid analysis of Vκ groups (Table 1). The DNA probes were used in combination with genomic DNA from 55 inbred strains. The final stringency used for the analysis was 0.2 x SSC (1 x SSC = 0.15 M NaCl, 0.015 M Na Citrate pH7.2), 1 mM EDTA, 0.1% SDS at 65°C which should indicate a sequence similarity of approximately 80% (Brodeur and Riblet, 1984).

In order to determine whether the different DNA probes detected non-overlapping sets of restriction endonuclease fragments (REFs), BamHI was used in the preliminary analysis. Although some of the REFs had

---

[1] Laboratory of Genetics, NCI, NIH, Bethesda, Maryland.
[2] currently at the Basel Institute for Immunology, Basel, Switzerland.
[3] University of Sherbrooke, Sherbrooke, Quebec, Canada.
[4] Netherlands Cancer Institute, Amsterdam, The Netherlands.

---

shared mobilities, intensity differences and REFs with unique mobilities indicated the DNA probes were detecting different sets of REFs (Figure 1A and 1B, data not shown for $V_\kappa1$, $V_\kappa9$, $V_\kappa22$ and $V_\kappa23$). The 13 V_κ probes were used to define 13 V_κ groups. Although these probes do not encompass the entire V_κ complex locus, greater than 90 REFs can be detected in a single inbred strain (Table 2). There seems to be a correspondence between the V_κ groups defined by amino acid comparisons and the V_κ allelic groups detected by specific DNA probes from these protein groups.

Allelic Polymorphism at Ig_κ

The C_κ plus 13 V_κ DNA probes were used, to screen the genomic DNA of 55 inbred strains (Table 3). Each probe detects 2 to 4 REF patterns among the inbred strains, and each of the inbred strains displayed only one of these patterns. Representative examples of the V_κ restriction endonuclease fragement length polymorphisms (RFLPs) detected are shown in Figure 1A and 1B. Each unique pattern (a, b, c or d) represents a different group of alleles. The $pV_\kappa T15-S$ $V_\kappa22$ probe detected a single nonpolymorphic 4.2 kilobase (kbp) BamH1 REF in all the mice examined. Other enzymes have not been used to establish RFLPs. The distribution of allelic groups among the prototype inbred strains (strain distribution pattern [SDP]) is listed in Table 2. Each of the probes detects from 1 to 9 intense hybridizing REFs and from 1 to 19 total fragments (Figure 1A and 1B). When the size of the REFs was estimated, each probe detected from 4.2 to 68.1 kbp of intensely hybridizing DNA fragments and a total of 4.2 to 107.7 kbp of hybridizing DNA.

Ig_κ Haplotypes Among Inbred Strains

The SDPs for the different V_κ allelic groups detected in the 55 inbred strains could be used to establish haplotypes of Ig_κ. Including the low intensity REFs, the inbred strains examined can be divided into 7 distinct haplotypes (Table 2 and 3) with the majority (67%) showing the BALB/c (IgK^c) distribution of allelic groups (Table 3). The NZB (IgK^b) and O20 (IgK^g) inbred strains were the only members of their respective haplotypes. The C58 and YBR inbred strains (IgK^d) differ from IgK^c at every V_κ allelic group tested (Table 2). The AKR, MRL, NFS, PL and RF inbred strains were found to be members of IgK^a and differ from IgK^b at ever V_κ allelic group (Table 2 and 3). IgK^e (SJL and MA inbred strains) differs from IgK^c only at Ig_κ-C, Ig_κ-J and Ig_κ-V21 (Table 2). IgK^f (represented by inbred strains BDP, CE, I and P) differs from IgK^b only at Ig_κ-V11, Ig_κ-V24 and Ig_κ-V9-26 and this same group of alleles (11, 24 and 9-26) was shared with IgK^g (Table 2). Because allelic groups are shared among the different haplotypes, the 7 haplotypes detected in the inbred strains examined may represent recombination events among a small number (2-4) of allelic groups. Within a given haplotype the numbers of intense or total REFs differs only slightly (57-61 and 91-99 respectively). The number of kbp detected also shows slight variation (438.8-465.5 kbp for intensely hybridizing DNA and 675.6-723.6 kbp for the total amount of hybridizing DNA).

Ig_κ Gene Order

Earlier studies have examined recombinant inbred and congenic strains of mice for crossing over within Ig_κ (Gibson and MacLean, 1979; Gibson et al., 1983, 1984; Lazure et al., 1981; Moynet et al., 1985; Goldrick et al., 1985; Boyd et al., 1986; and Taylor et al., 1985). Other studies involving backcross experiments have also detected crossing-over within Igκ (Gibson et al., 1984; D'Hoostelaere and Gibson, 1985; Moynet et al., 1985; Goldrick et al., 1985; Taylor et al., 1985; and Boyd et al., 1986). Table 4 summarizes these results and gives the distribution of allelic groups within the different Igκ haplotype. The NAK mouse was first described by Gibson et al (1984), and subsequently characterized for other genetic markers (Moynet et al, 1985; Goldrick et al., 1985; D'Hoostelaere and Gibson, 1985; Taylor et al., 1985 and Boyd et al., 1986). The original cross involved AKR and NZB (IgKα and IgKβ respectively), and the crossover event separated Vκ1, Vκ9, Vκ11, Vκ24 and Vκ9-26 from the other Vκ groups, Jκ. Ly-2 and a 7sRNA gene. We have added Vκ9-26 to the former group, and Vκ12,13 and Vκ19 to the later group of alleles (Table 4).

DNA from two B6.PL-Ly-2ᵃ congenics was also examined. A crossover event between Igκ-Ef1 and Ly-2 was first described by Gibson et al., (1983). The DNA from C57BL/6 and PL/J was the same for Vκ1, Vκ9, Vκ11, Vκ24 and Vκ9-26 BamHI REF patterns; therefore, the congenics were not tested for these groups. C57BL/6 DNA has the NZB patterns and PL/J DNA has the AKR patterns for Vκ4, Vκ8, Vκ10, Vκ12, 13, Vκ19, Vκ21 and Vκ23 (Figure 1A and 1B, Table 2, 3 and 4). The B6.PL (75NS) congenic was made homozygous for Ly-2ᵃ of PL origin after 10 backcross generations. Samples from the congenic were subsequently tested for chromosome 6 alleles and found to be homozygous for alleles of PL/J origin for Igκ-Ef1ᵃ (Vκ28) (Gibson et al., 1983; Goldrick et al., 1985), Igκ-Jᵃ (Boyd et al., 1986), Rn7s-6ᵃ (Taylor et al., 1985), Igκ-V21ᵃ (D'Hoostelaere and Gibson, 1985), and Igκ-V23ᵃ (Table 4). The congenic was shown to be homozygous for allele of C57BL/6 origin using DNA probes for Igκ-V4ᵇ, Igκ-V8ᵇ, Igκ-V10ᵇ (D'Hoostelaere and Gibson, 1985), and Igκ-V12-13ᵇ and Igκ-V19ᵇ (Table 4). The B6.PL (85NS) congenic was made homozygous for Ly-2ᵃ at the backcross generation 28. Samples from the congenic were subsequently tested for the above group of alleles, and found to be homozygous for alleles of PL/J origin using DNA probes for Igκ-Jᵃ (Boyd et al., 1986), Igκ-V21ᵃ (D'Hoostelaere and Gibson, 1985) and Igκ-V23ᵃ (Table 4). The remaining alleles examined were of C57BL/6 origin (Table 4).

Recombinant inbred strains of the AKXL series have been tested for Rn7s-6 (Taylor et al., 1985), Igκ-J (Boyd et al., 1986) and Igκ-Ef1 (Gibson et al., 1983; Goldrick et al., 1985). We have examined these lines using DNA probes for Vκ4, Vκ8, Vκ10, Vκ12,13 and Vκ21 and have found no discordancies with the published results (data not shown). We have also examined the OXA recombinant inbred strain series using DNA probes for Vκ1, Vκ9, Vκ10, Vκ19, Vκ21 and Vκ23 and found no discordancies (data not shown). We did detect a discordancy between the Vκ groups examined and Ly-3 in the OXAF or OXA6 recombinant inbred strain (Table 4).

We have conducted our own backcross experiments using a backcross population (C58.B6.C3-Hd/+) which carries the fully penetrant semi-dominant lethal locus hypodactyly (Hd) (Hummel, 1970) and tests homozygous for IgKᵈ of C58 origin, and the ABP/Le inbred strain from The Jackson Laboratory. The ABP/Le inbred strain carries the recessive locus waved 1 (wa-1), and DNA was tested and found to be IgKᶜ (Table 3 and 4). Both Hd and wa-1 are considered marker loci for chromosome 6 (Davidson and Roderick, 1986). The cross was made such that (C58.B6.C3-Hd/+ X ABP/Le)F₁ progeny which expressed the Hd heterozygous phenotype were mated with the ABP/Le parental strain. Samples from the progeny which expressed both phenotypes

(Hd/+, wa-1/wa-1) or lacked both phenotypes (+/+, +/wa-1) were examined for crossing-over within Igκ. DNA samples from 2 recombinants which gave results pertinent to the Igκ gene order (7255 and 5942) are listed in Table 4. These crossover samples could be used to establish a chromosomal orientation using the Hd and wa-1 loci. Animal 7255 displayed the hypoactyly and waved phenotypes; therefore, this animal was heterozygous on the centromere side and homozygous on the distal side of the crossover event on chromosome 6. The Vκ21 and .Jκ DNA probes detected the homozygous REF patterns and Jκ has been physically linked 2.3 kbp 5' of Cκ, and the remainder of the Vκ DNA probes detected the heterozygous REF patterns in DNA from animal 7255 (Table 4); therefore, the chromosomal orientation would be centromere-Hd-Igκ-V-Igκ-C-wa-1. Since the patterns for Igκ-V21 and Igκ-J were both homozygous, Igκ-V21 could still be distal to Igκ-C.

The second animal of interest (5942) did not express the hypodactyly or waved phenotypes; therefore, chromosome 6 was homozygous on the centromere side and heterozygous on the distal side of the crossover event. The DNA probes for the Vκ groups and Jκ detected homozygous REF patterns in the DNA of animal 5942 (Table 4). A sample of spleen cells from this animal was tested for the Ly-2 antigen, and both allelic forms were detected (personal communication, H.C. Morse III). This places Ly-2 distal to Igκ (Table 4).

The results from the chromosome 6 crossover animals [OXAF, NAK, B6.PL (75NS), B6.PL (85NS), ABP.C58 (7255) and ABP.C58 (5942)] predict the following gene order: centromere - Hd - (Igκ-V1, Igκ-V9, Igκ-V11, Igκ-V24, Igκ-V9-26) - (Igκ-V4, Igκ-V8, Igκ-V10, Igκ-V12,13, Igκ-V19) - (Igκ-V28, Rn7s-6) - Igκ-V23 - (Igκ-V21, Igκ-J, Igκ-C) - Ly-2, Ly-3) - wa-1. Gene groups within the parentheses could be interspersed, and only REFs with unique mobilities would be included in the gene order. The backcross experiments indicate all kappa genes are on chromosome 6.

The different haplotypes among inbred strains may represent the recombination of alleles during the establishment of these inbred strains. REF patterns of mitochondrial DNA suggest common ancestries among inbred strains of mice (Yonekawa et al., 1980; Ferris et al., 1982). Since mitochondrial DNA would have a maternal origin and the older inbred strains had identical REF patterns using several restriction endonucleases, the gene pool for the inbred strains may have mixed before inbreeding began and modern records were started (Morse, 1978; Altman and Katz, 1979). If the inbred strains represent a small founder population, recombination between a few Igκ haplotypes could be analyzed, and a gene order could be predicted (Table 4). Using the gene order derived from the recombiantion data, the haplotype results (Table 2) allow predictions of some smaller regions of cosegregation than could be derived from the crossover data. Starting from the Jκ-Cκ end of Igκ, four basic regions of cosegregation are seen: (Igκ-V4, Igκ-V8, Igκ-V10, Igκ-V19); (Igκ-V28, Rn7s-6); Igκ-V23; and (Igκ-V21, Igκ-J, Igκ-C). All of the NZB (IgKb), BALB/c (IgKc) and CE (IgKf) allelic groups for this larger region appear to be the same (V4, V8, V10, V19, V28, 7sRNA, V23, V21, J and C). AKR (IgKa) and C58 (IgKd) have the same distribution of allelic groups in this region, and O20 is unique except for Cκ. SJL (IgKe) displayed a new set of REFs for Igκ-V21, Igκ-J and Igκ-C and the change in the group of alleles corresponds to that seen in the 7255 crossover mouse. In SJL the remainder of this region is the same as IgKb, IgKc and IgKf (Table 4).

The other end of the Igκ complex locus includes Igκ-V11, Igκ-V24 and Igκ-V9-26. AKR (IgK^a), BALB/c (IgK^c) and SJL (IgK^e) share this group of alleles. NZB (IgK^b) and C58 (IgK^d) share alleles, and CE (IgK^f) and O20 (IgK^g) share alleles. This segregation (Igκ-V11, Igκ-V24 and Igκ-V9-26) was not seen in the crossover samples.

The Igκ-V1 allelic groups are defined by the different restriction endonucleases. Moynet et al., (1985) showed the AKR, BALB/c, SJL and CE strains shared REF patterns for BamHI and EcoRI and the NZB and C58 shared a different set of REF patterns using the same enzymes; however, using HindIII, BALB/c and SJL are different from AKR, and CE displayed an REF pattern similar to NZB and C58. When examining the Vκ1 IEF patterns NZB, C58 and CE are similar and AKR, BALB/c and SJL are similar (Gibson et al., 1983). The differences in REF patterns using different enzymes may be the result of crossing-over or mutation. For Igκ-V9 the AKR, BALB/c and SJL inbred strains share the Igκ-V9^a allelic groups and the NZB and C58 share the Igκ-V9^b allelic groups, similar to the results obtained with the Igκ-V11, Igκ-V24 and Igκ-V9-26 region, however the CE inbred strain is similar to NZB and C58 instead of O20. Both Igκ-V9 and Igκ-V1 were on the centromere side of the crossover in the NAK sample. NZB, BALB/c, SJL and CE share the Igκ-V12,13^b allelic group and AKR and C58 share the Igκ-V12,13^a allelic group, similar to the Igκ-V4, Igκ-V8, Igκ-V10, Igκ-V19 region; however the O20 inbred strain is similar to AKR instead of CE or producing a new allelic group. Igκ-V12,13 was on the distal side of the crossover in the NAK sample.

To recapitulate the results from crossover and haplotype data, which suggest a gene order: 1) the Hd and wa-1 markers provided a chromosomal orientation (centromere, Hd, Igκ-V, Igκ-C, wa-1); 2) the IgK^f and IgK^g similarities and results from the NAK crossover suggests Igκ-V11, Igκ-V24 and Igκ-V9-26 are together and proximal with respect to the centromere; 3) results from the NAK Igκ recombinant, the haplotype distribution (IgK^b, IgK^d and IgK^f), and the different allelic groups created by different enzymes suggests Igκ-V1 and Igκ-V9 are next and may be interspersed; 4) the NAK result and the presence of Igκ-V12,13^a in the O20 inbred strain suggest this group may come next; 5) the distribution of alleles and results from the two recombinants [NAK and B6.PL (75NS)] suggests Igκ-V4, Igκ-V8, Igκ-V10 and Igκ-V19 are next; 6) results from the two B6.PL congenics and the distribution of allelic groups in the prototype strains place Igκ-V28 and Rn7s-6 next; 7) results from the B6.PL (85NS) and the crossover mouse (#7255) separate Igκ-V23 from the other Vκ groups; 8) the allelic distribution and results from the two crossover mice (7255 and 5942) place Igκ-V21, Igκ-J and Igκ-C together proximal to Ly-2; 9) data from the OXAF recombinant inbred strain places Ly-3 distal to Igκ with Ly-2; 10) data from the two crossover mice (7255 and 5942) and other crossover samples (not shown) place wa-1 distal to Igκ and Ly-2.

SUMMARY AND CONCLUSIONS

The Igκ complex locus is on chromosome 6 of the mouse. DNA probes for 12 of the 18 Vκ protein groups and 1 DNA probe for a Vκ group not included in the protein analysis detect non-overlapping sets of REFs when stringencies are increased to detect heteroduplex hybridizations of 80% similarity or greater. Approximately 100 of these REFs representing greater than 700 kbp of hybridizable DNA can be detected in a single inbred strain of mice. When different inbred strains were examined 2 to 4 allelic forms for each probe were detected as determined by RFLPs except Vκ22 which was nonpolymorphic using BamH1. The 55 inbred strains examined could be divided into 7 haplotypes with 67% belonging to a single haplotype. This suggested restricted polymorphism among the inbred strains, which may be the result of a common ancestry. With the known polymorphisms the role of the Igκ complex locus and Igκ linked genes can be evaluated in humoral immune response mechanisms.

The results obtained from inbred strains, recombinant inbred strains, congenic strains and backcross populations of mice suggested a gene order. The predicted gene order is: centromere -Hd - (Igκ-V11, Igκ-V24, Igκ-V9-26) - (Igκ-V9, Igκ-V1) - Igκ-V12,13 - (Igκ-V4, Igκ-V8, Igκ-V10, Igκ-V19) - (Igκ-V28, Rn7s-6) - Igκ-V23 - (Igκ-V21, Igκ-J, Igκ-C) - (Ly-2, Ly-3) - wa-1. Gene groups within the parentheses could be interspersed, and only REFs with unique mobilities would be included in the predicted order. Igκ-V12,13; although separate from the other Vκ groups, may be included with Igκ-V4, Igκ-V8, Igκ-V10 and Igκ-V19 based on the crossover samples. The predicted gene order could be used in pulse field mapping, and to examine the hypothesis of ordered rearrangement during B cell ontogeny.

ACKNOWLEDGEMENTS

Animal breeding experiments were conducted at the Hazleton colony maintained under National Cancer Institute contract NO1-CB2-5584. The Basel Institute for Immunology was founded and is supported by F. Hoffmann-La Roche AG, Basel, Switzerland.

REFERENCES

Altman PL, Katz DD (eds) (1979) Inbred and genetically defined strains of laboratory animals. Part 1 Mouse and Rat. Federation of American Societies for Experimental Biology

Boyd RT, Goldrick MM, Gottlieb PD (1986) Genetic polymorphism at the mouse immunoglobulin Jκ locus (Igκ-J) as demonstrated by Southern hybridization and nucleotide sequence analysis. Immunogenetics 24: 150-157

Briles DE, Carroll RJ (1981) A simple method for estimating the probable number of different antibodies by examining the repeat frequencies of sequences or isoelectric focusing patterns. Molec Immuno 18:28-38

Brodeur PH, Riblet R (1984) The Immunoglobulin heavy chain variable (Igh-V) locus in the mouse. I. One hundred Igh-V genes comprise seven families of homologous genes. Eur J Immunol 14: 922-930

Coleclough C, Perry RP, Karjalainen K, Weigert M (1981) Aberrant rearrangements contribute significantly to the allelic exclusion of immunoglobulin gene expression. Nature 290: 372-378

Cory S, Tyler BM, Adams JM (1981) Sets of immunoglobulin Vκ sequences: Implications for the number of germline Vκ genes. Journal of Molecular and Applied Genetics 1: 103-116

Davisson MT, Roderick TH (1986) Mouse News Letter. No. 75

D'Hoostelaere LA, Gibson DM (1986) The Organization of immunoglobulin variable kappa chain genes on mouse chromosome 6.
Immunogenetics 23: 260-265

D'Hoostelaere LA, Jouvin E-M, Hüppi K (1985) Localization of $C_{T\beta}$
and C_κ on murine chromosome six. Immunogenetics 22: 277-283

Ferris SD, Sage RD, Wilson AC (1982) Evidence from mtDNA sequence
that common laboratory strains of inbred mice are descended from a
single female. Nature 295: 163-165

Gibson, DM (1984) Evidence for 65 electrophoretically distinct
groups of light chains in BALB/c and NZB myelomas. Mol Immunol
21: 421-432

Gibson DM, MacLean SJ (1979) Ef2: A new Ly-3-linked light chain
marker in normal mouse serum immunoglobulin. J Exp Med 149: 1477
1486

Gibson DM, MacLean SJ, Anctil D, Mathieson BJ (1984) Recombination
between kappa chain genetic markers in the mouse. Immunogenetics
20: 493-501

Gibson DM, MacLean SJ, Cherry M (1983) Recombination between kappa
chain genetic markers and the Lyt-3 locus. Immunogenetics 18:
111-116

Goldrick MM, Boyd RT, Ponath PD, Lou S, Gottlieb PD (1985)
Molecular genetic analysis of the V_κ Ser group associated with two
mouse light chain genetic markers. J Exp Med 162: 713-728

Heinrich G, Traunecker A, Tonegawa S (1984) Somatic mutation
creates diversity in the major group of mouse immunoglobulin κ
light chains. J Exp Med 159: 417-435

Hengartner H, Meo T, Mullen E (1978) Assignment of genes for
immunoglobulin κ and heavy chains to chromosome 6 and 12 in mouse.
Proc Natl Acad Sci USA 75: 4494-4498

Hummel KP (1970) Hypodactyly, a semideominant lethal mutation in
mice. The Journal of Heredity 61: 219

Jaenichen H, Peck M, Lindenmaier W, Wildgruber N, Zachau H (1984)
Composite human V_κ genes and a model of their evolution. Nucl
Acid Res 12: 5249-5263

Joho R, Weissman IL, Early P, Cole J, Hood L (1980) Organization of
κ light chain genes in germline and somatic tissue. Proc Natl
Acad Sci USA 77: 1106-1110

Kelley DE, Wiedmann LM, Pittet A-C, Strauss S, Nelson KJ, Davis J,
van Ness B, Perry RP (1985) Nonproductive kappa immunoglobulin
genes: recombinational abnormalities and other lesions affecting
transcription, RNA processing, turnover and translation. Mol Cell
Biol 5: 1660-1675

Lawler A (unpublished) pBC2-5 (4.8) is a pUC19 plasmid containing a
4.8 kbp HindIII fragment which was subcloned from a λ Charon 28
HindIII phage clone. The phage clone was made using size

selected (4.0-5.9 kbp) genomic DNA from a fetal liver $\mu^+\kappa^+$
hybridoma cell line from John Kearney. The partial sequence
indicates closest similarity to published $V_\kappa 12$ sequences. The
$V_\kappa 19$ subclone is a 260 bp HincII-MboII subclone of $p_\kappa(11)^{24}$
(Schibler et al., 1978) in pUC9. The PVKT15-S $V_\kappa 22$ subclone is a
400 bp HaeIII subclone of V_κS107A from P. Leder in pUC9.

Lazure C, Hum WT, Gibson D M (1981) Sequence diversity within a
subgroup of mouse immunoglobulin kappa chains controlled by the
Ig_κ-Ef2 locus. J Exp Med 154: 146-155

Morse HC III (ed) (1978) Origins of inbred mice. Academic Press
NY

Moynet D, MacLean SJ, Ng KH, Anctil D, Gibson DM (1985) Polymorphism
of κ variable region (V_κ-1) gene in inbred mice: Relationship to
the Ig_κ-Ef2 serum light chain marker. J Immunol 135: 727-732

Nishi M, Kataoka T, Honjo T (1985) Preferential rearrangement of
immunoglobulin κ chain joining regions $J_\kappa 1$ and $J_\kappa 2$ segments in
mouse spleen DNA. Proc Natl Acad Sci USA 82: 6399-6403

Osborne, B (unpublished) M167 cDNA from Joho (1980) was subcloned to
remove J_κ and C_κ sequences. The subclone is 310bp. Osborne University of Massachusetts.

Peck M, Smola H, Pohlenz H, Straubinger B, Gerl R, Zachau H (1985)
A large section of the gene locus encoding human immunoglobulin
variable regions of the kappa type is duplicated. J Mol Biol
183: 291-299

Potter M, Newell JB, Rudikoff S, Haber E (1982) Classification of
mouse V_κ groups based on the partial amino acid sequence to the
first invariant tryptophan: impact of 14 new sequences from IgG
myeloma proteins. Mol Immunol 19:1619-1630

Schibler U, Marcu KB, Perry RP (1978) The synthesis and processing
of the messenger RNAs specifying heavy and light chain immuno
globulins in MPC-11 cells. Cell 15: 1495-1509

Shapiro M (unpublished) A germline $V_\kappa 10$ by DNA sequencing. pC3386
is a 0.9 kbp EcoRI-HindIII fragment which ends approximately 2
amino acid codons from the V-J junction. pC3386 $V_\kappa 10$ non productive rearrangement is described in Kelley et al., 1985. The
$V_\kappa 10$ probe was used to isolate a phage clone from a genomic
library (pC9-26). A subclone 1.8 kbp was partially sequenced, and
the results compared with sequences of known V_κ exons. The closest similarity was found with $V_\kappa 9$; however, southern analysis
suggest the $V_\kappa 9$ probe and pC9-26 probe detect non-overlapping sets
of REFs. Shapiro M, ICR, Philadelphia

Smith-Gill SJ, Mainhart C, Lavoie TB, Feldman RJ, Drohan W, Brooks
BR (1987) A three-dimensional model of an anti-lysozyme antibody. J Mol Biol 194: 713-724

Stafford J, Queen C (1983) Cell-type specific expression of a
transfected immunoglobulin gene. Nature 306: 77-79

Taylor BA, Rowe L, Gibson DM, Riblet R, Yetter R and Gottlieb PD
(1985) Linkage of a 7S RNA sequence and kappa light chain genes
in the mouse. Immunogenetics 22: 471-481

Yonekawa H, Moriwaki K, Gotoh O, Watanabe J, Hayashi J-I, Miyashita N, Petras ML, Tagashira Y (1980) Relationship between laboratory mice and the subspecies Mus musculus musculus based on restriction endonuclease cleavage patterns of mitochondrial DNA. Japan J Genetics 55: 289

Table 1

Probes for Different Igκ Exon Groups

Probe	Vκ Gene Group	Source[*]	Type of probe and size	Hybridizes with Jκ-Cκ+/-
pECκ	N/A	M. Weigert	germline 6.6 kbp	+
T105	1	D. Gibson	rearranged genomic 3.7 kbp	+
H76K10	4,5	S. Cory	cDNA 1 kbp	+
M603K2	8	S. Cory	cDNA 1 kbp	+
M41	9	C. Queen	rearranged genomic 3.3 kbp	+
pC3386	10	M. Shapiro	rearranged genomic 0.9 kbp	-
p6684k-	11	R. Perry	rearranged genomic 4 kbp	+
pBC2-5(4.8)	12,13	A. Lawler	rearranged genomic 4.8 kbp	+
pK(11)^{24}-S	19	A. Lawler	cDNA 0.26 kbp	-
B61K16	21	S. Cory	cDNA 1 kbp	+
pVKT15-S	22	A. Lawler	rearranged genomic 0.4 kbp	-
HyHEL10	23	T. Lavoie	cDNA 1 kbp	+
M167	24	R. Joho	cDNA 0.3 kbp	-
pC9-26	9-26	M. Shapiro	germline 1.8 kbp	-

[*] Coleclough et al., 1981 for (pECκ); Moynet et al., 1985 for (Vκ1);
Cory et al., 1981; Stafford and Queen, 1983; Shapiro (unpublished); Kelley et al., 1985 for (Vκ11); Lawler (unpublished);
Smith-Gill et al., 1987 for (Vκ23); Joho et al., 1980 Osborne
subclone for (Vκ24).

Table 2
_____

Igκ Haplotypes

Prototype Strains	Igκ Haplo-types	Allelic Group V												Jκ [*]	Cκ	Number of Fragments Detected [§]		Kilobase Pair detected in Fragments [§]	
		24	11	9-26	9	1	12	4	8	10	19	23	21			intense	total	intense	total
AKR	a	a	a	a	a	a	a	a	a	a	a	a	a	a	b	60	91	465.5	701.5
NZB	b	b	b	b	b	b	b	b	b	b	b	b	b	b	b	60	98	464.3	706.7
BALB/c	c	a	a	a	a	c	b	b	b	b	b	b	b	b	b	60	95	453.3	675.8
C58	d	b	b	b	b	b	a	a	a	a	a	a	a	a	b	57	91	460.3	721.3
SJL	e	a	a	a	a	c	b	b	b	b	b	b	c	c	a	61	97	457.5	675.6
CE	f	c	c	c	b	b	b	b	c	b	b	b	b	b	b	60	99	438.8	723.6
O20	g	c	c	c	c	d	a	c	c	c	c	d	d	d	b	61	95	451.5	692.4

* = Data from Boyd et al (1986) was reproduced and only O20 displayed a new pattern.

§ = Fragments detected for the designated haplotypes were sized to the nearest 100 base pair.

Table 3

List of Inbred Strains within the Different Igκ Haplotypes

Haplotype	Inbred Strains
a	AKR/A, AKR/N, MRL/MpJ-lpr/lpr, NFS, PL/J, RF/J
b	NZB/B1NJ
c	129/J, A/HeJ, A/J, ABP/Le, AL/N, AU/SsJ, BALB/cAnPt, BALB/cJ, BALB/cWt, BSVS, BUB/BnJ, C3H/Fg, C3H/HeJ, C3H/HeN, C57BL/6N, C57BL/10N, C57BL/Ka, C57BL/Ks, C57BR/cdJ, C57L/J, CBA/H, CBA/J, CBA/N, DBA/1J, DBA/2J, DBA/2N, HRS/J, NH, NZW/N, PDB/Pt, RIIIS/J, SEA/GnJ, SEC/1REJ, SM/J-A*w, ST/bJ, STS/A, SWR/J
d	C58/J, YBR/Ei
e	SJL/J, SJL/JLwPt, MA/MyJ
f	BDP/J, CE/J, I/LnJ, P/J, P/N
g	O20/A

Table 4

Putative Gene Order Derived from Recombinants and Distribution of Allelic Groups with Igκ Haplotypes

DNA SAMPLE	Allelic Group *																	
	V11	V24	V9-26	V9	V1	V12	V4	V8	V10	V19	V28	Rn7s-6	V23	V21	Jκ	Cκ	Ly2	Ly3
AKR & PL	a	a	a	a	a	a	a	a	a	a	a	a	a	a	a	b	a	a
NZB	b	b	b	b	b	b	b	b	b	b	b	b	b	b	b	b	b	b
ABP, BALB/c & C57BL/6	a	a	a	a	c§	b	b	b	b	b	b	b	b	b	b	b	b	b+
C58	b	b	b	b	b	a	a	a	a	a	a	a	a	a	a	b	a	a
SJL	a	a	a	a	c§	b	b	b	b	b	b	b	b	c	c	a	b	b
CE	c	c	c	b	b	b	b	b	b	b	ND	b	b	b	b	b	a	b
O20	c	c	c	c	d	a	c	c	c	c	ND	ND	c	d	d	b	a	b
NAK	b	b	b	b	b	b	a	b	b	b	a	a	a	a	a	a	a	a
B6.PL(75NS)	a	a	a	a	ND	b	b	b	b	b	a	a	a	a	a	b	a	a
B6.PL(85NS)	a	a	a	a	ND	b	b	b	b	b	b	b	a	a	a	b	a	a
ABP.C58 7255	b/a	b/a	ND	b/a	b/c	ND	a/b	a/b	a/b	ND	ND	ND	a/b	b/b	b/b	b/b	ND	ND
ABP.C58 5942	ND	a/a	ND	a/a	c/c	ND	b/b	b/b	b/b	ND	ND	ND	b/b	b/b	b/b	b/b	b/a	ND
OXAF	ND	ND	ND	a	a	ND	ND	ND	a	a	ND	a	a	a	ND	b	a	b
OXA6	ND	ND	ND	a	a	ND	ND	ND	a	a	ND	b	a	a	a	b	a	b

* = The allelic groups are taken from: the current work; V28 (Goldrick et al 1985); Rn7s-6 (Taylor et al 1985); Jκ (Boyd et al 1986)

§ = The c allelic group is detected with HindIII. Using BamHI these strains show the AKR allelic group.

+ = The Ly3 type for ABP is not determined.

ND = Not Determined

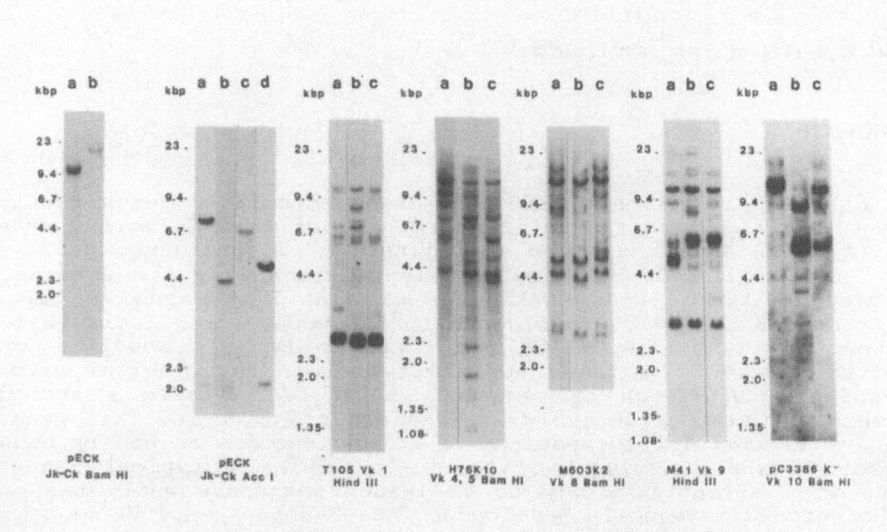

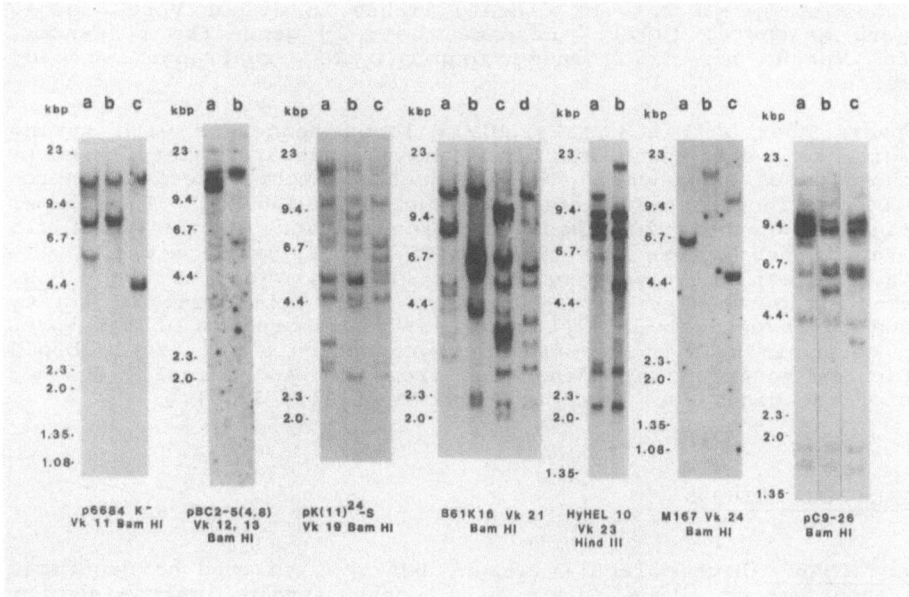

Figure 1

Genomic DNA was digested with the restriction endonuclease indicated, size separated on 0.7% agarose gels, gels were not acid treated prior to transfer, hybridized with the indicated DNA probe and the final stingency was 0.2 x SSC at 65°C. Representative REF patterns (a, b, c or d) are indicated. λ HindIII and ØX174 HaeIII standards are left of each panel.

Conservation of the Organization of the pre-B Cell Specific VpreB1/VpreB2/λ5 Loci in the Genus *Mus*

S. R. Bauer[1], L. A. D'Hoostelaere[2], and F. Melchers[1]

INTRODUCTION

During a search for B cell differentiation associated genes the λ5 gene was isolated by differential screening of a cDNA library made of poly(A)[+] RNA from the pre-B cell line 70-Z/3 (Sakaguchi et al., 1986a). The λ5 1.2 kb mRNA, selectivley expressed in pre B cells, is encoded by three exons (Sakaguchi et al., 1986b; Kudo et al., 1987b). Exon 3 is 70-78% homologous to the mouse $C\lambda_{1-4}$ loci, while the 3' part of exon 2 is 67-70% homologous to $J\lambda_{1-4}$. Exon 1 is not related to genes of the supergene family nor to any other reported DNA sequence. A search of sequences 5' of λ5 revealed a second gene, which is also selectively expressd in pre B cells. This gene, VpreB1, is located 4.2 kb upstream of λ5 and encodes an 850 bp mRNA made from 2 exons. Exon 1 of VpreB1 resembles a typical leader sequence with strong homology to Vλ leader sequences while the 5' region of exon 2 is equally homologous (46-48%) to Vκ and Vλ sequences. The 84 nucleotides at the 3' end of VpreB1 exon 2 do not resemble sequences of the Ig supergene family or any reported DNA sequence (Kudo and Melchers, 1987). The VpreB1 probe hybridizes strongly to a second gene, VpreB2, which was found to be over 95% homologous to VpreB1 but not closely linked to either VpreB1 or λ5 (Kudo and Melchers, 1987). Despite their Ig gene-like sequences, neither VpreB nor λ5 genes require DNA rearrangement for expression.

It appears that within the VpreB1/λ5 locus sequences with strong homologies to the Ig genes at the 5' and 3' ends are interspersed by Ig-nonhomologous sequences. These sequences might have been introduced by an insertional event (Kudo et al., 1987b). This paper investigates whether this peculiar organization of the VpreB1/λ5 locus originated within the (DBA/2 x C57BL/6)F_1 mouse strains, its parents, nearest relatives, or before speciation of the genus Mus. We report the results of a Southern blot hybridization survey designed to investigate the structure and polymorphism of the VpreB and λ5 genes in wild mouse strains representing a relatively broad evolutionary spectrum including mice from the biochemically defined groups of the genus Mus, Mus1-5 (Bonhomme et al., 1984).

MATERIALS AND METHODS

Mice and DNAs. High molecular weight DNA was isolated as described (Scott and Potter, 1984) from wild mouse strains maintained at Hazelton Laboratories in Rockville, MD, USA and described by Potter (1986).

[1] Basel Institute for Immunology, Basel, Switzerland
[2] Laboratory of Genetics, National Cancer Institute, Bethesda, MD 20892, USA

Strain Survey. 7 µg of DNA was digested to completion with HindIII, subjected to electrophoresis through 0.8% agarose gels in TAE buffer, transferred onto nitrocellulose filters, then probed first with a ^{32}P-labelled 600 bp EcoRI-HindIII fragment of λ5 cDNA plasmid pZ183-1a (Kudo et al., 1987b), exposed to film, then stripped and re-probed with a ^{32}P-labelled 650 bp EcoRI-AccI fragment of VpreB1 cDNA plasmid pZ121 (Kudo and Melchers, 1987). Random primed labelling, prehybridization, hybridization, and washing of non-specifically bound counts were done at high stringency (0.1 x SSC, 0.1% SDS, 65°C) essentially as described (Bauer et al., 1988).

RESULTS

DNA from at least two separate preparations of 32 different wild mouse strains were surveyed by Southern blot hybridization with both the λ5 and VpreB1 gene probes under high stringency conditions. In all cases one HindIII restriction fragment appeared to hybridize both to the λ5 probe and the VpreB1 probe (Figure 1) as would be expected if the λ5 and VpreB1 genes were maintained in close proximity in the genomes of wild mice as they are in inbred mice (Kudo and Melchers, 1987). Four VpreB1-λ5 HindIII RFLPs were distinguishable. All mice were homozygous. This defines 4 alleles,

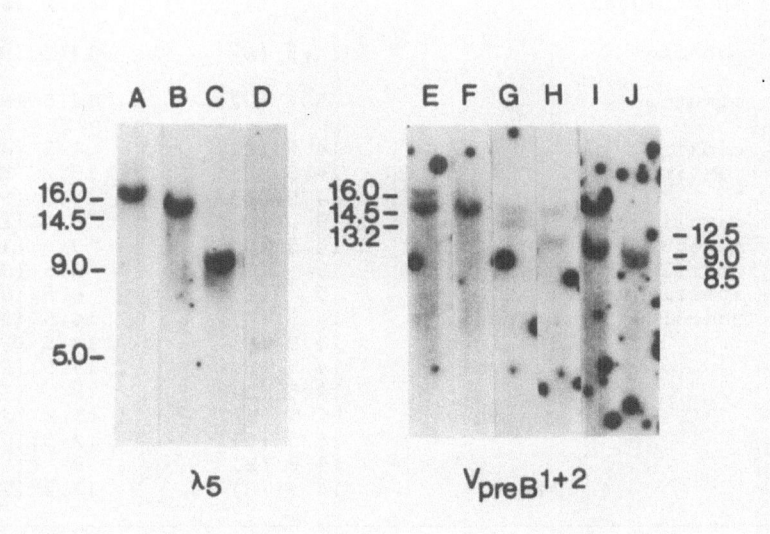

Fig. 1. Restriction fragment length polymorphism in wild mice. Southern blots of HindIII digested wild mouse DNAs probed with λ5 (lanes A-D) and VpreB1 (lanes E-J).

A-D, in the wild mice and inbred mice under survey. Figure 1, lanes A-D show representative samples of the 16.0, 14.5, 9.0 and 5.0 kb HindIII fragment which hybridized with λ5. Lanes E-J show representative samples of the bands which hybridized with the VpreB1 probe. In most mouse strains, two HindIII bands were seen with this probe. One of these HindIII bands always also hybridized to the λ5 probe while the second band presumably hybridized only to VpreB2. On this basis 6 alleles, E-J, were defined for the VpreB2 locus. The HindIII bands that hybridized only to the VpreB1 probe and not to the λ5 probe, thus representing the VpreB2 alleles, were 16.0, 14.5, 13.2, 12.5, 9.0 and 8.5 kb as shown in Figure 1, lanes E-J, respectively. Mice which showed allele F may actually lack a VpreB2 gene. Alternatively, the VpreB2 gene HindIII fragment fortuitously migrates with the VpreB1-λ5 14.5 kb HindIII allele B fragment. We have not yet digested these DNAs with other restriction enzymes which could possibly distinguish between the two possibilities.

Table 1. VpreB1/λ5 and VpreB2 HindIII RFLP patterns

Subgenera	Species		HindIII fragments (kb) and alleles	
			VpreB1/λ5	VpreB2
Pyromys	saxicola		14.5 (B)	12.5 (H)
	shortridgei		16 (A)	13.2 (G)
Coelomys	pahari		14.5 (B)	12.5 (H)
Nannomys	minutoides		5 (D)	12.5 (H)
Mus	cookii		14.5 (B)	8.5 (J)
	cervicolor		14.5 (B)	16 (E)
	"		14.5 (B)	14.5 (F)
	caroli		9 (C)	16 (E)
	spretus		14.5 (B)	9 (I)
	spicilegus	spicilegus	9 (C)	8.5 (J)
	spicilegus	tartaricus	9 (C)	8.5 (J)
	musculus	castaneus	14.5 (B)	14.5 (F)
		molossinus	14.5 (B)	14.5 (F)
		musculus*	14.5 (B)	14.5 (F)
		"	14.5 (B)	9 (I)
		domesticus‡	14.5 (B)	13.2 (G)
		"	14.5 (B)	12.5 (H)
		"	14.5 (B)	9 (I)
		inbred	14.5 (B)	13.2 (G)

* Survey included Mus musculus musculus samples trapped in 4 different locations.
‡ Survey included Mus musculus domesticus samples trapped in 14 different locations.

The organization of the λ5-VpreBl allele D (unique to Mus minu-
toides) may be different from all other alleles since its size (5 kb
containing both genes) is not large enough to carry the VpreBl-λ5
locus as it appears organized in the inbred DBA/2 and C57BL/6
strains where both genes span 9 kb of DNA.

We observed a striking conservation of the VpreBl/λ5 locus (Table
I). The λ5 and VpreB probes revealed a conserved λ5/VpreBl 14.5kb
HindIII fragment in all Mus musculus species and in 5 of the other
10 species examined which represent 3 additional subgenera. Of
these other 5 species, three have a 9kb HindIII fragment. The
VpreB2 locus was more polymorphic and showed no species-restricted
patterns of inheritance. The mice which displayed different alleles
(Table I) did not fall into different Mus genus subgroups as defined
by Bonhomme et al. (1984), or into the 4 Mus subgenera as described
by Marshall (1986).

Based on this survey, the assortment of alleles for λ5 and VpreB
genes (Table I) is apparently random relative to previously defined
subgroups of Mus. This may reflect a paucity of samples or may
indicate limited divergence preceeding stabilization of the present
day Mus subgroups.

DISCUSSION

The presence of single copy DNA fragments that hybridize to the
VpreB and λ5 genes at high stringency demonstrates a high degree of
conservation of these genes in the genus Mus. Apparently the
close physical linkage of the VpreBl and λ5 gene, and a separate
VpreB2 gene are also highly conserved. This suggests that some
functionally important constraint has kept the λ5 and at least one
VpreB gene together over long evolutionary periods since separation
of the Mus subgenera occurred between 9-12 (Bonhomme, 1986) or 10-12
(Thaler, 1986) million years ago. The observation that no HindIII
sites are found within the VpreB genes or the λ5 gene (Kudo et al.,
1987b; Kudo and Melchers, 1987) and thus must be in the flanking
regions, suggest that there is surprisingly little polymorphism,
with a preservation of the specific organization of both coding and
non-coding DNA sequences in the λ5-VpreB region.

This is in marked contrast to considerable restriction fragment
length polymorphism and gene amplification (Scott and Potter, 1984)
of the λL chain genes located an unknown distance away from
VpreBl/λ5 and VpreB2 which are all on chromosome 16 (Kudo et al.,
1987a; and unpublished data). It indicates that the unit of amplification of the λL chain genes does not include the VpreBl/λ5 or
VpreB2 gene loci. The difference in stringency of conservation between VpreBl/λ5 and λL chain genes is all the more surprising since
the 3' part of the second and all of the third exon of λ5 shows high
homologies to the corresponding sequences in J and C-regions of λL
chain genes. It suggests that there may be equal evolutionary
pressure on these parts of both λ5 and λL chains, possibly due to an
equivalent, so far unknown function, while a stronger pressure for
evolutionary conservation appears to exist for the first, 5' exon of
λ5, for the 4.2 kb intervening sequences, and for VpreBl, when compared to the corresponding sequences of λL chains, i.e. the V-

segments. The greater number of flanking region polymorphisms observed for VpreB2 may also indicate that there is relatively less evolutionary pressure on this separate gene and that the high degree of conservation in the VpreB1/λ5 flanking regions may be imposed by a required physical linkage.

In addition to the studies reported in this paper, we have observed a widespread conservation of VpreB-hybridizing sequences in several mammalian species, including man (Bauer et al., 1988). Cloning of the human VpréB gene and subsequent structural analysis of its organization show a remarkably high degree of homology and conservation of structure of the VpreB genes in mouse and man. As with the mouse gene, the human VpreB gene is expressed only in pre-B cell lines. These observations, together with the wild mouse VpreB1-λ5 survey of this paper, support the idea that VpreB and λ5 are members of the Ig gene family that are highly conserved in structure and serve the same funtion of being expressed selectively in pre B cells of mammals. These genes are useful as markers of normal pre B cells and their related malignancies in mouse and man, and promise to be useful tools for studying differentiation of cells in the early stages of the B cell lineage.

ACKNOWLEDGEMENTS

The Basel Institute for Immunology was founded and is supported by F. Hoffmann-La Roche Limited Company, Basel, Switzerland.

REFERENCES

Bauer SR, Kudo A, Melchers F (1988) Structure and pre B lymphocyte-restricted expression of the VpreB gene in humans, and conservation of its structure in other mammalian species. EMBO J, in press.

Bonhomme, F (1986) Evolutionary relationships in the genus Mus. Current Topics in Microbiology and Immunology 127:19-34.

Bonhomme F, Catalan J, Britton-Davidan J, Chapman VM, Moriawaki K, Nevo E, Thaler L (1984) Biochemical diversity and evolution in the Genus Mus. Biochem. Gen, 22:275-303.

Kudo A, Melchers F (1987) A second gene, VpreB, in the λ5 locus of the mouse, which appears to be selectively expressed in pre B lymphocytes. EMBO J 6:2267-2272.

Kudo A, Pravtcheva D, Sakaguchi N, Ruddle FH, Melchers F (1987a) Localization of the murine λ5 gene on chromosome 16. Genomics, in press.

Kudo A, Sakaguchi, N, Melchers F (1987b) Organization of the λ5 gene transcribed selectively in pre B lymphocytes. EMBO J 56:103-107.

Marshall JT (1986) Systematics of the genus Mus. Current Topics in Microbiology and Immunology 127:12-18.

Potter M (1986) Listing of stocks and strains of mice in the genus Mus derived from the feral state. Current Topics in Microbiology and Immunology 127:373-395.

Sakaguchi N, Berger CN, Melchers F (1986a) Isolation of a cDNA copy of an RNA species expressed in murine pre B cells. EMBO J 5:2139-2147.

Sakaguchi N, Melchers F (1986b) λ5, a new light chain-related locus selectively expressed in pre B lymphocytes. Nature 324:579-582.

Scott CL, Potter M (1984) Polymorphism of Cλ genes and units of duplication in the genus Mus. J Immunol 5:2630-2637.

Thaler L (1986) Origin and evolution of mice: an appraisal of fossil evidence and morphological traits. Current Topics in Microbiology and Immunology 127:3-11.

The Omega and Iota Surrogate Immunoglobulin Light Chains

S. Pillai and D. Baltimore

INTRODUCTION

A major activity of a pre-B lymphocyte is the stepwise rearrangement of immunoglobulin heavy and light chain genes. When a pre-B
cell has successfully completed the process of rearrangement at
both heavy and light chain loci, this dividing lymphocyte under-
goes a cellular transition into a mature B cell whereby it stops
dividing and expresses membrane immunoglobulin tetramers (μm2L2)
on its surface which will function as the antigen receptor. The
process of rearrangement is of central importance to the generation of immunological diversity. However, it is imperative that
in any given lymphocyte only a single heavy chain allele be pro-
ductively rearranged (allelic exclusion), and that only a single
κ or λ light chain allele be correctly rearranged (allelic and
isotypic exclusion). These processes of allelic and isotypic
exclusion are unique to the immune system and ensure that any
lymphoid clone expresses only a single antigen receptor. A considerable body of evidence exists to support the view that an in-
frame rearrangement at the heavy chain locus and the consequent
intracellular synthesis of μm protein provides a "feedback" signal during differentiation; this signal leads to the shut-off of
rearrangement at the H-chain locus and permits a pre-B cell to
move on to the stage of light chain gene rearrangement (Weaver et
al., 1984; Nussenzweig et al., 1987; Reth et al., 1985; 1987).
The formation of complete H-L tetramers is in turn believed to
provide a feedback signal leading to the shut-off of L-chain gene
rearrangement (Ritchie et al., 1984). We asked the question --
how does the μm protein in a pre-B cell provide a feedback signal
during differentiation? Does μm associate with any pre-B specific proteins to generate a feedback signal? Is there a pre-B
specific subset of genes which help mediate the feedback process?

Pre-B Cells Synthesize Either or Both of Two Surrogate Ig Light
Chains

Three distinct intracellular forms of the μm protein may be
identified in B cells and we have designated these sequential
forms of μm as μm1, μm2 and μm3 (Pillai and Baltimore 1987a).
Although in B cells μm has a long half-life and the acylated,
terminally glycosylated μm3 form reaches the cell surface, in the
majority of pre-B cell lines μm has a brief existence and the
μm2 and μm3 forms are never observed during biosynthetic studies
(Pillai and Baltimore 1987a and unpublished observations). The
rapid turnover of μm is pre-B specific; in non-lymphoid cells
expressing a transfected μm gene the μm protein has a relatively
long half-life (Pillai and Baltimore, unpublished observations).
The pre-B specific degradation of μm takes place in an acidic
compartment and is correlated with the association of μm in pre-B
cells with either one or both of two surrogate immunoglobulin
light chains. The omega chain (Pillai and Baltimore, 1987b) is
an 18 kd protein which forms disulfide linked tetramers with μm.

Whitehead Institute for Biomedical Research, Cambridge, MA 02142
and Department of Biology, Massachusetts Institute of Technology,
Cambridge MA 02139

A preliminary sequence analysis (unpublished) of this pre-B
specific protein suggests that it is the product of the λ-5 gene
(Sakaguchi and Melchers, 1986; Sakaguchi et al., 1987). In
certain pre-B cell lines (e.g. NFS 5.3, Hardy et al. 1986;
dextran sulfate induced 70Z/3, Paige et al., 1981) that express
μm on the cell surface in the absence of the synthesis of
"conventional" κ or λ light chains, μm on the cell surface is
stoichiometrically associated with the disulfide linked omega
chain and with the non-disulfide linked iota chain. The iota
surrogate light ⁻chain is a 14 kd pre-B specific protein which on
peptide mapping and preliminary sequence analysis is clearly
unrelated to the omega chain; its possible sequence identity to
the V-preB1 gene (Kudo et al., 1987) remains to be established.
Upon cell surface iodination of the (unusual) surface μm positive

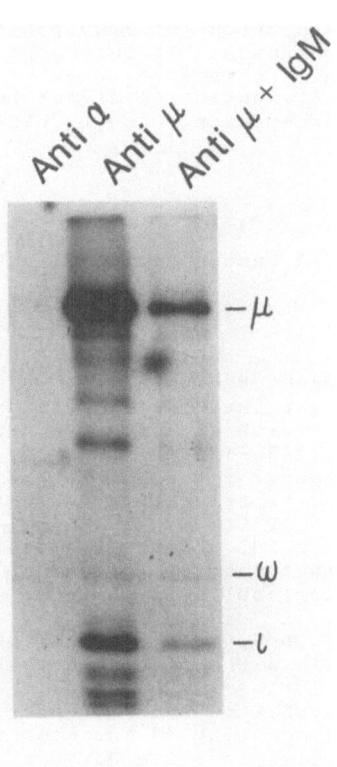

Fig. 1: Cell surface iodination of NFS 5.3 followed by
immunoprecipitation of cell lysate with a monoclonal anti-mouse
IgM antibody and analysis on a 12.5 % polyacrylamide/sodium
dodecyl sulfate gel (Pillai and Baltimore 1987b and unpublished
observations). Lane 1: immunoprecipitation with an irrelevant
antibody. Lane 2: immunoprecipitation with anti-μ antibody
reveals μ, ω and ι proteins and other members of the "μm
activation complex". Lane 3: competition with unlabelled IgM
demonstrates that ω, ι, and the other observed polypeptides are
associated with μm.

pre-B cell lines referred to above, iota is more readily iodinated than omega; iota, omega and μm are all specifically inhibited from binding to a monoclonal anti-μ antibody by an excess of
unlabelled IgM (Fig. 1, lanes 2 and 3).

An "Activated Receptor" Model for Feedback Regulation

Our working model for the mechanism of feedback regulation
mediated by the μm protein is as follows: in pre-B cells μm
associates with and forms tetramers with a surrogate light chain
protein (omega or iota). These tetramers are in turn tightly
associated with 6 other polypeptides, 2 of which are phospho-
proteins (unpublished observations). This μm associated complex
presumably functions from an intracellular transmembrane location
as a ligand-independent "activated receptor", providing a cue
that signals further differentiation. A detailed characterization of the proteins that make up the μm associated "activated
receptor" complex (which is degraded in an acidic compartment
with kinetics similar to the "downregulation" of many polypeptide
hormone receptors) is currently in progress. If indeed this
model proves correct in broad outline, it remains to be
ascertained whether the requisite differentiation signal is
provided by the generation of a second-messenger or by direct
nuclear translocation of μm itself.

ACKNOWLEDGEMENT

This work was supported by an American Cancer Society Grant to
D.B.

REFERENCES

Hardy RR, Dangl IL, Hayakawa K, Jager G, Herzenberg LA,
  Herzenberg LA (1986) Frequent λ light chain gene rearrangement
  and expression in a Ly-1 B lymphoma with a productive κ chain
  allele. Proc Natl Acad Sci USA 83,1438-1442
Kudo A, Melchers F (1987) A second gene V pre-B 1 in the λ-5
  locus of the mouse which appears to be selectively expressed in
  pre-B lymphocytes. EMBO J 6,2267- 2272.
Nussenzweig M, Shaw AC, Sinn E, Danner DB, Holmes KL, Morse HC,
  Leder P (1987) Allelic Exclusion in transgenic mice that
  express the membrane form of immunoglobulin μ. Science
  236,816-819
Paige CJ, Kincade PW, Ralph P (1981) Independent control of
  immunoglobulin heavy and light chain expression in a mouse pre-
  B cell. Nature 292,631-632
Pillai S, Baltimore D (1987a) Myristoylation and the post-
  translational acquisition of hydrophobicity by the membrane
  immunoglobulin heavy chain polypeptide in B lymphocytes. Proc
  Natl Acad Sci USA 84,7654-7658
Pillai S, Baltimore D (1987b) Formation of disulphide-linked μ2ω2
  tetramers in pre-B cells by the 18 K ω-immunoglobulin light
  chain. Nature 329,172-174
Reth MG, Ammirati P, Jackson S, Alt FW (1985) Regulated
  progression of a cultured pre-B cell line to the B cell stage.
  Nature 317,353-355.
Reth MG, Petrac E, Wiese P, Lobel L, Alt FW (1987) Activation of
  Vκ gene rearrangement in pre-B cells follows the expression of
  membrane-bound Ig heavy chain.   EMBO J
Ritchie KA, Brinster RL, Storb U (1984) Allelic exclusion and
  control of endogenous immunoglobulin gene rearrangement in κ
  transgenic mice. Nature 312,517-520

Sakaguchi N, Melchers F (1986) λ-5, a new light chain related
  locus selectively expressed in pre-B lymphocytes. Nature
  324,579-582)
Sakaguchi N, Berger C-N, Melchers F (1987) Isolation of a cDNA
  copy of an RNA species selectively expressed in pre-B
  lymphocytes. EMBO J 5,2134-2137
Weaver D, Costantini F, Imanishi-Kari T, Baltimore D (1984) A
  transgenic Immunoglobulin μ gene prevents rearrangement of
  endogenous genes. Cell 42,117-127

MHC Class I Gene Expression by Tumors: Immunotherapeutic Implications

J.S. Weber[1] and G. Jay[2]

An anti-tumor role has been established for macrophages (Fidler 1974; Fernandez-Cruz et al. 1985), NK cells (Talmadge et al. 1980; Kawase et al. 1982), and helper T cells (Fugiwara et al. 1984; Greenberg et al. 1985) in various experimental systems, but an optimal immune defense against tumor cell growth in vivo depends on the ability of cytotoxic T lymphocytes (CTLs) to recognize and destroy malignant cells (Dailey et al. 1984; Rosenstein et al. 1984). This recognition involves an interaction between the effector cell and antigens present on the tumor cell in association with MHC class I molecules (Zinkernagel et al. 1979). The MHC class I molecules are composed of a heavy glycoprotein chain of 45 kilodaltons (kD) and a noncovalently-associated beta-2 microglobulin molecule of 15 kD (Hood et al. 1983). The heavy chain is highly polymorphic and is encoded by the H-2K, D and L loci in the mouse, and by the HLA-A, -B and -C loci in human. Virtually all normal cells display class I molecules (Daar et al. 1984), as do many tumor cells. Active immunosurveillance in vivo may select for tumor variants with altered or down-regulated class I antigens, and reduced class I gene expression by tumors may provide a means of avoiding destruction by cytotoxic T lymphocytes.

The expression of MHC class I genes is not tightly controlled in human tumors. Numerous studies have described altered levels of class I antigen expression in tumors (Tanaka et al. 1988). Most small cell lung cancers (Doyle et al. 1985), skin basal cell carcinomas (Turbitt et al. 1981), neuroblastomas (Lampson et al. 1983) and embryonal tumors (Jones et al. 1980) are devoid of class I molecules. Significant numbers of newly diagnosed colon carcinomas (Csiba et al. 1984; Momberg et al. 1986) or melanomas (Reuter et al. 1984) either lack class I expression or show altered expression. Metastatic lesions from primary melanomas that express class I molecules have been shown to be class I negative (Natali et al. 1985). Many ovarian, breast and cervical carcinomas also show little or no class I expression (Fleming et al. 1981; Ferguson et al. 1985). Thus, reduced expression of class I antigens is characteristic of a variety of human malignancies.

In experimental murine systems, spontaneously-derived tumors like B16 melanoma (Nanni et al. 1983) or line 1 lung carcinoma (Bahler et al. 1985) lack class I antigens. Carcinogen-induced tumor lines such as MCA 101 (Weber et al. 1987), cells transformed by human adenovirus 12 (Schrier et al. 1983) or simian virus 40 (Rogers et al. 1983), or AKR virus induced leukemia cells (Festenstein et al. 1981) express few or no class I molecules. In contrast, virtually all normal mouse or human cells express class I antigens with the exception of renal tubular cells (Paul et al. 1982; Halloran et al. 1985), hepatocytes (Fukusata et al. 1986), some neuronal cells and cells of pancreatic exocrine origin (Hart et al. 1983).

Both normal and tumor cells have evolved mechanisms to specifically modulate MHC expression. Several naturally-occurring macromolecules can modulate class I gene expression on tumors. Both alpha interferon, a leukocyte product, and gamma interferon, derived from macrophages, can up-regulate class I expression

[1]Surgery Branch and [2]Laboratory of Molecular Virology
National Cancer Institute
Bethesda, Maryland 20892

Current Topics in Microbiology and Immunology, Vol. 137
© Springer-Verlag Berlin · Heidelberg 1988

on murine or human tumor cells in culture (Lindahl et al. 1973; Gracomini et al. 1984). A 30-basepair sequence located 5' of the class I transcriptional promoter has been shown to be responsive to alpha or gamma interferon by increasing RNA transcription of class I genes (Israel et al. 1986). Alpha TNF, a macrophage-derived glycoprotein with potent anti-tumor properties, can augment class I expression in tumor cells in synergy with alpha or gamma interferon in vitro (Scheurich et al. 1986). A 19-kD glycoprotein (E19K) encoded by the early region of adenovirus 2, can down-regulate MHC expression by binding nascent class I molecules in the endoplasmic reticulum and impeding their transport to the cell surface (Burgert et al. 1985). A protein encoded by the early 1A region of adenovirus 12 can decrease the amount of steady-state mRNA encoding class I antigens (Schrier et al. 1983). The complex transcriptional and post-transcriptional regulatory network for class I genes suggests that pharmacologic intervention may be appropriate for modulating class I antigen expression on tumor cells in vitro and on tumors in vivo.

Control of class I gene expression may be part of a coordinated genetic program associated with progression from a normal to a malignant phenotype. Expression of a transfected n-myc oncogene in rat neuroblastoma cells in vitro is associated with down-regulation of the class I loci, as well as faster growth in vivo and a metastatic phenotype (Bernards et al. 1986). Revertants that lose n-myc expression become high expressors of class I antigens. F9 teratocarcinoma cells, which undergo morphologic differentiation upon exposure to retinoic acid in vitro, lose expression of c-myc and n-myc oncogenes at the same time that they begin to express MHC class I antigens (Solter et al. 1979). In cell lines derived from patients with Burkitt's lymphoma, selective down-regulation of the HLA-A locus by transfection of the adenovirus E19K gene correlated with loss of an Epstein-Barr virus (EBV) membrane protein and a more malignant phenotype; reversion of cell lines to a less malignant lymphoblastoid cell type correlates with increased HLA-A and EBV membrane protein expression (Masucci et al. 1987). Tumor growth due to escape from immune surveillance may be a result of MHC down-regulation in malignancies induced under the control of viral or cellular oncogenes.

A number of experiments have suggested that the ability to form tumors in mice varies inversely with the expression of class I antigens. Clones of T10, a methylcholanthrene-induced sarcoma of ($H-2^b$ x $H-2^k$) F_1 origin, are deficient in H-2K gene expression and readily metastasize to the lung. The ability to metastasize was abolished by transfecting T10 with either the $H-2K^b$ or $H-2K^k$ gene (Wallich et al. 1985). $H-2K^b$ expressing clones were also less tumorigenic. An AKR leukemia subline, K36.16, has no $H-2K^k$ antigen present on its surface. Transfection of this subline with the gene for $H-2K^k$ resulted in decreased tumorigenicity in AKR mice (Hui et al. 1984). The oncogenic adenovirus 12 can transform mouse cells which invariably become low expressors of class I antigens. Transfection of either the H-2K or H-2L gene into an adenovirus 12-transformed cell line, originally lacking class I expression, resulted in decreased tumorigenicity (Tanaka et al. 1985). Treatment of another clone of adenovirus 12 transformed cells with a combination of alpha and beta interferon resulted in increased class I antigen expression and decreased tumorigenicity in syngeneic C3H/HeJ mice (Hayashi et al. 1985). A subline of a spontaneous murine melanoma, B16BL6, normally expresses very low levels of $H-2K^b$ molecules. Transfection of the $H-2K^b$ gene results in decreased tumor growth in syngeneic mice and fewer metastases to the lung (Weber et al. 1987). Murine lung carcinoma line 1 cells, derived from a spontaneous tumor, have been transfected with the $H-2D^P$ gene. In semi-syngeneic mice that have been primed with tumor, the transfected clone is less tumorigenic (Baker et al. 1987).

These data suggest that the growth of a variety of spontaneous, carcinogen-induced and virally-transformed tumors is determined by the level of expression of MHC encoded antigens by the tumor cell. However, the presence of

class I molecules is by no means an exclusive determinant of oncogenicity.
Among the adenoviruses, types 2 and 5 will not form tumors in mice, yet
express low levels of class I molecules (Haddada et al. 1986). Presumably
tumor-specific antigens are epitopes recognized in association with class I
molecules. If one or the other is diminished or absent, tumor growth may
result from lack of immune host recognition.

Further evidence that increased levels of class I antigens augment host tumor
recognition is shown in the previous studies with the T10, AKR, Ad12-transformed
and B16 tumor lines transfected with H-2K genes. In each case, augmentation of
class I antigen levels results in increased immunogenicity. Syngeneic animals
immunized with the transfected clones are protected against subsequent challenge
by the class I-deficient parental line (Hui et al. 1984; Wallich et al. 1985;
Tanaka et al. 1986). These data strongly suggest that loss of class I antigen
expression permits tumors to escape immune recognition, and that immunoselection
in vitro may generate populations of tumor cells heterogeneous for class I
expression.

Not all immune effectors show increased activity against class I expressing
tumor cells. Lymphokine-activated killer (LAK) cells have been shown to
mediate regression of a variety of murine and human tumors when administered
with IL-2 (Mule et al. 1986; Rosenberg et al. 1987). LAK cell anti-tumor
activity in vivo or in vitro is neither class I-restricted (Shiloni et al.
1986) nor does anti-tumor activity in vivo depend on the level of class I
antigens present on the tumor cells (Mule et al. 1987). Natural killer (NK)
cells are present in normal hosts that have not been sensitized to tumor.
They show broad anti-tumor reactivity in vitro and will kill normal fibroblasts
or bone marrow cells less readily than tumor cells. In contrast to cytotoxic
T lymphocytes, their ability to destroy a cell in vitro varies inversely
with the expression of class I antigens (Ljunggren et al. 1985, 1986). While
the importance of NK activity in anti-tumor surveillance is unclear, NK cells
may eliminate class I-deficient tumor variants that arise in vivo in a nonspecific manner.

The level of class I antigen expression by tumor cells may affect their
sensitivity to biological response modifiers that modulate the host immune
system. Interleukin-2 (IL-2) is a T-cell derived glycoprotein that stimulates
T-cell growth (Smith 1980), and generates promiscuous anti-tumor activity
in normal peripheral blood lymphocytes after a three-day in vitro incubation
(Grimm et al. 1982). IL-2 alone also mediates regression of lung metastases
generated by a variety of spontaneous and carcinogen-induced murine tumors
(Donohue et al. 1984; Mule et al. 1987). The anti-tumor activity of IL-2
on established lung metastases is mediated via the action of Lyt-2$^+$ lymphocytes.
Tumors that express low or undetectable levels of class I antigens are
resistant to the effects of IL-2, whereas lung metastases generated by high
class I expressors are eliminated by IL-2 immunotherapy (Weber et al. 1987).
B16BL6 is a murine melanoma resistant to the anti-tumor effects of IL-2. Its
transfection with the H-2K^b gene generates clones of B16BL6 expressing the
H-2K^b antigen that are susceptible to IL-2. The regression of advanced high
class I-expressing B16BL6 lung metastases was shown to be mediated by Lyt-2
bearing cells.

Subcutaneous tumors generated by high class I-expressor B16BL6 clones are
also sensitive to alpha TNF, a lymphokine secreted by macrophages that can
mediate its biological effects via Lyt-2$^+$ cells. Tumors generated by low or
non-class I expressing B16BL6 clones, or methylcholanthrene-induced sarcomas
devoid of class I expression, do not regress after alpha TNF treatment (Ascher
et al., unpublished). IL-2 and alpha TNF appear to stimulate Lyt-2$^+$ immune
cells that recognize the presence of a tumor antigen. The Lyt-2 molecule
as well as the clonotypic T-cell receptor are required for targeting of a
cytolytic T cell to antigen in association with MHC class I products (Yague

et al. 1985). For any given level of tumor antigen, augmented class I expression should potentiate specific cytolytic T-cell recognition. The ability to modulate tumor class I expression in vitro may provide a means of augmenting immune recognition in vivo.

Exposure to alpha or gamma interferon or alpha TNF in vitro can induce tumor cells to express increased levels of class I antigens (Hayashi et al. 1985; Tanaka et al. 1986). These tumor cells can be utilized in different ways to potentiate immune recognition. The modified tumor cells may be used with non-specific immune stimulators to actively immunize tumor-bearing patients or patients after surgical resection of a tumor. The data accumulated from murine transfection experiments suggest that immunization with high class I-expressors can protect animals from subsequent challenge by parental low class I expressors. Cytolytic T cells generated in the presence of high class I-expressing tumor cells may recognize the parental cells whose weak tumor antigens could not previously stimulate a CTL reaction in vivo.

High, but not low, class I-expressing murine sarcoma cells ordinarily act as good stimulators in an in vitro sensitization reaction with syngeneic splenocytes or lymph node cells from tumor-bearing mice (Shu et al. 1986). Incubation of tumor-bearer lymphocytes with high class I expressor tumor cells results in activation of lymphocytes that can be adoptively transferred to tumor-bearing mice and have potent anti-tumor activity when administered with IL-2 (Shu et al. 1985). A strategy to improve the anti-tumor effect of in vitro sensitized lymphocytes might involve addition of interferon-treated tumor cells to the lymphocyte/tumor reaction in order to boost immune reactivity. Conceivably, draining lymph node cells from target-bearing patients can be exposed to tumor cells treated in short term in vitro culture with alpha or gamma interferon to induce class I expression. Interferon-treated tumor cells may act as better stimulators for the in vitro sensitization reaction, resulting in specific, potent cytolytic cells.

Tumor-infiltrating lymphocytes (TILs) have been shown to proliferate when incubated in vitro in the presence of autologous tumor and IL-2, and are capable of anti-tumor activity in vitro, as well as in vivo after adoptive transfer in mice and humans (Rosenberg et al. 1986). Addition of autologous tumor cells with augmented class I expression to the incubation mixture may improve the proliferation and cytolytic activity of TILs. The murine TIL population is composed almost exclusively of Lyt-2^+ T cells. Improved recognition of poorly immunogenic tumor antigens via association with increased class I molecules may select a TIL subpopulation that reacts more strongly and specifically with tumor determinants.

The interferons or alpha TNF may function in vivo to modulate class I antigen expression, in which case they would represent an excellent priming treatment prior to tumor resection for TIL preparation or prior to immunotherapy with TILs and IL-2. Exposure of the TIL population to tumor cells with increased class I expression ex vivo during proliferation and in vivo after adoptive transfer may maximize their anti-tumor potency. A tumor with class I expression induced in vivo by interferons may become more immunogenic, attracting more infiltrating lymphocytes that are capable of specifically recognizing tumor antigens and exerting an anti-tumor effect after expansion with IL-2 and adoptive transfer.

The transfer of new genetic information to tumor cells by DNA transfection may have important implications for human immunotherapy. Increased expression of HLA class I or II antigens in human tumor cells in short term culture or as tumor lines may be achieved by transfection of HLA genes. Stable HLA transfectants may function as strong stimulators in an in vitro sensitization with lymphocytes from tumor-bearing patients or with TILs from a low class

I-expressing tumor. A product of a single gene may be up-regulated by DNA transfection, whereas alpha or gamma interferon may induce the expression of multiple gene products, not all of which may cause increased immunogenicity or better immune recognition. The use of alpha or gamma interferon in vitro in a TIL/tumor cell culture may also affect lymphocyte activation directly, whereas modulation of HLA expression by transfection only impacts directly on the target cell.

The adenovirus-derived proteins that down-regulate class I gene expression may be useful in vitro to eliminate class I antigens on cloned potent allo-geneic human LAK cells that can be grown and purified in large quantities and may constitute a 'universal donor' cell while leaving its capability to recognize and lyse tumor cells intact. The availability of an 'off the shelf' LAK effector would eliminate patient-to-patient variability in numbers of cells generated and anti-tumor potency.

A decreased level of MHC class I expression by tumor cells has an important effect on their ability to grow and metastasize in an immunocompetent host. This effect is achieved through decreased immunogenicity and escape from recognition and destruction by cytolytic T cells. The ability to specifically modulate MHC class I gene expression may improve the clonotypic T cell receptor interaction with tumor antigens, leading to proliferation in vitro of specific cytolytic lymphocytes capable of eliminating tumor cells in vivo with heterogeneous MHC expression. As our definition of tumor-associated antigens and molecules that determine susceptibility to various immunotherapies improves, the ability to modulate specific target genes will yield enormous dividends in tumor regression. Up-regulation of tumor class I genes is a step in that direction.

REFERENCES

Ascher A, Mule JJ, Weber JS, Krosnick J, Rosenberg SA. (unpublished results)

Bahler DW, Lond EM. (1985) Dimethyl sulfoxide induces expression of H-2 antigens on mouse lung carcinoma cells. J Immunol 134: 2790.

Baker DW, Frelinger JG, Harwell LW, Lord EM. (1987) Reduced tumorigenicity of a spontaneous mouse lung carcinoma following H-2 gene transfection. Proc Natl Acad Sci USA 84: 4562

Bernards R, Dessain SK, Weinberg RA. (1986) N-myc amplification causes down-modulation of MHC class I antigen expression in neuroblastoma. Cell 47: 667

Burgert HG, Kvist S. (1985) An adenovirus type 2 glycoprotein blocks cell surface expression of human histocompatibility class I antigens. Cell 41: 987.

Csiba A, Whitwell HL, Moore M. (1984) Distribution of histocompatibility and leucocyte differentiation antigens in normal human colon and in benign and malignant colonic neoplasms. Br J Cancer 50: 699

Daar AS, Fuggle SU, Fabre JW, Ting A, Morris PJ. (1984) The detailed description of HLA-A, -B and -C antigens in normal human organs. Transplant 38: 287

Dailey MO, Pillemer E, Weissman IL. (1984) Protection against syngeneic lymphoma by a long lived cytotoxic T cell alone. Proc Natl Acad Sci USA 79: 5384

Donohue JH, Rosenstein M, Chang AE, Lotze MT, Robb RJ, Rosenberg SA. (1984) The systemic administration of purified interleukin-2 enhances the ability of sensitized murine lymphocytes to cure a disseminated syngeneic lymphoma. J Immunol 132: 2123

Doyle A, Martin WJ, Funa K, Gazdar A, Carney D, Martin SE, Linnoila I, Cuttita F, Mulshine J, Binon P, Minna J. (1985) Markedly decreased expression of class I histocompatibility antigens, protein and mRNA in human small cell lung cancer. J Exp Med 161: 1135

Ferguson A, Moore M, Fox H. (1985) Expression of MHC products and leuco-cyte differentiation antigens in gynaecological neoplasms: An immunohis-tochemical analysis of the tumor cells and infiltrating lymphocytes. Br

J Cancer 52: 551

Fernandez–Cruz E, Ulich T, Schreiber RD. (1985) In vivo activity of lymphokine-activated macrophages in host defense against neoplasia. J Immunol 134: 3489

Festenstein H, Schmidt W. (1981) Variation in MHC antigenic profiles of tumor cells and its biologic effects. Immunol Rev 60: 85

Fidler IJ. (1974) Inhibitors of pulmonary metastases by intravenous injection of specifically activated macrophages. Cancer Res 34: 1074

Fleming KA, McMichaeal A, Morton JA, Woods J, McGee JOD. (1981) Distribution of HLA class I antigens in normal human tissue and in mammary cancer. Clin Path 34: 779

Fujiwara H, Fukuzawa M, Yoshioka T, Nakajima H, Hamaoka T. (1984) The role of tumor specific Lyt-1$^+$2$^-$ T cells in eradicating tumor cells in vivo. J Immunol 133: 1671

Fukusato T, Gerber MA, Thung ST, Ferrone S, Schaffner F. (1986) Expression of HLA class I antigens on hepatocytes in liver disease. Am J Pathol 123: 264

Gracomini P, Aguzzi A, Pestka S, Fisher PB, Ferrone S. (1984) Modulation by recombinant DNA leucocyte (alpha) and fibroblast (beta) interferons of the expression and shedding of HLA and tumor associated antigens by human melanoma cells. J Immunol 133: 1649

Greenberg PD, Kern DF, Cheever MA. (1985) Therapy of disseminated murine leukemia with cyclophosphamide and Lyt1$^+$2$^-$ T cells. J Exp Med 161: 1122

Grimm EA, Mazumder A, Zhang HZ, Rosenberg SA. (1982) Lymphokine activated killer phenomenon: lysis of natural killer-resistant fresh solid tumor cells by interleukin-2 activated autologous human peripheral blood lymphocytes. J Exp Med 155: 1823

Haddada H, Lewis AM, Sogn JA, Coligan JE, Cook JL, Walker TA, Levine AS. (1986) Tumorigenicity of hamster and mouse cells transformed by adenovirus types 2 and 5 is not influenced by the level of class I major histocompa tibility antigens expressed on the cells. Proc Natl Acad Sci USA 83: 9684

Halloran PF, Jephthah-Ochola J, Urmson J, Farkas S. (1985) Systemic immunologic stimuli increase class I and class II antigen expression in mouse kidney. J Immunol 135: 1053

Hart DNJ, Newton MR, Reece-Smith H, Fabne JW, Morris PJ. (1983) Major histocompatibility complex antigens in the rat pancreas, isolated pancreatic islets, and adrenal glands. Transplant 36: 431

Hayashi H, Tanaka K, Jay F, Khoury G, Jay G. (1985) Modulation of the tumorigenicity of human adenovirus-12 transformed cells by interferon. Cell 43: 263

Hood L, Steinmetz B, Malissen B. (1983) Genes of the major histocompatibility complex of the mouse. Ann Rev Immunol 1: 529

Hui K, Grosveld F, Festenstein H. (1984) Rejection of transplantable AKR leukaemia cells following MHC DNA-mediated cell transformation. Nature 311: 750

Israel A, Kimura A, Fournier A, Fellous M, Kourilsky P. (1986) Interferon response sequence potentiates activity of an enhancer in the promoter region of a mouse H-2 gene. Nature 322: 743

Jones EA, Bodmer WF. (1980) Lack of expression of HLA antigens on choriocarcinoma cell lines. Tissue Antigens 16: 195

Kawase I, Urdahl DL, Brooks CG, Henney CS. (1982) Selective depletion of NK cell activity in vivo and its effect on the growth of NK sensitive and NK resistant tumor cell variants. Int J Cancer 29: 567

Lampson LA, Fisher CA, Whelan JP. (1983) Striking paucity of HLA-A, B, and C and B$_2$-microglobulin on human neuroblastoma cell lines. J Immunol 130: 2471

Lindahl P, Leary P, Gresser I. (1973) Enhancement by interferon of the expression of surface antigens of murine leukemia L1210 cells. Proc Natl Acad Sci USA 70: 2785

Ljunggren HG, Karre K. (1985) Host resistance directed selectively against H-2 deficient lymphoma variants. Analysis of the mechanism. J Exp Med

162: 1745

Ljunggren HG, Karre K. (1986) Variations in MHC Antigen expression on tumors and its significance. Experimental strategies and interpretations in the analysis of changes in MHC gene expression during tumour progression opposing influences of T cell and natural killer mediated resistance. J Immunogenet 13: 141

Masucci MG, Torsteindottin S, Colombani J, Brautbai C, Klein E, Klein G. (1987) Down-regulation of class I HLA antigens and of the Epstein-Barr virus-encoded latent membrane protein in Burkett lymphoma lines. Proc Natl Acad Sci ÛSA 84: 4567

Momberg F, Degeher T, Bacchus E, Moldenhauer G, Hammerling GJ, Moller P. (1986) Loss of HLA-A, -B, -C and de novo expression of HLA-D in colorectal cancer. Int J Cancer 37: 179

Mule JJ, Yang JC, Shu S, Lafreniere R, Rosenberg SA. (1987) Identification of cellular mechanisms operational in vivo during the regression of established pulmonary metastases by the systemic administration of high-dose recombinant interleukin-2. J Immunol 139: 285

Mule JJ, Yang J, Shu S, Rosenberg SA. (1986) The antitumor efficacy of lymphokine-activated killer cells and recombinant interleukin-2 in vivo: Direct correlation between reduction of established metastases and cytolytic activity of lymphokine-activated killer cells. J Immunol 136: 3899

Nanni P, Colombo M, DeGiovanni C, Lollini P, Nicoletti G, Parmiani G, Prodi G. (1983) Impaired H-2 expression in BL6 melanoma variants. J Immunogenet 10: 361

Natali PG, Bigotti A, Cavaliere R, Liao S-K, Taniguchi M, Matsui M, Ferrone S. (1985) Heterogeneous expression of melanoma associated antigens and HLA antigens by primary and multiple metastatic lesions removed from patients with melanoma. Cancer Res 45: 2883

Natali PG, Bigotti A, Nicotra NR, Viona M, Manfredi D, Ferrone S. (1984) Distribution of human class I (HLA-A, -B, -C) histocompatibility antigens in normal and malignant tissues of non-lymphoid origin. Cancer Res 44: 4679

Paul LC, Paradyusz JM, Milford EM, Kunz HW, Carpenter CB. (1982) Expression of RT 1.A and RT 1.B/D antigens on endothelium of rat kidneys. Transplant 34: 121

Reuter DJ, Bergman W, Welaart K, Scheffer E, Van Vloten WA, Russo C, Ferrone S. (1984) Immunohistochemical analysis of malignant melanomas and nevocellular revi with monoclonal antibodies to distinct monomorphic determinants of HLA antigens. Cancer Res 44: 3930

Rogers M, Gooding LR, Margulies DH, Evans GA. (1983) Analysis of a defect in the H-2 genes of SV40 transformed C3H fibroblasts that do not express H-2K^k. J Immunol 130: 2418

Rosenberg SA, Lotze MT, Muul LM, Chang AE, Avis FP, Leitman S, Linehan WM, Robertson CN, Lee RE, Rubin JT, Seipp CA, Simpson CG, White DE. (1987) A progress report on the treatment of 157 patients with advanced cancer using lymphokine activated killer cells and interleukin-2 or high dose interleukin-2 alone. New Engl J Med 316: 891

Rosenstein M, Rosenberg SA. (1984) Generation of lytic and proliferative lymphoid clones to syngeneic tumor: in vitro and in vivo studies. J Natl Cancer Inst 72: 1161

Scheurich P, Kronke M, Schluter C, Ucer U, Pfizenmaier K. (1986) Non-cytocidal mechanisms of action of tumor necrosis factor on human tumor cells: enhancement of HLA gene expression synergistic with IFN-gamma. Immunobiol 172: 291

Schrier PI, Bernards R, Vaessen RTMJ, Houweling A, van der Eb AJ. (1983) Expression of class I major histocompatibility antigens switched off by highly oncogenic adenovirus 12 in transformed rat cells. Nature 305: 771

Seigler HD, Kremer WB, Metzgar RS, Ward FE, Hwang AT, Amos DB. (1971) HLA antigenic loss in malignant transformation. J Natl Cancer Inst 46: 577

Shiloni E, Lafreniere R, Mule JJ, Schwarz SL, Rosenberg SA. (1986) Effect of immunotherapy with allogeneic lymphokine-activated killer cells and recombinant interleukin-2 on established pulmonary and hepatic metastases in mice. Cancer Res 46: 5633 .

Smith KA. (1980) T-cell growth factor. Immunol Rev 51: 337

Solter D, Shevinsky L, Knowles BB, Strickland S. (1979) The induction of antigenic changes in a teratocarcinoma stem cell line (F9) by retinoic acid. Develop Biol 70: 515

Talmadge JE, Myers KM, Prieur DJ, Starkley JR. (1980) Role of NK cells in tumor growth and metastases in beige mice. Nature 284: 622

Tanaka K, Hayashi H, Hamada C, Khoury G, Jay G. (1986) Expression of major histocompatibility complex class I antigens as a strategy for the potentiation of immune recognition of tumor cells. Proc Natl Acad Sci USA 83: 8723

Tanaka K, Isselbacher KJ, Khoury G, Jay G. (1984) Reversal of oncogenesis by the expression of a major histocompatibility complex class I gene. Science 228: 26

Tanaka K, Yoshioka T, Bieberich C, Jay G (1988) Role of the MHC class I antigens in tumor growth and metastasis. Ann. Rev. Immunol. (in press).

Turbitt ML, Mackie RM. (1981) Loss of beta-2-microglobulin from the cell surface of cutaneous malignant and premalignant lesions. Brit J Dermatol 104: 507

Wallich R, Bulbuc N, Hammerling GJ, Katsav S, Segal S, Feldman M. (1985) Abrogation of metastatic properties of tumour cells by de novo expression of H-2K antigens following H-2 gene transfection. Nature 315: 301

Weber JS, Jay G, Tanaka K, Rosenberg SA. (1987) Immunotherapy of a murine tumor with interleukin-2: increased sensitivity after MHC class I gene transfection. J Exp Med (in press)

Yague J, White J, Coleclough C, Kappala J, Palmer E, Marrack P. (1985) The T cell receptor: the alpha and beta chains define idiotype, antigen and MHC specificity. Cell 42: 81

Zinkernagel RM, Doherty PC. (1979) MHC restricted cytotoxic T cells: studies on the biological role of polymorphic major transplantation antigens determining T-cell restriction-specificity, function and responsiveness. Adv Immunol 27: 51

Identification of Regulatory Elements Associated with a Class I MHC Gene

D.S. Singer and R. Ehrlich

INTRODUCTION

The class I genes of the major histocompatibility complex (MHC) comprise a family of homologous DNA sequences, some of which encode the heavy chain moiety of classical transplantation antigens. The major functions of the transplantation antigens are mediation of graft rejection and serving as restriction elements for antigen presentation (Klein, 1979; Klein, 1975; Klein, 1977). Although class I molecules are expressed on all nucleated cells, with the exception of neurons and mature trophoblasts (Faulk et al, 1977; Lampson et al, 1983), their level of expression varies. Lymphoid cells express the highest levels, while other tissues express much lower amounts. Exogenous and endogenous factors, such as tumor necrosis factor, α/β-interferon or γ-interferon (Burrone & Milstein, 1982; Collins et al, 1986; Imai et al, 1981; Lindhal et al, 1973; Satz & Singer, 1984; Wallach et al, 1982) increase the levels of class I expression, whereas other agents, such as oncogenic viruses (Meruelo et al, 1984; Schrier et al, 1983), cause reduction in these levels.

In both mouse and man, the class I MHC gene families contain between 20 and 40 homologous DNA sequences (Cohen et al, 1983; Orr et al, 1982; Steinmetz et al, 1982; Weiss et al, 1984). In contrast, the genome of the miniature swine, unlike mouse or man, consists of only 7 members (Singer et al, 1982; Singer et al, 0). One of these genes, PD1, encodes a classical transplantation antigen. PD1 has been isolated (Singer et al, 1982), and its structure determined (Satz et al, 1985). Introduction of PD1 into mouse L cells results cell surface expression of the PD1-encoded product (Singer et al, 1982). PD1 expression in mouse L cells is regulated and transcription is enhanced by treatment of transfected L cells with α/β-interferon (Satz & Singer, 1983; Satz & Singer, 1984). Introduction of PD1 into transgenic mice results in cell surface expression of the gene product in a variety of lymphoid tissues (Frels et al, 1985).

The molecular mechanisms regulating class I MHC gene expression are largely unknown. The transcriptional promoter and DNA sequence elements involved in the interferon response have been identified in some cases (Friedman & Stark, 1985; Kimura et al, 1986; Israel et al, 1986; Korber et al, 1987). An enhancer element has also been identified in the murine K^b gene (Kimura et al, 1986). In order to further characterize the regulatory elements associated with class I MHC genes, we have undertaken a detailed analysis of the in vivo patterns of expression and regulation of expression of PD1. In the present paper, we will summarize the evidence that expression of PD1 is regulated both in vivo and in the transgenic mouse and that the PD1 5' flanking sequences contain both positive and negative regulatory elements.

RESULTS AND DISCUSSION

Expression of PD1 In Vivo and in Transgenic Mice

PD1 is expressed in transgenic mice and in swine in a variety of tissues, as shown in Table I. In both cases, the over-all patterns of expression are similar. Thus,

Immunology Branch, NCI, NIH, Bldg. 10, Room 4B-17, Bethesda, Md. 20892

Current Topics in Microbiology and Immunology, Vol. 137
© Springer-Verlag Berlin · Heidelberg 1988

expression of PD1 is highest in lymphoid tissues, such as lymph node and spleen and much lower in kidney and heart. Expression in other tissues is intermediate. In vivo, PD1 is preferentially expressed in B cells, relative to T cells. Recent data suggest that the same bias is seen in transgenic animals as well (Ehrlich and Singer, in preparation). The variations in level of PD1 RNA in the different tissues indicate that PD1 expression is actively regulated. Furthermore, the parallel patterns of expression of PD1 observed in vivo and in transgenic animals suggest that any trans acting regulatory elements have been sufficiently conserved between the species to allow regulation of a porcine gene in a mouse cell.

Table 1. Expression of PD1 In Vivo and in Transgenic Mice[a]

Tissue	Swine	B10.PD1
Kidney	1	1
Heart	2	0.1
Testis	1.3	3.9
Liver	1.7	ND
Lung	3.8	2.7
Lymph Node	5.2	12.9
Thymus	1.8	3.0
Spleen	3.7	10.8
PBL	11.4	ND
B cells	4.8	ND
T cells	1.8	ND
Bone Marrow	ND	3.5
Muscle	ND	0.7

[a]Levels of specific RNA were determined for the transgenic (B10.PD1) RNA samples by direct Northern analysis and for swine tissue RNA samples by S1 nuclease analysis using a DNA probe which had been shown to be PD1-specific. Intensities of specific bands were determined by densitometry. RNA samples from the tissues were processed in parallel, using the same hybridizing probe. The data presented are the average values of two experiments using separate RNA preparations. Data have been normalized to the intensity of the kidney specific bands. ND, not determined.

Identification and Mapping of Regulatory DNA Sequence Elements in the 5' Flanking Region of PD1.

In order to identify regulatory DNA sequence elements governing the in vivo patterns of expression of PD1, a series of deletion mutants was constructed within the 5' end of PD1 (Figure 1). The 5' termini of the mutants were located either at a Hind III site at -1121 (pH series) or at an Nde I site at -528 (pN series). A nested set of deletions (spanning nucleotides +15 to -236) was generated by Bal 31 exonuclease digestion. The deletion mutants were cloned into the promoter assay vector, pSVOCAT, which lacks eukaryotic promoters or enhancers, and tested for their ability to promote the synthesis of chloramphenicol acetyl transferase (CAT) following transfection into either mouse L cells or monkey Cos-7 cells. Using these constructs, the PD1 promoter can be mapped to the region between -220 bp and -38 bp (Table 2). Thus, a construct containing this region is able to promote CAT synthesis; more extensive deletions do not support CAT synthesis. This is true for both transient and stable transfectants of mouse L cells. Similar results were obtained with Cos-7 cells (data not shown). Contained within this region of the DNA are three sequence elements which have been associated with promoter function in other gene systems (Dierks et al, 1983). These elements are TCTAA, CCAAT, and ACCC; it is presumed that these elements function as necessary components of the PD1 promoter.

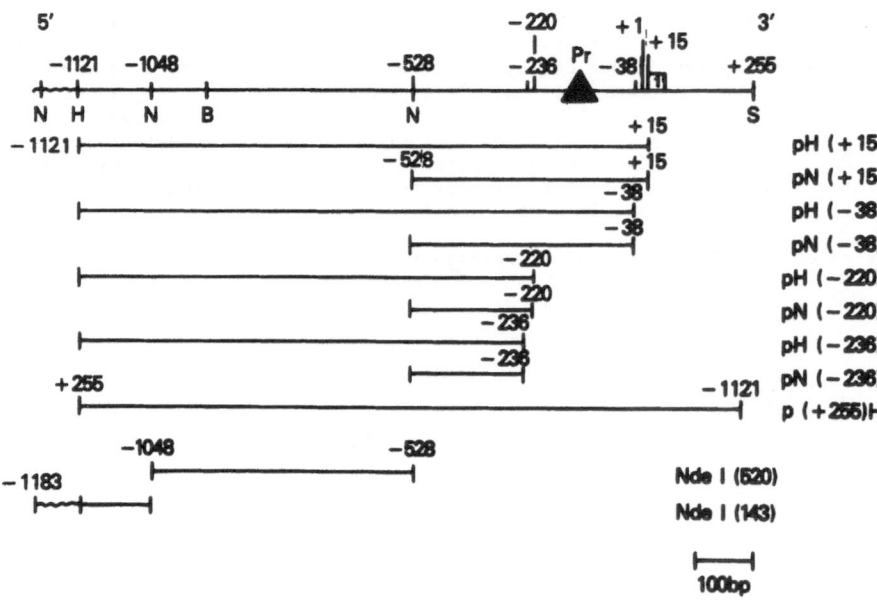

Figure 1. Map of DNA sequence of PD1 5' flanking region. DNA deletion fragments
containing PD1 5' flanking sequence, indicated by a solid line, were
inserted into the Hind III site of pSV0. Solid triangle indicates position
of promoter. N, Nde I; H, Hind III; B, Bgl II; S, Sac I.

Table 2. Mapping of the PD1 Promoter[a].

	DNA:	pH(-38)	pH(-220)	pH(-236)	pH(+255)	pSV0
Transfection:						
Transient		4.2+2	1.2+0.03	1.2+0.03	0	1
Stable						
Net Activity		2.0+0.03	0	ND	0	1
DNA Copy Number		13	6	ND	14	29
CAT Activity/copy		15	0	ND	0	3
(x 102)						

[a]Each of the deletion mutants was introduced into mouse L cells, either in transient
or stable transfections. CAT activity was assayed and quantitated by densitometry.
The transient transfection results are from 5 separate experiments; the stable transfections are from 3 separate experiments. In the transient assay, an aliquot of cells
from each transfection was used to determine the amount of DNA present; there was no
detectable difference in the gross level of DNA among the different transfections.

PD1 has been shown to respond to treatment by α/β-interferon: treatment of PD1-
transfected L cells with α/β-interferon results in increased transcription of the PD1
gene (Satz & Singer, 1984). The ability of PD1 to respond to interferon can be mapped
to a region between -38 bp and -528 bp, since both pH(-38) and pN(-38), which is

truncated an Nde I site (see Figure 1), are able to respond to interferon (Table 3). The magnitude of this increase, although relatively modest, corresponds to that seen on the surface of PD1-transfectants. Thus, all of the interferon response can be accounted for by sequences contained within this region. That the response is pro- moter dependent and specific is seen by the findings that none of the promoter- deleted constructs respond to interferon, nor does the SV40 promoter contained in pSV1.

Table 3. Mapping of the Interferon Response Element and Negative Regulatory Element

DNA	CAT Activity[a]	Ratio of CAT Activity +IFN/-IFN[b]
pN(-38)	8.9	1.6
pH(-38)	1.0	1.5
pN(+15)	4.5	1.4
pH(+15)	0.8	1.4
pN(-236)	1.2	ND
pH(-236)	2.0	ND
pH(-220)	ND	0
p(+255)H	0	0
pSV0	1.4	ND
pSV1	ND	1.0

[a]CAT activity was assayed following a 48 hour transfection of Cos cells with 1 ug of plasmid DNA. Densitometric results were normalized to pH(-38). Representative results of one of five experiments are given.
[b]Stably transfected L cells were treated for 24 hours with 800 u/ml α/β-interferon. Ratios of CAT activities in treated and untreated samples were determined following densitometry and represent the average of three experiments.

In addition to the interferon response element (IRE), we have identified two addition regulatory elements: a positive and a negative one. The positive element increases the activity of an SV40 promoter and appears to be a classical enhancer (Ehrlich et al, submitted for publication). In contrast, the negative element reduces the acti- vity of the homologous PD1 promoter. As shown in Table 3, the plasmid pN(-38) gener- ates approximately 9 times the CAT activity as the parent pH(-38) plasmid from which it is derived. A similar increase in CAT activity is observed following truncation of the pH(+15) plasmid. No effect is observed following truncation of the promoterless construct, pH(-236), indicating that this effect is PD1-promoter dependent. These data suggest that the DNA segment -1120 bp to -528bp contains a negative regulatory element which reduces the activity of the PD1 promoter. This has been confirmed by demonstrating that cells transfected with pH(-38) contain lower steady state levels of CAT RNA than pN(-38) transfectants (data not shown). Furthermore, introduction of the -1120 bp to -528 bp segment upstream of the SV40 promoter also reduces the activity of that promoter. However, this reduction is only observed if the viral enhancer is contained within the construct (Ehrlich et al, submitted). Thus, the activity of the PD1 negative regulatory element is dependent on the presence of a postive enhancer element.

Cell Specificity of PD1 Promoter and Negative Regulatory Element

The level of PD1 gene expression was been shown to vary among adult tissues both in vivo and in transgenic mice (Table 1). To begin to assess the possible role of the PD1 5' region in regulating cell-specific levels of expression, the PD1CAT constructs were transfected into various adult and embryonic cell lines. The efficiency of the PD1 promoter was compared among two fibroblast lines (L and ETH21), a kidney-derived line (Cos 7), and an embryonic teratocarcinoma (F9). Striking differences in the levels of CAT activity directed by the PD1 promoter were observed (Table 4). Since the different cells displayed very different efficiencies of transfection, the amount of CAT activity directed by the PD1 promoter was standardized relative to the background level of pSVO. pSVO, although lacking a eucaryotic promoter, still promotes low level CAT transcription from a cryptic promoter located within the pBR322 DNA sequences. This promoter is not affected by eucaryotic regulatory elements. Rather, the amount of CAT activity directed by pSVO is proportional to the amount of transfected DNA and is largely independent of any tissue specificity of the promoter (data not shown). When compared following such standardization, the efficiencies of the PD1 promoter, as assessed by pN(-38), in the various cell lines differed substantially. The highest promoter activity was observed in fibroblast L cells, whereas the lowest level occurred in the kidny-derived Cos cells. F9 teratocarcinoma cells express low levels of endogenous class I H-2 mRNA. Introduction of pN(-38) in F9 cells similarly resulted in low levels of CAT activity. Treatment of F9 cells with retinoic acid induces cell differentiation; concomitantly, class I H-2 expression increases twofold. Following treatment of F9 cells with retinoic acid, the level of CAT activity directed by pN(-38) also increased two-fold. Microscopic examination of these treated F9 cells revealed the presence of embryoid bodies. Cell surface analysis by FACS of these cells revealed a two-fold increase in H-2 expression. Thus, the response of the exogenous PD1 promoter to the induction of differentiation of the F9 cells is indistinguishable from that of the endogenous H-2 genes. Taken together, these results suggest that the 490 bp DNA fragment containing the PD1 promoter displays different levels of transcription in different cell types.

Table 4. Efficiency of PD1 Promoter and Repressor Elements in Various Cell Types[a].

Cell Line	Origin	Species	pN(-38)	pH(-38)	N/H
L Cells	Fibroblast	Mouse	100	27	3.7
F9	Teratocarcinoma	"	32	4.9	6.7
F9RA	"	"	65	8.6	7.5
Cos 7	Kidney	Monkey	19	2.7	7.0
ETH21	Fibroblast	Pig	N.D.	222	N.D.

[a]The relative efficiency of transcription of each of the PD1CAT fusion plasmids in the various cell types was determined by correcting its activity relative to that of pSVO in the same cell line. The table summarizes the results of 2-5 separate experiments for each cell type. N/H column represents the relative activity of pN to pH fusion plasmids. F9RA = F9 cells treated with retinoic acid and cAMP.

The ability of the PD1 negative regulatory element to function in these various cell types was assessed by comparing the relative CAT activities directed by pH(-38), which contains the negative element with those of pN(-38), which does not (Table 4). In all of the cell types examined, the presence of the negative element reduces the amount of CAT activity generated. The magnitude of the inhibitory effect varies somewhat, suggesting that the negative element may function with different efficiencies in different cell types. The extent to which this reflects cell specificity, as opposed to species specificity, remains to be determined.

The in vivo function of the PD1 negative regulatory element is unknown. When tested in cell lines derived from different lineages, the magnitude of the suppression observed varies by two0fold. Whether these are biologically significant differences remains to be established. However, the greatest reduction is observed in kideny-derived Cos cells. The in vivo level of expression of PD1 in the kidney is one of the lowest observed. Nevertheless, it is clear the the negative regulatory element alone does not regulate PD1 expression. Rather, the cumulative activities of the negative and positive elements, as well as the promoter are probably responsible. Further detailed analysis of the 5' flanking region of PD1, as well as other SLA genes which display distinct patterns of expression, should contribute significantly to an understanding of the mechanisms regulating class I gene expression.

REFERENCES

Burrone OH and Milstein C (1982) Control of HLA-A, B, C synthesis and expression in interferon treated cells, EMBO Journal 1:345-349

Cohen D, Paul P, Font M, Cohen O, Sayagh B, Marcadet A, Busson M, Majory G, Cann H and Dausset J (1983) Analysis of HLA class I genes with restriction endonuclease fragments. Implications for polymorphism of the human major histocompatibility complex, Proc Natl Acad Science (USA) 80:6289-6292

Collins T, Lapierre LA, Fiers W, Strominger JL and Pober JS (1986) Recombinant human tumor necrosis factor increases mRNA levels and surface expression of HLA-A,B antigens in vascular endothelial cells and dermal fibroblasts in vitro, Proc Natl Acad Sciences (USA) 83:446-450

Dierks P, Van Ooyen A, Chochran MD, Dobkin C, Reiser J and Weissman C (1983) Three regions upstream from the cap site are requied for efficient and accurate transcription of the rabbit beta globin gene in mouse 3T6 cells, Cell 32:695-706

Faulk WD, Sanderson AR and Temple A (1977) Distribution of MHC antigens in human placental chorionic villi, Transplant Proc 9:1379-1384

Frels WI, Bluestone JA, Hodes R, Capecchi M and Singer DS (1985) Expression of a microinjected porcine class I MHC gene in transgenic mice, Science 228:577-580

Friedman RL and Stark GR (1985) Alpha interferon induces transcription of HLA and metallothionein genes which have homologous upstream sequences, Nature 314:637-639

Imai K, Pellegrino MA, Ng AK and Ferron S (1981) Role of antigen density in immune lysis of interferon-treated human lymphoid cells, Scand J Immunol 14:529-535

Israel A, Kimura A, Fournier A, Fellous M and Kourilsky P (1986) Interferon response sequence potentiates activity of an enhancer in the promoter region of a mouse H-2 gene, Nature 322:743-746

Kimura A, Israel A, LeBail O and Kourilsky P (1986) Detailed analysis of the mouse H-2K^b promoter: Enhancer-like sequences and their role in the regulation of class I gene expression, Cell 44:261-272

Klein J (1975) Biology of the mouse histocompatibility complex Springer Verlag, New York

Klein J (1977) In Gotze E Major Histocompatibility Complex Springer Verlag, New York

Klein J (1979) The major histocompatibility complex of the mouse, Science 203:516:521

Korber B, Hood L and Stroynowski I (1987) Regulation of murine class I genes by interferons is controlled by regions located both 5' and 3' to the transcriptional initiation site, Proc Natl Acad Sciences (USA) 84:3380-3384

Lampson LA, Fisher CA and Whelan JP (1983) Striking paucity of HLA-ABC and beta$_2$-microglobulin on human neuroblastoma cell lines, J Immunol 130:2471-2478

Lindhal P, Leary P and Gresser I (1973) Enhancement by interferon of the expression of histocompatibility antigens of mouse lymphoid cells, Eur J Immunol 4:779-784

Meruelo D, Kornreich R, Rossomondo A, Pampeno C, Mellor AL, Weis EH, Flavell RA and Pellicer A (1984) Murine leukemia virus sequences are encoded in the murine MHC, Proc Natl Acad Sciences (USA) 81:1804-1808

Orr H, Bach R, Ploegh H, Strominger JL, Kavathas P and DeMars R (1982) Use of HLA
    loss mutants to analyse the structure of the human MHC, Nature 296:454-456
Satz ML and Singer DS (1983) Differential Expression of Porcine Major
    Histocompatibility DNA Sequences Introduced into Mouse L cells, Molec Cell Biol
    3:2006-2016
Satz M and Singer DS (1984) Effect of mouse interferon on the expression of the
    porcine MHC gene introduced into mouse L-cells, J Immunol 132:496-501
Satz M, Wang LC, Singer DS and Rudikoff S (1985) Structure and expression of two
    porcine genomic clones encoding class I MHC antigens, J Immunol 135:2167-2175
Schrier P, Bernard R, Vaseen MJ, Howeling AH and Vander Eb AJ (1983) Expression of
    class I MHC switched off by highly oncogenic adenovirus 12 in transformed rat
    cells, Nature 305:771-775
Singer Dinah S, Ehrlich R, Golding H, Satz L, Parent L and Rudikoff S   no year
    Structure and expression of class I MHC genes in the miniature swine, In Warner C,
    Rothschild M and Lamont S Molecular Biology of the Major Histocompatibility
    Complex of Domestic Animal Species Iowa State University press
Singer DS, Camerini-Otero M, Satz M, Osborne B, Sachs D and Rudikoff S (1982)
    Characterization of a porcine genomic clone encoding a major transplantation
    antigen; expression in mouse L-cells, Proc Natl Acad Sciences (USA) 79:1403-1407
Steinmetz M, Winoto A, Minard K and Hood L (1982) Clustering of genes encoding mouse
    transplantation antigens, Cell 28:489-498
Wallach DM, Fellous M and Revel M (1982) Preferential effect of gamma interferon on
    the synthesis of HLA antigens and their mRNA's in human cells, Nature 299:833-836
Weiss EH, Golden L, Fahrner K, Mellor A, Devlin H, Tiddens H, Bud H and Flavell RA
    (1984) Organization and evolution of the class I gene family in the MHC of the
    C57BL/10 mouse, Nature 310:650-655

Tind, Tsu and Tthy form a Trimolecular Complex Encoded Within the Tsu Locus on Chromosome 12 of the Mouse

G.M. Peterman, R. Singhai, A. Dean, and F.L. Owen

INTRODUCTION

Greater than 90% of AKR mice spontaneously develop thymic lymphomas by 8-10 months of age (Gross 1977). Thymic leukemia in these mice is caused by mink cell focus-forming (MCF) viruses that arise by recombination between ecotropic and nonecotropic MuLV (Hartley 1977). Although up to 90% of thymocytes in the preleukemic AKR mice may be infected by MCF viruses, as manifested by viral antigen expression, AKR thymomas have been reported to originate from only one clone of thymocytes (Pederson 1980; Chattopadhyay 1982). Therefore, infection and replication of these viruses in an immature thymocyte does not necessarily lead to transformation, and a particular leukemia-susceptible subpopulation of thymocytes may exist which represents the target cells of transformation by these polytropic viruses.

As an approach to identify such a target-cell population, we examined AKR thymic leukemias using monoclonal antibodies specific for a series of alloantigens encoded by genes distal to the immunoglobulin (Igh-1) locus on chromosome 12 (Owen 1983). These antibodies recognize products of multiple linked genes which are expressed by thymus-derived lymphocytes at characteristic stages of development.

In the present report we show in a series of immunoprecipitation studies that Igh-1 linked T-cell alloantigens encoded by the Tsu region are expressed by AKR thymic leukemias. These results suggest that the cell susceptible to leukemogenesis may lie within the subset of T cells which express these determinants and will be useful in the design of strategies for cloning the genes encoding these proteins.

MATERIALS AND METHODS

Source of Cells

AKRL tumor cells were adapted to in vitro growth by H. Hiai (Aichi Cancer Center Research Institute, Nagoya, Japan). Briefly, cell lines were established from spontaneous thymic leukemias in AKR/Ms mice by removal of leukemic thymus fragments as previously described (Kaneshima 1983).

Metabolic Labeling

Cells were labeled with [^{35}S]methionine as previously described.[1] Usually 1x10^7 cells in log phase were washed and resuspended in 1-2 ml of methionine free media for 1 hour at 37°C. [^{35}S]methionine (200-400 uCi, S.A. = 1120 Ci/mmol, NEN, Boston, MA) was then added and the

---

Department of Pathology, Tufts University School of Medicine, Boston, MA 02111

cells incubated an additional 3-4 hours at 37°C with occasional
shaking. The cell pellet was washed in PBS containing 0.02% NaN3 and
2 mg cold methionine/ml and then lysed by the addition of 1-2 ml cold
lysis buffer. After ultracentrifugation at 35,000 rpm for 30 min at
4°C (Beckman model L3-50 ultracentrifuge with a 50 Ti head) the
supernatant was collected and used for immunoprecipitation.

Subcellular Fractionation

Cells to be fractionated were washed in PBS and resuspended in 0.5 ml
cold 10 mM Tris, pH 7.4 containing 1 mM $MgCl_2$ and 1 mM KCL. The cells
were subjected to 2 cycles of freeze-thawing and an additional 0.5 ml
of the above buffer was added. The suspension was then centrifuged at
800 xG for 15 minutes at 4°C, the supernatant was removed, an
additional 0.5 ml Tris buffer was added to the cell pellet, and the
suspension was recentrifuged. This step was repeated twice and 0.8 ml
of Tris buffer was added to the final pellet which contained the cell
nuclei. The pooled supernatants were then centrifuged at 100,000 x G
for 1 hour at 4°C (Beckman L3-50 Preparative Ultracentrifuge). The
supernatant contained cell cytosol; cell membranes were obtained by
resuspending the pellet in lysis buffer. In order to assess the
purity of isolated subcellular components, 5'-nucleotidase and lactic
dehydrogenase (LDH) activity was analyzed in each fraction (Quigley
1976).

Iodination of Subcellular Fractions

Subcellular fractions were isolated from log phase cells. Isolated
membranes, cytosol and nuclei were then labeled with ^{125}I by the
iodogen bead method. Briefly, 0.5 mCi [125]I (high pH, high
concentration, S.A. = 17.4 Ci/mg, NEN Products, Boston, MA) was added
to each subcellular component in a total volume of 0.4-0.6 ml 10 mM
Tris, pH 7.4 containing 1 mM $MgCl_2$ and 1 mM KCL. Two iodobeads
(Pierce Chemical Co., Rockford, IL) were added to each subcellular
fraction and all fractions were placed on a rocker platform for 1 hour
at 4°C. The beads were then removed and 200-400 ul of each fraction
was immunoprecipitated as described below.

Immunoprecipitations

Radiolabeled whole cell lysates, subcellular fractions or cell free
supernatants were immunoprecipitated as previously described.[2]
Briefly, affinity purified monoclonal antibodies specific for Tsu
linked alloantigens were added to radiolabeled cell fractions for
16-18 hours at 4°C. In most experiments 12-25 ug/ml affinity purified
monoclonal antibody was added to radiolabeled cell lysates or
subcellular fractions. Isotype identical negative control antibodies
used included anti-Thy 1.2 (uk), myeloma proteins MOPC-21 (γ_1 k) and
TEPC-183 (uk). In some experiments, polyclonal goat anti-MuLV gp70
was used as a positive control. Fifteen microliters of affinity
purified rabbit anti-mouse Ig (Jackson Immunoresearch, Avondale, PA)
was then added to each cell extract for 2 hours at 4°C followed by the
addition of Protein A beads (Sigma) for 2 hours at 4°C on a rocker
platform. The beads were then washed 3 times in cold lysis buffer and
boiled for 5 minutes in the presence of 2x sample buffer (0.125M
Tris-HCl, pH 6.8, 4% SDS, 20% glycerol, 10% 2-mercaptoethanol, 0.004%

bromphenol blue). All samples were then centrifuged for 10 minutes and the supernatants were analyzed by SDS-PAGE.

Peptide Mapping

Limited proteolysis was performed by the method of Cleveland (1977). Briefly, individual polypeptides identified after iodination and immunoprecipitation with anti-Tthy, anti-Tind or anti-Tsu were analyzed by SDS-PAGE and cut from the dried gel. Each piece was then rehydrated in sample buffer for 1 hour at room temperature and individual pieces containing equal CPM were analyzed by SDS-PAGE either in the absence or presence of Staphylococcus aureus V8 protease (Miles Labs).

Silver Stain

Supernatants were collected from cell lines incubated overnight in serum-free media. The supernatants were then concentrated and aliquots of concentrated supernatant were immunoprecipitated with anti-Tind or a negative control antibody and analyzed by SDS-PAGE. The gels were then visualized after silver staining (Bio-Rad).

RESULTS AND DISCUSSION

Owen and co-workers (Owen 1983) have identified a cluster of murine T cell specific genes approximately 4 map units distal to the Igh locus and proximal to the locus for serum prealbumin on chromosome 12 (Fig. 1).

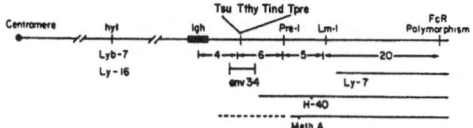

Figure 1 and Legend: Map of chromosome 12 of the mouse demonstrating the map position of the Tsu region and the presumed retroviral insertion site env 34 which may act as an LTR for Tsu region molecules.

This gene complex has been designated Tsu (Owen 1983) and the protein products of this locus have been identified by monoclonal antibodies derived following immunization of Balb/C mice with T cells from the Igh allotype congenic strain C.AL-20 as previous described (Owen 1983). More recently, we have demonstrated that spontaneous leukemia in AKR mice results in the transformation of thymocytes which express elevated levels of Tsu gene products (Owen and Peterman 1984). In the present report we identify the protein products of this gene complex and present evidence that these proteins may be the products of separate genes which form a trimolecular complex.

The results shown in Fig. 2 indicate that monoclonal anti-Tthy and anti-Tind recognize similar components present on plasma membranes obtained from AKR thymus and the cloned AKR thymic leukemia cell 92.1.

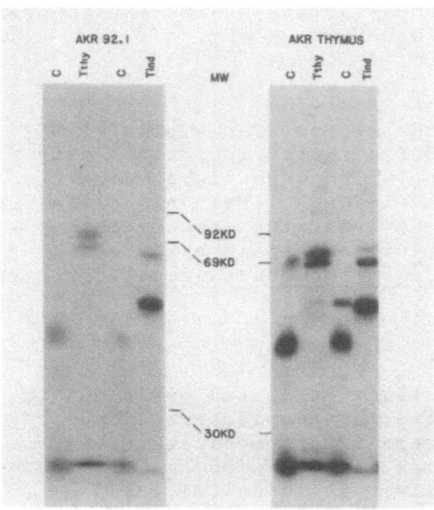 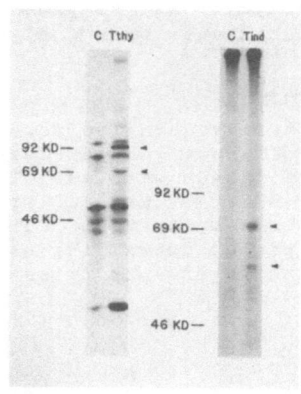

Figure 2 and Legend: SDS-PAGE of 6-month-old AKR thymus and the
cloned AKR cell line 92.1.   Plasma membranes were obtained by
alternate cycles of freeze-thawing, labeled with ^{125}I and
immunoprecipitated with anti-Tthy, anti-Tind or isotype identical
negative control antibodies.   Immunoprecipitates were analyzed on 12%
acrylamide gels under reducing conditions.

Figure 3 and Legend: SDS-PAGE of AKR thymic leukemias 79 and 225.
Cells (1×10^7) were labeled with (^{35}S)-methionine for 3 hours at 37°C.
The cells were then washed and lysed as described.   Cell lysates were
immunoprecipitated with anti-Tthy, anti-Tind or an isotype matched
negative control and analyzed by SDS-PAGE under reducing conditions ol
12% acrylamide gels.

Anti-Tthy immunoprecipitates polypeptides of 69-72 Kd, and anti-Tind
weakly recognizes a polypeptide of similar mobility on SDS-PAGE and a
second polypeptide of 52 Kd.   These results were obtained by
immunoprecipitation of iodinated plasma membranes.   Similar results
were obtained by metabolic labeling and SDS-PAGE of AKR thymic
leukemia lysates (Fig. 3), however, an additional 93 Kd polypeptide is
recognized by monoclonal anti-Tthy, which is not evident after
iodination of isolated plasma membranes.

The results of subcellular fractionation experiments indicate that the
93 Kd polypeptide identified by anti-Tthy remains localized to the
cell cytosol (data not shown).   These polypeptides form a complex of

130-150 Kd identified by SDS-PAGE under non-reducing conditions (data
not shown). The focus of the present communication is to address the
similarity among the polypeptides recognized by anti-Tthy, anti-Tind
and anti-Tsu using peptide maps obtained by limited proteolysis
(Cleveland 1977). We first examined the possibility that the 69 Kd
polypeptide recognized by anti-Tthy and the 52 Kd polypeptide
recognized by anti-Tind are processed determinants on the same
polypeptide. Using proteolytic cleavage with Staphylococcus aureus V8
protease, peptide maps were obtained and are shown in Fig. 4. In
these experiments the 69 Kd and 52 Kd polypeptides immunoprecipitated
by anti-Tthy and anti-Tind, respectively, were cut from the gel and
rehydrated. The gel slices were then divided into two pieces and
reanalyzed by SDS-PAGE, either in the presence or absence of V8
protease.

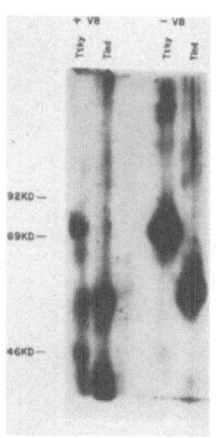

<u>Figure 4 and Legend</u>:   Proteolytic cleavage analysis of membrane
polypeptides from AKR 79 recognized by anti-Tthy and anti-Tind.
Specific polypeptides were cut from dried gels and reanalyzed by SDS-
PAGE on 12% gels under reducing conditions, either in the absence or
presence of 2 ug V8 protease per lane.

These results indicate the polypeptide recognized by anti-Tthy and
anti-Tind share peptides of similar apparent molecular weight;
however, additional peptides are visualized in the Tthy lane, which
are absent after digestion of the anti-Tind immunoprecipitates. We
conclude that the 69 Kd polypeptide recognized by anti-Tthy is not
identical to the 52 Kd polypeptide recognized by anti-Tind, although
the possibility that they share a common 52 Kd peptide cannot be
excluded.

Because anti-Tind and anti-Tsu identify polypeptides with similar
mobility in SDS-PAGE, limited proteolytic cleavage was used to
determine the degree of similarity between the determinants recognized
by these antibodies. These results are shown in Fig. 5 and indicate
the 50-52 Kd polypeptides recognized by these monoclonal antibodies
have characteristic cleavage sites identified by exposure to
<u>Staphylococcus aureus</u> V8 protease.

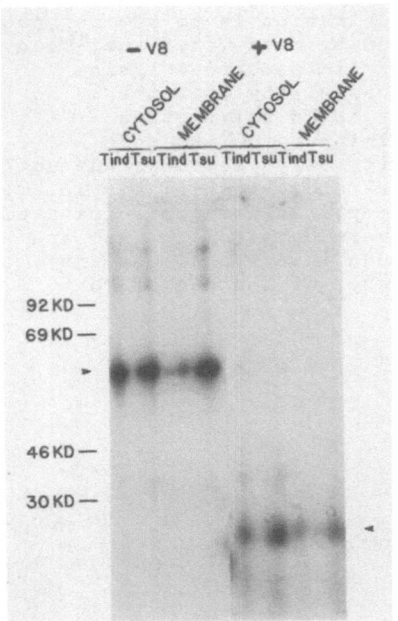

Figure 5 and Legend: Proteolytic cleavage analysis of cytosol and membrane polypeptides from AKR 225 recognized by anti-Tind and anti-Tsu. Specific polypeptides recognized by anti-Tind and anti-Tsu were cut from dried gels and reanalyzed by SDS-PAGE on 12% gels under reducing conditions either in the absence or presence of 2 ug Staphylococcus aureus V8 protease per lane.

Although these results indicate that the determinants recognized by anti-Tind and anti-Tsu have a similar composition, the results shown in Fig. 6 indicate the polypeptide recognized by anti-Tsu possesses additional sites which are more resistant to V8 protease than the determinants recognized by anti-Tind. Although both polypeptides migrate with similar mobility in SDS-PAGE in the presence of 1 ug V8 protease, exposure to increasing concentrations of protease markedly increased the mobility of the determinants recognized by anti-Tind obtained after iodination of either serum-free cell supernatants or purified plasma membranes. These results indicate that the peptide composition of the determinants recognized by anti-Tind and anti-Tsu are not identical, since different patterns of digestion were observed in the presence of V8 protease.

The determinants recognized by anti-Tind were then quantitated by silver staining as shown in Fig. 7. Monoclonal anti-Tind or an isotype identical negative control were incubated with aliquots of Amicon-concentrated, serum-free cell supernatant obtained after 24 hour culture of 2.5×10^6 cells. Immunoprecipitates were then analyzed by SDS-PAGE and visualized by silver staining. These results indicate that AKR thymic leukemias spontaneously release polypeptides in sufficient quantity (70-90 ng from 2.5×10^6 cells) to be sequenced as a prelude to efforts to clone the components of the Tsu genomic region.

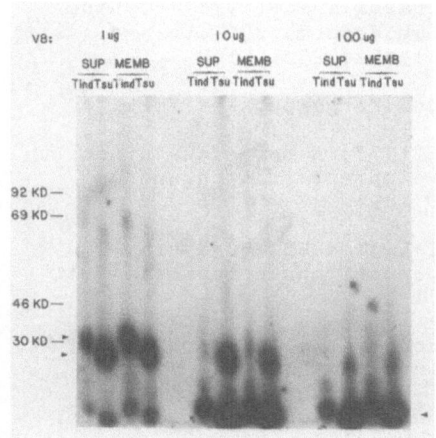

<u>Figure 6 and Legend</u>: Proteolytic cleavage analysis of supernatant and membrane polypeptides recognized by anti-Tind and anti-Tsu from AKR 225. Specific polypeptides were removed after SDS-PAGE and incubated with 1, 10 or 100 ug V8 protease per lane and reanalyzed by SDS-PAGE.

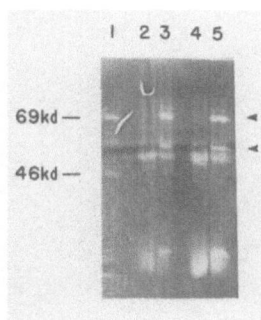

<u>Figure 7 and Legend</u>: SDS-PAGE of polypeptides recognized by anti-Tind from AKR thymoma 79 supernates developed with silver stain (Bio Rad). Lane 1, protein mw markers; Lane 2, BGV cell line supernatant immunoprecipitated with control antibody or, Lane 3, with anti-Tind; Lane 4, cell line supernatant immunoprecipitated with control antibody or, Lane 5, with anti-Tind.

REFERENCES

Chattopadhyay SK, Cloyd MW, Linemeyer DL, Lander MR, Rands E, Lowy DR (1982) Cellular origin and role of mink cell focus-forming viruses in murine thymic lymphomas. Nature 295: 25

Cleveland DW, Fischer SG, Kirschner MW, Laemmli VK (1977) Peptide
    mapping by limited proteolysis in sodium dodecyl sulfate and
    analysis by gel electrophoresis. J Biol Chem 252: 1102

Gross L (1977) Oncogenic viruses, 2nd edn. Pergamon, New York

Hartley JW, Wolford NK, Old LJ, Rowe WP (1977) A new class of murine
    leukemia virus associated with the development of spontaneous
    lymphomas. Proc Natl Acad Sci USA 74: 789

Kaneshima H, Hiai H, Fujiki H, Oguro YB, Lijima SB, Sugimura T,
    Nishizuka Y (1983) Tumor promotors-dependent mouse leukemia cell
    line. Leukemia Res 43: 4676

Owen FL (1983) T-cell alloantigens encoded by the IgT-C region of
    chromosome 12 in the mouse. Adv in Immunol 34: 1

Owen FL, Peterman G (1984) Neoplastic model for differentiation of
    cells bearing Igh-1 linked products. Immunol Rev 82: 29

Quigley J (1976) Association of a protease (plasminogen activator)
    with a specific membrane fraction isolated from transformed cells. J
    Cell Biol 71: 472

III. Allelomorphic and Mutant Phenotypes

Lps Gene-Associated Functions

S.N. Vogel and M.J. Fultz

SENSITIVITY TO LPS IS GENETICALLY CONTROLLED

As a result of a spontaneous mutation estimated to have occurred between 1960 and 1965, the C3H/HeJ mouse strain now exhibits a profound state of hyporesponsiveness to endotoxin, the ubiquitous lipopolysaccharide (LPS) cell wall component of Gram negative bacteria. The failure of C3H/HeJ mice to respond to LPS in vivo is reflected by the failure of a variety of cell types derived from these mice (i.e., B cells, T cells, macrophages, and fibroblasts) to respond to LPS in vitro (reviewed in Rosenstreich 1985). Based on genetic analyses using the C3H/HeJ mouse in crosses with other fully LPS-responsive strains, it is now recognized that the capacity to respond to LPS is controlled by a single, autosomal gene, Lps, for which a normal allele (Lps^n) and a defective allele (Lps^d) have been defined (reviewed in Rosenstreich 1985). The in vivo or in vitro responses to LPS exhibited by F_1 progeny of Lps^n/Lps^n X Lps^d/Lps^d crosses have been found to be intermediate, indicating that the Lps gene is codominantly expressed (Sultzer 1972; Glode and Rosenstreich 1976; Watson et al. 1977b; Rosenstreich et al. 1978; McGhee et al. 1979). Using recombinant inbred strains derived from LPS-responsive and hyporesponsive strains, as well as backcross linkage analyses, Watson et al. (1977,1978,1980) demonstrated that the gene which controlled both in vivo responsiveness to LPS and the capacity of spleen cells to respond proliferatively to LPS in vitro, was located on Chromosome 4 between the Mup-1 (major urinary protein) and the Ps (polysyndactyly) loci, near the brown coat color locus (b). The recombination frequency between Mup-1 and Lps was estimated in these studies to be 0.06 ± 0.02 (Watson et al. 1978). To date, the product of the Lps gene has not been identified. However, it has been postulated that C3H/HeJ mice fail to respond to LPS due to the faulty expression of a membrane-associated element (Forni and Coutinho 1978) or from an impaired capacity to process LPS into a suitably stimulatory form (Truffa-Bachi et al. 1977).

Two other mouse strains have also been characterized as endotoxin-hyporesponsive: the C57BL/10ScCR strain (Coutinho et al. 1977) and its progenitor strain, C57BL/10ScN (Vogel et al. 1979). The LPS-hyporesponsiveness exhibited by C57BL/10ScCR mice has also been mapped to Chromosome 4 (Coutinho and Meo 1978) and F_1 progeny derived from C3H/HeJ X C57BL/10ScCR crosses fail to respond to LPS (i.e., they possess non-complementary mutations; Coutinho and Meo 1978; Watson et al. 1980). The mutation which led to the Lps^d phenotype in the C57BL/10ScN strain has been estimated to have arisen some time between 1947 and 1961 (Vogel et al. 1979).

C3H/HeJ MACROPHAGES EXHIBIT DIFFERENTIATION DEFECTS

The differentiation of macrophages to a fully activated state is driven in a step-wise fashion by environmental signals, such as

Dept. of Microbiology, U. S. U. H. S., Bethesda, MD 20814.

cytokines and LPS (reviewed in Rosenstreich 1981). The finding that administration of potent macrophage activating agents greatly increased LPS responsiveness in normal (Lps^n) mice, and resulted in a transient reversal of LPS-hyporesponsiveness in C3H/HeJ (Lps^d) mice, led to the hypotheses that: (i) the degree of LPS responsiveness exhibited by a particular strain was correlated with the level of activation exhibited by their macrophages, and (ii) macrophages derived from C3H/HeJ mice might exhibit a lower state of differentiation than macrophages derived from fully LPS-responsive strains. To test the latter hypothesis, macrophages from fully LPS-responsive C3H/HeN or C3H/OuJ mice were compared with C3H/HeJ macrophages for their ability to bind and phagocytose ^{51}Cr-labeled, opsonized sheep erythrocytes as a measure of Fc receptor expression, a well-characterized marker of macrophage differentiation. Macrophages from C3H/HeN (Lps^n) mice were found to increase their Fc receptor capacity in vitro, in striking contrast to macrophages derived from C3H/HeJ mice. By 48 hr in culture, C3H/HeJ macrophages (resident peritoneal or thioglycollate-elicited) exhibit a profound deficit in their capacity to bind and phagocytose via Fc receptors (Vogel and Rosenstreich 1981; Fig.1, Medium). These findings were confirmed using a second Lps^n (C57BL/10Sn) vs. Lps^d (C57BL/10ScN) strain pair. The defect in Fc receptor capacity was found to be fully correctable by treatment of macrophages with crude lymphokine supernatants, and subsequent biochemical and serological characterization of the active factor supported the conclusion that the active factor was interferon-γ (IFN-γ). These findings have since been extended by the demonstration that various purified and recombinant IFN (rIFN) preparations (i.e., highly purified murine IFN-α/β, murine rIFN-γ, some human rIFN-α species (Fertsch and Vogel, 1984), and murine rIFN-β (unpublished)) augment Fc receptor capacity in C3H/HeJ macrophages. Treatment of C3H/HeJ macrophages with purified IFN-α/β resulted in an increase in the number and density of Fc receptors, with no change in affinity (Vogel et al. 1983).

The finding that exogenous interferons could normalize the Lps^d phenotype with respect to Fc receptor expression, led to the hypothesis that the failure of C3H/HeJ mice to respond to naturally occurring levels of LPS results in a failure to produce adequate levels of endogenous, macrophage-derived IFN. This LPS-induced cytokine might provide an essential autocrine signal for the maintenance of the macrophage at a certain "normal" (i.e., Lps^n-like) level of differentiation. Since macrophages have been shown to produce IFN-α/β in response to LPS (Ho 1980), C3H/HeN and C3H/HeJ macrophages were treated with anti-IFN-α/β antibody and assessed for their ability to phagocytose via Fc receptors. Figure 1 illustrates that treatment of C3H/HeN macrophages with anti-IFN-α/β antibody, but not with a control antibody, reduced their capacity to phagocytose to levels exhibited by C3H/HeJ macrophage cultures.

This hypothesis was further supported by the findings that: (i) co-culture of C3H/HeN and C3H/HeJ macrophages resulted in greater Fc receptor expression than expected; (ii) culture supernatants from unstimulated C3H/HeN macrophages induced a significant increase in C3H/HeJ Fc receptor capacity; and, (iii) expression of a second differentiation marker, Mac-1, decreased spontaneously in C3H/HeN macrophage cultures with time; C3H/HeJ macrophages had to be treated with exogenous IFN-α/β to inhibit Mac-1 to comparable levels.

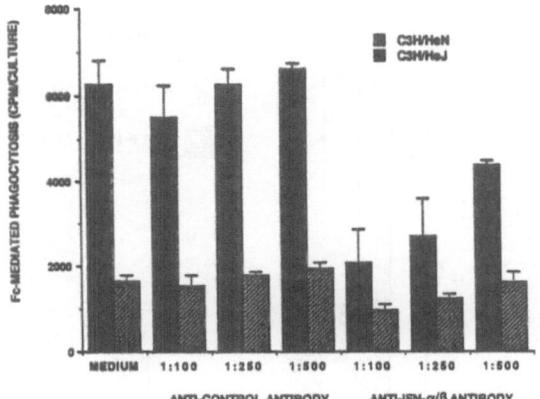

Fig. 1.   Fc-mediated phagocytosis in C3H/HeN ($\underline{Lps}^n$) and C3H/HeJ ($\underline{Lps}^d$) macrophages treated with medium only, anti-control antibody, or anti-IFN-α/β. Data taken from Vogel and Fertsch (1984).

In light of the well-characterized antiviral activity of interferons, the hypothesis was tested further by comparing macrophages from LPS-responsive and hyporesponsive mouse strains for susceptibility to infection with Vesicular Stomatitis Virus (VSV; Vogel and Fertsch 1987).   Thioglycollate-elicited, peritoneal exudate macrophages derived from fully LPS-responsive mouse strains (C3H/OuJ or C57BL/10J) were refractory to VSV infection (MOI = 0.1) in vitro, whereas macrophages derived from C3H/HeJ or C57BL/10ScN mice were permissive for VSV and replicated virus to high titers, resulting in complete destruction of the macrophage monolayer within 24 hr of infection.   Levels of the enzyme 2'5'-oligoadenylate synthetase, an IFN-inducible marker, were approximately 10-fold higher in LPS-responsive macrophages. Susceptibility to VSV could be partially induced in LPS-responsive macrophages by exposure to anti-IFN-α/β antibody in vitro (Figure 2).   The concentration of antibody used in these studies (1:400) was chosen based on the capacity of this same antibody to inhibit Fc-mediated phagocytosis half maximally (Figure 1). Taken collectively, these findings strongly support the hypothesis that in genetically "normal" ($\underline{Lps}^n$) animals, LPS provides a naturally occurring stimulus that results in the production of IFN-α/β by macrophages.   This endogenous IFN, in turn, is utilized by the macrophage as an autostimulatory differentiation signal (e.g, for the maintenance of Fc receptor expression).   In many ways the $\underline{Lps}^d$ macrophages are phenotypically very comparable to macrophages derived from mice injected with high titered anti-IFN-α/β antibody (i.e., they are sensitive to virus infection in vitro and exhibit depressed 2'5'-oligoadenylate synthetase levels; Gresser et al. 1985). The recent findings of Gessani et al. (1987), that freshly explanted, resident peritoneal cells from $\underline{Lps}^n$ strains, but not $\underline{Lps}^d$ strains, can confer an antiviral state upon peritoneal macrophages which have been "aged" in culture to induce virus susceptibility, are also consistent with this hypothesis.

168

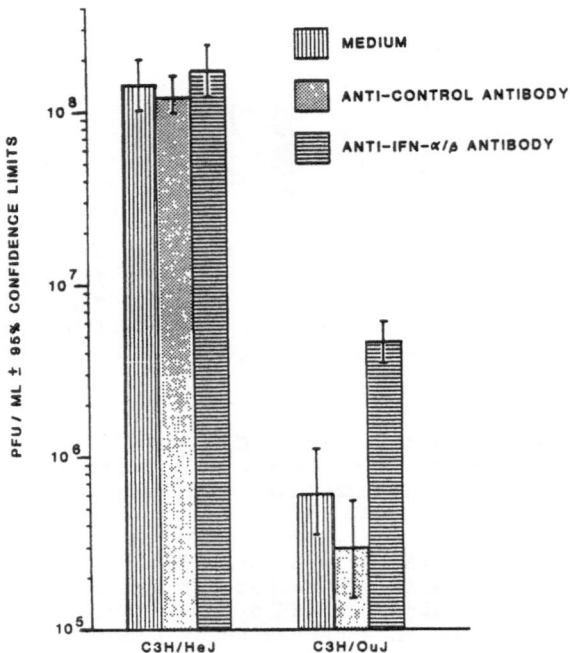

Fig. 2. Effect of anti-IFN-α/β antibody on VSV replication in
C3H/OuJ (Lps^n) and C3H/HeJ macrophages (Vogel and Fertsch 1987).

POSSIBLE RELATIONSHIP BETWEEN THE Lps GENE AND THE Ifa LOCUS

Based on the combined results of backcross linkage analyses and
linkage analyses using recombinant inbred strains, Watson et al.
(1978) estimated the precent recombination frequency between Mup-1
and Lps to be 6 ± 2, and the recombination frequency between Lps and
Ps to be 13 ± 7 (Figure 3). In a recent study by DeMaeyer and
Dandoy (1987), two three point crosses were carried out (Figure 3).
In the first analysis (using Mup-1, the interferon-α locus (Ifa),
and misty coat color (m) as markers), the percent recombination
frequency between Mup-1 and Ifa was determined to be 13.6 ± 3.6.
However, when a second analysis was carried out in which the gene
order and recombination frequencies were determined using Mup-1,
brown coat color (b), and Ifa, the map distance between Mup-1 and
Ifa was determined to be 5.3 ± 3.0. Thus, the positions of Lps
relative to Mup-1 and of Ifa relative to Mup-1 may be coincidental.

Since the Ifa locus has been shown to be comprised of approximately
15 structural genes (reviewed in DeMaeyer and Dandoy 1987), it is
possible that the endogenous IFN defect exhibited by Lps^d mice is
the result of a mutation within the Ifa locus. To test this
hypothesis, Southern blot analysis of DNA derived from C3H/HeJ
(Lps^d) and C3H/OuJ (Lps^n) mice was carried out using IFN-α_2 cDNA
(kindly provided by Dr. Paula Pitha-Rowe) as a probe. Our
preliminary findings indicate that when Bgl I was used as the

restriction endonuclease, strain specific banding patterns were
detected. This suggests several possibilities: (i) the ability of
mice to respond to LPS may be dependent upon the induction of an
endogenous IFN-α, the gene for which is defective in Lps^d mice, or
(ii) separate, but closely linked mutations exist in
LPS-hyporesponsive mice, one within the Lps^d allele and one within
the IFN-α gene cluster. Additional experiments are underway to
distinguish between these possibilities.

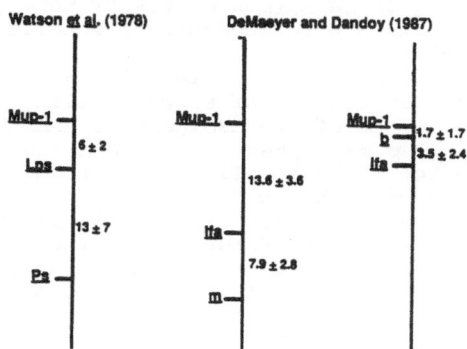

Fig. 3. Comparison of the linkage analyses performed on chromosome
4 markers by Watson et al.(1978) and DeMaeyer and Dandoy (1987).

Since the failure of macrophages to produce IFN endogenously results
in a lowered state of macrophage differentiation, as observed in
macrophages derived from Lps^d mice, this may also underlie the
observations that susceptibility to Salmonella typhimurium (O'Brien
et al. 1980) and the failure to respond to BCG to develop
macrophages activated to a tumoricidal state (Ruco et al. 1978) have
been formally linked to the expression of the Lps^d allele.

REFERENCES

Coutinho A, Forni L, Melchers F, Watanabe T (1977) Genetic defect in
    responsiveness to the B cell mitogen lipopolysaccharide. Eur J
    Immunol 7:325-328
Coutinho A, Meo T (1978) Genetic basis for unresponsiveness to
    lipopolysaccharide in C57BL/10Cr mice. Immunogenetics 7: 17-24
DeMaeyer E, Dandoy F (1987) Linkage analysis of the murine
    interferon alpha locus (Ifa) on chromosome 4. J Hered 78:204-209
Fertsch D, Vogel SN (1984) Recombinant interferons increase
    macrophage Fc receptor capacity. J Immunol 132:2436 - 2439
Forni L, Coutinho A (1978) An antiserum which recognizes
    lipopolysacchride reactive B cells in the mouse. Eur J Immunol
    8:56-62
Gessani S, Belardelli F, Borghi P, Boraschi D, Gresser I (1987)
    Correlation between the lipopolysaccharide response of mice and
    the capacity of mouse peritoneal cells to transfer an antiviral
    state. J Immunol 139:1991 - 1998
Glode LM, Rosenstreich DL (1976) Genetic control of B cell
    activation by bacterial lipopolysaccharide is mediated by

multiple distinct genes or alleles. J Immunol 117:2061-2066

Gresser I, Vignaux F, Belardelli F, Tovey MG, Maunoury M-T (1985) Injection of mice with antibody to mouse interferon alpha-beta decreases the level of 2'5'-oligoadenylate synthetase in peritoneal macrophages. J Virol 53:221-227

Ho M (1980) Cellular sources of endotoxin-induced interferons. In: Schlessinger D (ed) Microbiology 1980. ASM Publ, Wash.,DC, p 128

McGhee JR, Michalek SM, Moore RN, Mergenhagen SE, Rosenstreich DL (1979) Genetic control of in vivo sensitivity to lipopolysaccharide: Evidence for codominant inheritance. J Immunol 122:2052-2058

O'Brien AD, Rosenstreich DL, Scher I, Campbell GH, MacDermott R, Formal SB (1980) Genetic control of susceptibility to Salmonella typhimurium in mice: Role of the LPS gene. J Immunol 134:20-14

Rosenstreich DL (1981) The macrophage. In: Oppenheim JJ, Rosenstreich DL, Potter M (eds) Cellular functions in immunity and inflammation. Elsevier, NY, p 127

Rosenstreich DL (1985) Genetic control of endotoxin response: C3H/HeJ mice. In: Berry LJ (ed) Handbook of endotoxin, Vol. 3: Cellular biology of endotoxin. Elsevier, Amsterdam, p 82

Rosenstreich DL, Vogel SN, Jacques AR, Wahl LM, Oppenheim JJ (1978) Macrophage sensitivity to endotoxin: Genetic control by a single codominant gnen. J Immunol 121: 1664-1670

Ruco LPS, Meltzer MS, Rosenstreich DL (1978) Macrophage activation for tumor cytotoxicity: Control of macrophage tumoricidal capacity by the LPS gene. J Immunol 121:543-548

Sultzer B (1972) Genetic control of host responses to endotoxin. Infec Immun 5:107-113

Truffa-Bachi P, Kaplan JG, Bona C (1977) The mitogenic effect of lipopolysaccharide. Metabolic processing of lipopolysaccharide by mouse lymphocytes. Cell Immunol 30:1-11

Vogel SN, Fertsch D (1984) Endogenous interferon production by endotoxin-responsive macrophages provides an autostimulatory differentiation siganl. Infec Immun 45:417-423

Vogel SN, Fertsch D (1987) Macrophages from endotoxin-hyporesponsive (Lps^d) mice are permissive for Vesicular Stomatitis Virus because of reduced levels of endogenous interferon: possible mechanism for natural resistance to virus infection. J Virol 61:812-818

Vogel SN, Finbloom DS, English KE, Rosenstreich DL, Langreth SG (1983) Interferon-induced enhancement of macrophage Fc receptor expression: β-interferon treatment of C3H/HeJ macrophages results in increased numbers and density of Fc receptors. J Immunol 130: 1210-1214

Vogel SN, Hansen CT, Rosenstreich DL (1979) Characterization of a congenitally LPS-resistant athymic mouse strain. J Immunol 122: 619-622

Vogel SN, Rosenstreich DL (1981) LPS-unresponsive mice as a model for analyzing lymphokine-induced differentiation in vitro. Lymphokines 3: 149-180

Watson J, Kelly K, Largen M, Taylor BA (1978) The genetic mapping of a defective LPS response gene in C3H/HeJ mice. J Immunol 120:422-424

Watson J, Kelly K, Whitlock C (1980) Genetic control of endotoxin sensitivity. In: Schlessinger D (ed) Microbiology 1980. ASM Publ, Washington, DC, p 4

Watson J, Largen M, McAdam KPWJ (1977) Genetic control of endotoxic responses in mice. J Exp Med 147:39-48

Supported by NIH Grant #AI-18797.

The Immunobiology of the T Cell Response to *Mls* Locus Disparate Stimulator Cells

C.A. Janeway, Jr.

INTRODUCTION

The *Mls* locus described by Festenstein (1973) is a murine locus at which polymorphism leads to unidirectional stimulation in mixed lymphocyte reactions (MLR). Initially, four alleles were described, but recent analysis has shown that these original assignments probably reflect two segregating loci, each with two alleles (Abe et al, 1987). In describing the immunobiology of the T cell response to *Mls* locus disparities, I will consider only those mapping to chromosome 1, originally termed Mls^a and Mls^b for the stimulating and responding alleles respectively. Disparities at this locus stimulate the most potent and reproducible responses in primary MLR, and are consequently the most interesting for immunobiological analysis.

RESULTS

In this section, I will briefly describe the salient features of the T cell response to stimulator cells disparate at the *Mls* locus, using published data to make each point. Once the characteristics of this response are defined, the implications of these findings will be discussed and used to make predictions about the nature of the product of the *Mls* locus.

Primary T Cell Responses to *Mls* Locus Disparate Stimulator Cells Are Unidirectional

When T cells from an Mls^b strain are mixed with mitomycin C-inactivated stimulator cells of an Mls^a strain in MLR, a potent primary T cell proliferative response is obtained. When the reciprocal combination is used, no significant T cell proliferation is observed (Festenstein, 1973; Janeway and Katz, 1985). This unidirectionality in the primary T cell proliferative response to Mls^a stimulator cells is a unique feature of this MLR. MLR carried out between lymphocytes from strains differing at the MHC are always bi-directional, with the sole exception of responses of T cells from I-E negative strains to stimulator cells from I-E positive strains that are otherwise MHC identical, such as B10.A(4R) anti-B10.A(2R) (Lerner et al, 1980).

The Frequency of T Cells Responding to *Mls* Locus Disparate Stimulator Cells is Greater than the Frequency of T Cells Responding to MHC Disparate Stimulator Cells

The intensity of the primary MLR induced by *Mls* locus disparate stimulator cells suggested that the number of T cells responding in such cultures was very high. In fact, several groups have measured the precursor frequency of T cells responding to *Mls* locus disparate stimulator cells (Janeway et al, 1980; Lutz et al, 1981; Miller and Stutman, 1982), and all have found that about five-fold more T cells respond to such differences than respond to MHC differences in MLR. As the frequency of T cells responding to an MHC difference has been estimated to be 3-5%, this places the frequency of T cells responding to *Mls* locus disparate stimulators at approximately 20% of all T cells.

Department of Pathology and Section of Immunobiology, Howard Hughes Medical Institute at the Yale University School of Medicine, New Haven, CT 06510

The T Cells Responding to *Mls* Locus Disparate Stimulator Cells are CD4 Positive

T cells respond more potently to *Mls* locus disparate stimulator cells than do whole spleen cells, and CD4$^+$ T cells respond more potently than unfractionated T cells (Janeway et al, 1980). The T cell blasts recovered from primary MLR responding to *Mls* locus disparities are 85-90% CD4$^+$ and only 10-15% CD8$^+$ (Janeway et al, 1980; Jones et al, 1986). Cloned T cell lines that respond to *Mls* locus disparities are also CD4$^+$ (Katz et al, 1986).

T Cells Responding to *Mls* Locus Disparate Stimulator Cells Are not MHC Restricted, but MHC Polymorphism Does Affect Such Responses

There has been controversy about the role of the MHC in T cell responses to *Mls* locus disparate stimulator cells. Originally, using the response to *Mls^c* disparate stimulator cells, Peck et al (1977) described what appeared to be MHC restriction in this response. This was extended to *Mls^a* by Janeway et al (1980) and by Gress et al (1981). However, Molnar-Kimber andl Sprent (1980) did not observe MHC restriction in such responses, and lines (Janeway et al, 1980) and clones (Webb et al, 1981; Jones and Janeway, 1982) of T cells responsive to *Mls^a* stimulator cells did not show MHC restricted recognition. Nevertheless, using recombinant inbred strains of mice, an influence of MHC on the intensity of the response of both normal T cells and cloned T cell lines was reported by Jones and Janeway (1982) and confirmed by Lynch et al (1985). In particular, strain DBA/1 (*Mls^a, H-2^q*) is ineffective as a stimulator for cloned T cells lines responsive to *Mls^a* stimulator cells, while congenic lines D1.LP (*Mls^a, H-2^b*) and D1.C (*Mls^a, H-2^d*) are effective stimulators of these same cloned T cell lines. Thus, MHC genotype does significantly affect the ability of *Mls^a* stimulator cells to induce T cell proliferative responses.

T Cell Proliferative Responses to *Mls* Locus Disparate Stimulator Cells are Inhibited by Antibodies Specific for Class II MHC Molecules Borne by the Stimulator Cells

To examine the role of MHC molecules in T cell proliferative responses to *Mls* locus disparate stimulator cells more directly, anti-MHC monoclonal antibodies were tested for their ability to inhibit these responses. Anti-class II MHC monoclonal antibodies were found to inhibit such responses by both normal T cells and cloned T cell lines (Janeway et al, 1980; Debreuil et al, 1982; Janeway and Katz, 1985; Katz and Janeway, 1985), with anti-I-E antibodies inhibiting most responses more effectively than anti-I-A antibodies. However, inhibition is observed using either anti-I-A or anti-I-E antibodies, and complete inhibition is usually achieved with very low concentrations of a mixture of anti-I-A and anti-I-E antibodies. Inhibition of responses to *Mls* locus disparate stimulator cells is more readily achieved relative to inhibition of responses to MHC disparate stimulator cells. These data, taken together with the influence of MHC on primary responses and responses of cloned T cell lines, strongly implicate the class II MHC molecules in such responses.

T Cell Responses to *Mls* Locus Disparate Stimulator Cells are Inhibited by Antibodies Directed at the CD4:T Cell Receptor Complex

To examine the structures on the T cell that are involved in the response to *Mls* locus disparate stimulator cells, monoclonal antibodies specific for CD4 and the variable region of the T cell receptor have been tested for their ability to inhibit such responses. Anti-CD4 potently inhibits all such responses (Janeway and Katz, 1985). When cloned lines expressing V regions reactive with the monoclonal antibody KJ-16 were tested, this antibody also inhibited responses of such cells to *Mls* locus disparate stimulator cells (Katz and Janeway, 1985). As CD4 appears to be functionally a part of the T cell receptor complex specific for class II MHC ligands (Saizawa et al, 1987; Janeway et al, 1988), these data strongly implicate the CD4:T cell receptor complex in responses to *Mls* locus disparate stimulator cells.

Cloned T Cell Lines Specific for a Wide Variety of Different Antigen:Class II MHC Differences Respond to *Mls* Locus Disparate Stimulator Cells

Cloned T cell lines normally show strict specificity for a peptide fragment of a protein antigen and a particular self class II MHC molecule; about 3% also respond to a given class II MHC alloantigen (Janeway et al, 1982). When similar analyses are carried out using Mls^a stimulator cells to activate Mls^b cloned T cell lines, about 20% respond (Katz and Janeway, 1985). These figures accord well with the precursor frequencies observed using normal T cells in similar responses, and suggest that responsiveness to *Mls* locus disparate stimulator cells is distributed independently of specificity for antigen and self class II MHC. Similar results have been obtained in studies from several laboratories (Braciale and Braciale, 1981; Janeway et al, 1983; Abromson-Leeman and Cantor, 1983; Ben-Nun et al, 1983).

Mls^a Stimulator Cells Present Antigen More Efficiently to Cloned, Class II MHC Restricted T Cells than Do Mls^b Stimulator Cells

When cloned T cell lines that lack overt reactivity to Mls^a stimulator cells are examined for their ability to respond to antigen presented by stimulator cells from Mls^a or Mls^b strains, one finds that stimulator cells from Mls^a strains present antigen about 10 fold more efficiently than stimulator cells from Mls^b strains (Janeway et al, 1983). This is true for antigens presented in association with I-A or I-E molecules, of various MHC genotypes. This result suggests that *Mls* stimulatory alleles expressed on antigen presenting cells somehow promote the stimulation of the T cell through its receptor by antigen:class II MHC complexes.

DISCUSSION

The findings cited above clearly implicate recognition of class II MHC molecules by the CD4:T cell receptor complex in the unidirectional response of T cells to *Mls* locus disparate stimulator cells. This finding increases the fascination of this locus, as *Mls* locus disparity has a remarkable effect on the interaction of the T cell receptor with its class II MHC ligand. Normally, T cell receptors respond to class II MHC molecules with exquisite specificity. That a single locus could encode a change in stimulator cells that leads to responses with little specificity for MHC polymorphism, including the relatively equal role of I-A and I-E complexes in these responses, suggests that whatever the product of the *Mls* locus may be, understanding it will lead to a clearer understanding of the recognition of class II MHC molecules by the T cell receptor.

Several models have been proposed to account for the behavior of the *Mls* locus. It has been proposed that the *Mls* locus encodes a minor H antigen that associates with class II MHC. However, this model is unlikely since minor H antigen recognition is usually precisely MHC restricted. A second proposal is that the *Mls* locus encodes a translocated class II MHC molecule. This is also unlikely, since antibodies to conventional class II MHC molecules inhibit this response, and do so in a fashion that is specific for the MHC of the stimulator cell. A third proposal is that the *Mls* locus encodes a cellular mitogen that acts on a mitogen receptor on the T cell. This proposal would require that T cells from strains bearing stimulatory alleles at *Mls* would lack this receptor, either genetically or through ontogenetic selection. It would also require that the mitogen somehow require class II MHC interaction with the T cell receptor.

The three proposals on which most attention is presently focused all accomodate readily the observation that the T cell receptor and its class II MHC ligand must interact for *Mls* locus disparities to be effective in stimulating T cell responses. The first is that the product of the *Mls* locus encodes or regulates the expression of a molecule expressed on the antigen presenting cell that promotes effective interaction of the T cell receptor with its class II MHC ligand. This molecule could be an adhesion strengthening molecule or a ligand for an undefined T cell surface receptor. This receptor would have to work in concert with the conventional T3 associated receptor to account for the effect of anti-receptor antibody on the response. However, this proposal does have the virtue of accounting for the augmented presentation of antigen associated with *Mls*^{a} antigen presenting cells.

A second possibility is that the *Mls* locus encodes a peptide that associates with class II MHC molecules very effectively, and also has affinity for a wide variety of T cell receptors. This would account for the ability of *Mls* locus disparate stimulator cells to signal via the T cell receptor, and for the role of class II MHC molecules in *Mls* locus responses. It could also be argued that such signals are delivered to all T cells, only some of which are overtly responsive, the others showing a lowered threshold for responsiveness, which would again account for the augmented antigen presentation by *Mls*^{a} stimulator cells. This proposal is of interest, as such peptides could also be envisioned as playing a role in the selection of the self class II MHC recognizing repertoire, as has been proposed (Janeway et al, 1983). Such a universal class II binding and T cell receptor stimulating peptide would be unique, and would have to be able to drive the T cell receptor away from its normal high degree of specificity for self class II MHC. This possibility is particularly interesting in light of some bacterial mitogens that appear to have this behavior (Lynch et al, 1986; Buxser and Janeway, unpublished observations).

Finally, it has been proposed that the *Mls* locus encodes a molecule with a regulatory function, the inhibition of autoreactivity. By this hypothesis, *Mls*^{a} stimulators would signal down-regulation less effectively than *Mls*^{b} stimulators. This proposal is outlined in detail by Hammerling (this volume). The main problem with this hypothesis is that one has to argue that genetically, down regulation is recessive.

SUMMARY AND CONCLUSIONS

The *Mls* locus is of great interest to immunobiologists because it encodes an unknown product whose expression causes a very potent T cell proliferative response. The stimulating cells present *Mls* locus disparities via class II MHC molecules, and the responding T cells utilize the CD4:T cell receptor complex to recognize such differences. What is not known is the nature of the gene product of this locus. Three leading hypotheses are that it encodes a cell adhesion protein or receptor, that it encodes a peptide that interacts with class II MHC and the T cell receptor in an unusual fashion, or that it encodes regulatory signals. All three hypotheses have interesting implications that make unravelling this mystery well worth achieving.

ACKNOWLEDGEMENTS

The author wishes to thank Michael Katz, Pat Conrad, and Barry Jones for much of the work described here. The work was supported by NIH grant AI-14579.

REFERENCES

Abe R, Finkelman FD, Hodes RJ (1987) T cell recognition of Mls. T cell clones demonstrate polymorphism between Mls^a, Mls^c, and Mls^d. J Immunol 138: 373

Abromson-Leeman S, Cantor H (1983) Specificity of T cell clones for antigen and autologous major histocompatibility complex products determines specificity for foreign major histocompatibility complex products. J Exp Med 158: 428

Ben-Nun A, Lando Z, Dorf ME, Burakoff S (1983) Analysis of cross-reactive antigen-specific T cell clones. Specific recognition of two major histocompatibility complex (MHC) and two non MHC antigens by a single clone. J Exp Med 157: 2147

Braciale VL, Braciale TJ (1981) *Mls* locus recognition by a cloned line of H-2 restricted influenza virus specific cytotoxic T lymphocytes. J Immunol 127: 859

Debreuil PC, Caillol DH, Lemonnier FA (1982) Analysis of unexpected inhibitions of T lymphocyte proliferation to soluble antigen, alloantigen and mitogen by unfragmented anti-I-A^k or anti-I-E/C^k monoclonal antibodies. J Immunogenetics 9: 11

Festenstein H (1973) Immunogenetic and biological aspects of *in vitro* lymphocyte allotransformation (MLR) in the mouse. Transplant Rev 15: 62

Gress RE, Wesley MN, Hodes RJ (1981) The role of H-2 in T cell recognition of *Mls*. J Immunol 127: 1763

Janeway CA Jr, Lerner EA, Jason JM, Jones B (1980) T lymphocytes responding to *Mls* locus antigens are Lyt-1$^+$, 2$^-$ and I-A restricted. Immunogenetics 10: 481

Janeway CA Jr, Lerner EA, Conrad PJ, Jones B (1982) The precision of self and non-self major histocompatibility complex encoded antigen recognition by cloned T cells. Behring Inst Mitteilungen 70: 200

Janeway CA Jr, Conrad PJ, Tite JP, Jones B, Murphy DB (1983) Efficiency of antigen presentation differs in mice differing at the *Mls* locus. Nature 306: 80.

Janeway CA Jr, Katz ME (1985) The immunobiology of the T cell response to *Mls* locus disparate stimulator cells. I. Unidirectionality, new strain combinations and the role of Ia antigens. J Immunol 134: 2057

Janeway CA Jr, Carding S, Jones B, Murray J, Portoles P, Rasmussen R, Rojo J, Saizawa K, Bottomly K (To be published) CD4+ T cells: Specificity and function. Immunol Rev 101

Jones B, Janeway CA Jr (1982) MHC recognition by clones of *Mls* specific T lymphocytes. Immunogenetics 16: 243

Jones B, Mjolsness S, Janeway CA Jr, Hayday A (1986) Transcription of functionally rearranged gamma genes in primary T cells of adult immuno-competent mice. Nature 323: 635

Katz ME, Janeway CA Jr (1985) The immunobiology of T cell responses to *Mls* locus disparate stimulator cells. II. Effects of *Mls* locus disparate stimulator cells on cloned, protein antigen specific, Ia restricted T cell lines. J Immunol 134: 2064

Katz ME, Tite JP, Janeway CA Jr (1986) The immunobiology of T cell responses to *Mls* locus disparate stimulator cells. III. Helper and cytolytic functions of cloned, *Mls* reactive T cell lines. J Immunol 136: 1

Lerner EA, Matis LA, Janeway CA Jr, Jones PP, Schwartz RH, Murphy DB (1980) Monoclonal antibody against an Ir gene product. J Exp Med 152: 1734

Lynch DH, Gress RE, Needleman BW, Rosenberg SA, Hodes RJ (1985) T cell responses to Mls determinants are restricted by cross-reactive MHC determinants. J Immunol 134: 2071

Lynch DH, Cole BC, Bluestone JA, Hodes RJ (1986) Cross-reactive recognition by antigen-specific, major histocompatibility complex-restricted T cells of a mitogen derived from *Mycoplasma arthritidis* is clonally expressed and I-E restricted. Eur J Immunol 16: 747

Lutz CT, Glasebrok AL, Fitch FW (1981) Enumeration of alloreactive helper T lymphocytes which cooperate with cytolytic T lymphocytes. Eur J Immunol 11: 726

Miller RA, Stutman O (1982) Estimation of IL-2 secreting helper T cells by limiting dilution analysis, and demonstration of unexpectedly high levels of IL-2 production per responding cell. J Immunol 128: 2258

Molnar-Kimber K, Sprent J (1980) Absence of H-2 restriction in primary and secondary mixed lymphocyte reactions to strong *Mls* determinants. J Exp Med

Peck AB, Janeway CA Jr, Wigzell H (1977) T lymphocyte responses to *Mls* locus antigens involve recognition of H-2 I region gene products. Nature 266: 840

Saizawa K, Rojo J, Janeway CA Jr (1987) Evidence for a physical association of CD4 and the CD3:α:β T cell receptor. Nature 328: 260

Webb SR, Molnar-Kimber K, Bruce J, Sprent J, Wilson DB (1981) T cell clones with dual specificity for *Mls* and various major histocompatibility complex determinants. J Exp Med 154: 1970

Genetic Analysis of Serologically Undefined Determinants: A T Cell "Clonological" Analysis of the *Mls* System

R. Abe and R.J. Hodes

INTRODUCTION

Just as the development of B cell hybridization techniques and the availability of B cell monospecific products (monoclonal antibody) have revolutionized basic immunological approaches, recently established techniques for T cell cloning have provided another powerful tool. Experiments utilizing T cell clones have provided information relevant to T cell specificity, function, and the biochemistry of the T cell receptor which had been difficult to obtain with polyclonal T cell populations. In this communication, we describe a "clonological analysis", i.e. the use of cloned T cells for genetic analysis of the strongly stimulatory, yet serologically undefined, T cell stimulatory determinants of the Mls (minor lymphocyte stimulatory locus) system.

Mls System

In the murine system, one set of determinants in addition to major histocompatibility complex (MHC) gene products is known to be strongly stimulatory for naive T cells. The gene locus encoding these determinants was designated as Mls (Festenstein 1973) and the Mls^a locus was mapped on chromosome 1 (Festenstein et al. 1977). While genetic, biochemical and molecular biological analysis of MHC genes and their products have been extensive and their biologic importance has been well documented, characterization of the nature of Mls remains extremely limited. One example is the formal genetic analysis of Mls. Although Mls was originally described as having four alleles, a, b, c, and d, each of which encodes polymorphic cell-surface determinants, a number of recent observations, such as the high degree of crossreactivity between Mls^a and Mls^d, and the absence of any formal mapping of the genes encoding Mls^c and Mls^d, have led several investigators to question this original concept (Webb et al. 1981; Katz et al. 1985). Inasmuch as it is currently impossible to approach these essential genetic questions serologically, because of the lack of appropriate reagents, T cell clones specific for putatively different allelic Mls products have been employed in the analysis of Mls genetics.

T CELL CLONOLOGICAL ANALYSIS OF THE Mls SYSTEM

Overview

Because of the characteristics of cloned T cells, this analysis has several unique advantages and disadvantages which must be considered.

Immunology Branch, National Cancer Institute, National Institutes of Health, Bethesda, MD 20892, U.S.A.

Advantages:
1) Each cloned T cell recognizes a single specific determinant.
Therefore reactivity to a specific determinant can be assessed
without being obscured by T cell reactivities to other determinants
which are also present.
2) Since T cell clones are selected for proliferative response to
relevant determinants, they represent a uniform population of
strongly responding cells. Therefore T cell responses to a given
determinant are usually sensitive and stable, and nonspecific
background responses are usually low.
3) Cloned T cells permit the direct assessment of responses to a
given determinant in the absence of regulatory influences such as
those mediated by suppressor T cells.

Disadvantages:
1) Multiple crossreactivities of cloned T cells are often observed.
2) The process of generating cloned T cells might select certain
populations. Therefore, in terms of function and repertoire,
cloned T populations are not necessarily representative of
heterogeneous T cell responses.
3) In general, T cells recognize antigenic determinants in
conjunction with MHC gene products. Therefore, unlike serological
analysis with antibodies which detect non-MHC determinants
directly, in an analysis with cloned T cells, influences of MHC-
gene products on T cell response must be considered .

Approach
1) MHC compatible and Mls disparate strain combination were
selected for establishment of each Mls-specific cloned T cell line
(Abe et al. 1987a, 1987b).
2) The specificity of cloned T cells was determined based upon
patterns of reactivity to inbred strains, backcross animals and
recombinant inbred strains (see below).
3) In order to avoid skewing of conclusions based upon the use of
cloned populations, primary MLR using heterogeneous T cell
populations were performed in parallel, and at least three
different clones of each Mls specificity were employed for
determination of Mls type.

Generation and Identification of Mls-specific Cloned T Cells

Generation of Mls-specific cloned T cells has been described in
detail elsewhere (Abe et al. 1987a, 1987b). Briefly, Lyt-2$^-$nylon
wool nonadherent T cells isolated from unprimed B10.BR (H-2^k, Mls^b)
were cultured in the presence of H-2 identical, Mls disparate
stimulators, such as AKR/J (Mls^a), C3H/HeJ (Mls^c) or CBA/J (Mls^d)
for generation of Mls^a-, Mls^c- and Mls^d-specific T cell clones,
respectively. After four cycles of stimulation, the T cell lines
were cloned by limiting dilution in the presence of 10% lectin-free
culture supernatant from Con A-stimulated BALB/c spleen cells as a
source of IL-2.

In order to employ cloned T cell populations in a genetic analysis
of the Mls system, it was first critical to establish the
specificities of these clones. Since the gene encoding Mls^a
determinants has been mapped by using BXD RI strains, the
specificity of anti-AKR clones for Mls^a could be directly tested by
the pattern of responses to 21 BXD RI strains in addition to a
number of independent inbred strains (Table 1). All 11 BXD strains
of the Mls^a genotype stimulated anti-AKR/J clones but none of the

10 Mls^b stains was stimulatory. This pattern of responsiveness was consistent with Mls^a specificity of these T cell clones.

Table 1. Identification of specificities of anti-AKR/J clones

Strain	Mls genotype	Response of clones[*]
AKR/J,DBA/2,D1.LP	a	+[=]
B10.BR, B10.D2, C57L/J	b	-
BXD[+] 5,8,9,11,22,24,25, 27,28,29,30,	a	+
BXD 1,6,12,13,14,15, 16,18,19,23,	b	-

[*] BARC1, BARB2, BARB12, AND BARC12
[+] (C57BL/6xDBA/2J) recombinant inbred strains
[=] + or - indicates the presence or absence of response

Unlike Mls^a, the Mls^c gene has not yet been formally mapped. Therefore, the only available means to determine whether T cell clones are Mls^c specific was to compare the pattern of proliferative responses of potential Mls^c-reactive clones with the primary anti-Mls^c responses of unprimed T cells to different stimulators.

Table 2. Identification of specificities of anti-C3H/HeJ clones

Strain	Primary MLR by non-Mls^c strain[*]	Response of anti-C3H clones[+]
C3H/HeJ, A/J	+	+
B10.BR, B10.A	-	-
BXH[=] 3,6,12,14	+	+
BXH 7	-	-
AKR x (AKRxC3H)F$_1$		
2,3,5,6,7,8,9,10,12,13,14, 15,16,19,20,22,23,24,	+	+
1,4,11,17,18,21,	-	-

[*] Response of unprimed AKR/J or B10.A T cells
[+] BC3C6, BC3B13 and BC3C13
[=] (C57BL/6xC3H/HeJ) recombinant inbred strains

Comparisons were made by stimulating unprimed T cells and cloned T cells derived from B10.BR ($H-2^k$) anti-C3H/HeJ ($H-2^k$, Mls^c) with 3 different groups of mice (Table 2). C3H/HeJ and A/J, which have previously been typed as Mls^c strains, stimulated strong proliferative responses by clones as well as unprimed MHC compatible T cells; while B10.BR and B10.A, which have been typed Mls^b, stimulated neither clones nor unprimed T cells. In a second group, BXH RI strains which originated from a combination of B6 and C3H/HeJ were employed and it was found that BXH 3,6,12, and 14, but not BXH 7, stimulated both unprimed B10.BR and anti-C3H/HeJ clones. Finally, and most conclusively, experiments were performed using AKR/J x (C3H/HeJxAKR/J)F$_1$ [Mls^a x (Mls^{a}x Mls^c)F$_1$] backcross animals. In the progeny of this backcross, there should be Mls$^{a/a}$

and $Mls^{a/c}$ animals. Therefore, if potential Mls^c-reactive clones are in fact Mls^c specific, these clones should respond to those stimulator cells that can stimulate unprimed AKR/J (Mls^a) T cells. On the basis of this hypothesis, responses of unprimed AKR/J T cells and clones to stimulator cells from a total of 24 backcross animals were studied. The response pattern of unprimed heterogeneous AKR/J T cells and anti-C3H/HeJ T cell clones were precisely concordant as shown in Table 2. Thus it appears that these clones recognize the determinants that define the Mls^c response.

Analysis of Polymorphism in Mls

Once the specificities of these Mls^a-reactive and Mls^c-reactive clones were defined, these clones were used as "reagents" for clonological analysis to address the question of Mls polymorphism.

Table 3. Proliferative responses of Mls^a-and Mls^c-reactive clones to Mls-different stimulator cells

Stimulator strain	Genotype		Responses of T cell clones				
	H-2	Mls	Anti-Mls^a		Anti-Mls^c		
			BARC1	BARB12	BC3C6	BC3B13	BC3C13
AKR/J	k	a	+	+	−	−	−
B10.BR	k	b	−	−	−	−	−
C3H/HeJ	k	c	−	−	+	+	+
CBA/J	k	d	+	+	+	+	+

As shown in Table 3, AKR/J (Mls^a) stimulated Mls^a-specific T cell clones and C3H/HeJ (Mls^c) stimulated Mls^c-specific T cell clones but not vice versa, indicating that Mls^a and Mls^c determinants recognized by T cells are antigenically different. From this point of view, the Mls system is truly polymorphic. However, experimental results also indicated that CBA/J (Mls^d) stimulated both Mls^a- and Mls^c-specific clones, suggesting the coexistence of both Mls^a and Mls^c determinants on CBA/J cells. From this pattern of responses, two different interpretations appeared possible. First, different alleles of a single Mls locus might encode at least three polymorphic stimulatory molecules, Mls^a, Mls^c and Mls^d. The Mls^d cells would express both Mls^a and Mls^c determinants on a unique Mls^d molecule. An alternative explanation is that Mls^d is not a unique Mls molecule but that Mls^d stimulators simply express both Mls^a and Mls^c. In order to address this question, a clonological analysis was performed of Mls^d reactive T cell responses.

A panel of B10.BR (Mls^b) anti-CBA/J (Mls^d) clones were tested for their responses to 4 Mls-different stimulators (Table 4). Each of these clones responded to CBA/J stimulators but not to syngeneic B10.BR, indicating that these clones were not self MHC-reactive. In addition to their reactivities to CBA/J, seven of nine clones responded to AKR/J (Mls^a) and two clones responded to C3H/HeJ (Mls^c). None of these clones reacted with both AKR/J and C3H/HeJ. Further analysis of specificities of these clones using inbred strains, RI strains and backcross animals as described above indicated that determinants recognized by AKR/J-reactive and C3H/HeJ-reactive clones are in fact, Mls^a and Mls^c, respectively.

Although this clonal distribution of anti-Mls^d crossreactivity with Mls^a or Mls^c appeared to favor the idea that no unique Mls^d determinants exist, cloned T cell populations do not necessarily represent the whole repertoire of B10.BR for CBA/J. Therefore heterogeneous T cell responses were also studied. Since unprimed (AKR/JxC3H/HeJ)F$_1$ [(Mls^{a}xMls^c)F$_1$] T cells did not significantly respond to CBA/J (Mls^d) (data not shown; Abe et al. 1987b; Ryan et al. 1987), no evidence was obtained for the existence of unique stimulatory determinants expressed on CBA/J (Mls^d) which are distinct from Mls^a and Mls^c.

Table 4. Responses of clones from a B10.BR anti-CBA/J line to stimulator cells from Mls-different strains

| T cell clones | Response of T cell clones with stimulator cells from | | | |
	AKR/J (Mls^a)	B10.BR (Mls^b)	C3H/HeJ (Mls^c)	CBA/J (Mls^d)
BCAC1	-	-	+	+
BCAC2	+	-	-	+
BCAC3	+	-	-	+
BCAC4	+	-	-	+
BCAC5	-	-	+	+
BCAC6	+	-	-	+
BCAC10	+	-	-	+
BCAC12	+	-	-	+
BCAC17	+	-	-	+

Table 5. Response patterns of Mls^a-and Mls^c-specific T cell clones to stimulators from (AKRxC3H) x B10.BR offspring

| Pattern of Mls expression in offspring | Responses of clones | | No. of mice |
	Mls^a-specific	Mls^c-specific	
Group 1	+	-	
Group 2	-	+	} 33
Group 3	+	+	
Group 4	-	-	} 37
			Total 70

Allelism of Mls

Since no inbred mouse can express the product of more than one allele encoded by a single locus, the coexistence of Mls^a and Mls^c on CBA/J led us to ask whether the genes encoding these two determinants are in fact allelic. In order to address this question, a segregation analysis was carried out by testing the stimulatory capacity of spleen cells from progeny of (AKR/Jx C3H/HeJ)F$_1$ x B10.BR [(Mls^{a}xMls^c)F$_1$ x Mls^b] breedings for Mls^a- and Mls^c-specific cloned T cells. The hypothetical basis of this segregation analysis was the following: If the Mls^a and Mls^c

determinants were encoded by allelic genes, as originally proposed, all of the offspring from this breeding would be either $Mls^{a/b}$ or $Mls^{c/b}$ genotypically and phenotypically Mls^a or Mls^c, respectively. However, as shown in Table 5, Mls^a- and Mls^c-specific clones exhibited 4 different patterns, corresponding phenotypically to Mls^a, Mls^c, $Mls^{a/c}$ and Mls^b. This observation was confirmed by testing primary MLR to these animals. Of a total of 70 progeny from this breeding tested, 37 exhibited either coexpression or nonexpression of both Mls^a and Mls^c determinants, indicating that the genes encoding Mls^a and Mls^c determinants are not allelic or linked (Abe et al. 1987c).

CONCLUDING REMARKS

Through the use of Mls specific T cell clones, the genetic and antigenic relationships among products of the stimulatory Mls^a, Mls^c and Mls^d phenotypes were analyzed. Results from these experiments indicated that the stimulatory Mls phenotypes, Mls^a, Mls^c and Mls^d, in fact represent the expression of the products of at least two independent and unlinked gene loci with no evidence to date of structual polymorphism within the products of any one locus. Furthermore, it would appear that a similar clonological analysis using monoclonal T cells with defined specificities could be a powerful tool for analysis of other non-MHC genetic systems, in most of which gene products are serologically undefined and which may play important roles in transplantation.

The authors wish to thank Drs. R.E. Gress and N. Shinohara for their critical reviews of this manuscript.

REFERENCES

Abe R, Ryan JJ, Finkelman FD, Hodes RJ (1987a) T cell recognition of Mls: T cell clones demonstrate polymorphism and allelism among Mls^a, Mls^c, and Mls^d. J Immunol 138:373-379

Abe R, Ryan JJ, Hodes RJ (1987b) Clonal analysis of the Mls system: A reappraisal of polymorphism and allelism among Mls^a, Mls^c, and Mls^d. J Exp Med 165:1113-1129

Abe R, Ryan JJ, Hodes RJ (1987c) Mls is not a single gene, allelic system: Different stimulatory Mls determinants are the products of at least two nonallelic, unliked genes. J Exp Med 166:1150-1155

Festenstein H (1973) Immunological and biological aspects of in vitro lymphocyte allotransformation (MLR) in the mouse. Transplant Rev 15:62-88

Festenstein H, Bishop C, Taylor BA (1977) Location of Mls locus on mouse chromosome 1. Immunogenetics 5:357-361

Katz ME, Janeway CA Jr (1985) The immunobiology of T cell responses to Mls locus-disparate stimulator cells on cloned, protein antigen-specific, Ia-restricted T cell lines. J Immunol 134:2064-2070

Ryan JJ, Mond JJ, Finkelman FD (1987) The Mls^d-defined primary mixed lymphocyte reaction: a composite response to Mls^a and Mls^c determinants. J Immunol 138:4085-4092

Webb SR, Molnar-Kimber K, Jennifer B, Sprent J, Wilson DB (1981) T cell clones with dual specificity for Mls and various major histocompatibility complex determinants. J Exp Med 154:1970-1974

X-Chromosome Linked Mutations Affecting Mosaic Expression of the Mouse X Chromosome.

V. M. Chapman, S. G. Grant, R. A. Benz, D. R. Miller, and D. A. Stephenson

INTRODUCTION

In eutherian females one of the two sex chromosomes is inactive (Lyon, 1961; Russell, 1961). The inactive status is established relatively early during embryogenesis and is somatically heritable within a cell lineage throughout development (see Chapman, 1987). The inactivation event is generally random with respect to the parental origin of an X chromosome such that equal numbers of cells expressing the paternal (X^p) and maternal (X^m) chromosome can be seen as a mosaic mixture in adult tissues using a variety of direct and indirect measures of X chromosome gene function (see reviews by West, 1982; Gartler and Riggs, 1983; Chapman, 1987)

Using allelic variants of ubiquitous X-linked enzymes that are separable electrophoretically the relative contributions of X^m and X^p gene product can be qualitatively identified. Electrophoretic variants for both hypoxanthine phosphoribosyltransferase (HPRT) and phosphoglycerate kinase-1 (PGK-1) have been previously established as alleles for the Hprt and Pgk-1 loci on the mouse X chromosome (Nielsen and Chapman, 1977; Chapman et al., 1983). With the exception of HPRT-A expression in the erythrocytes (Johnson et al., 1985) both allelic forms of each enzyme do not differ in specific activity so that the relative abundance of electrophoretic forms present in homogenates of tissues provides a measure of the relative proportion of cells which express either X^m or X^p in tissues of heterozygous females. Furthermore, the different alleles are overtly neutral with respect to the viability of cells which express either allelic gene product. Thus, these enzyme markers were used in a screening system to identify mutations that affect the randomness of the inactivation event.

Deviations from the equal occurrence of cells which express X^m and X^p could occur by either non-random inactivation or by random inactivation followed by selection for cells which express one kind of X chromosome. The X-chromosome controlling element (Xce) is one examples of non-random inactivation that has been reported in the mouse (Cattanach and Williams, 1972; West and Chapman, 1978) and is thought to map to a central position on the mouse X chromosome (Cattanach et al., 1970). In addition, several X-linked mutations have also been described which lead to altered mosaic expression within specific cell lineages. Some prominent examples of human disorders or mutations that produce an imbalance in mosaic expression of the X chrommosome include: Wiskott-Aldrich syndrome (Gealy et al., 1980) X-linked agammaglobinemia (Conley et al., 1986), Lesch-Nyhan syndrome (Nyhan et al., 1970), PGK deficiency (Krietsch et al., 1985), and X-linked congenital hyperuricosuria (Dancis et al., 1968). The X-linked immune deficiency mutation (xid) in the mouse also leads to unbalanced mosaic expression in B-cells (Nahm et al., 1983; Forrester et al., 1987).

Significant advances in the production of germ-line mutations using ethyl-nitrosourea (ENU) in the mouse have been reported by several laboratories (Russell et al., 1979; Johnson and Lewis, 1981; Bode 1984). These reports demonstrate that mutations can be recovered at frequencies greater than 1 mutation per 2000 loci tested. We have, therefore, used ENU as a mutagen to ask whether we could induce X-linked mutations that alter the mosaic expression of X chromosomes in heterozygous females as a consequence of either altering the process of inactivation itself or by inducing mutations which would cause a selective growth of cells expressing only one kind of X chromosome. In this report we describe our initial findings of nine non-mosaic female progeny of ENU-treated male mice. Further, we demonstrate the heritability of

Molecular and Cellular Biology Department, Roswell Park Memorial Institute, 666 Elm Street, Buffalo, N.Y. 14263

this phenotype from two of these progeny and show that the effect is primarily limited to blood lineages.

PROTOCOL FOR THE PRODUCTION AND IDENTIFICATION OF X CHROMOSOME MUTATIONS

The protocol for ENU treatment of males carrying variant alleles of the indicator loci Hprt and Pgk-1 is shown in figure 1. These males were mated with females carrying different alleles at the X-chromosome indicator genes. The first generation (G_1) heterozygous female progeny were tested for deviations from normal mosaic expression of HPRT and PGK-1 in hemolysates and tissues from the tail. The use of two separate sampling procedures allowed us to establish whether an observed non-mosaic expression was specific to a lineage or whether it was likely to be generalized to all tissues. By using both Hprt and Pgk-1 we had an internal control to distinguish between specific mutations at the indicator loci and those that were less specific but perturb normal mosaicism. Furthermore, the indicator loci map to a central portion of the X chromosome separated by a distance of approximately 20 centiMorgans (Chapman et al., 1983) thus providing an important X-chromosome marker system for subsequent genetic analysis of any new mutations that might be recovered using this procedure.

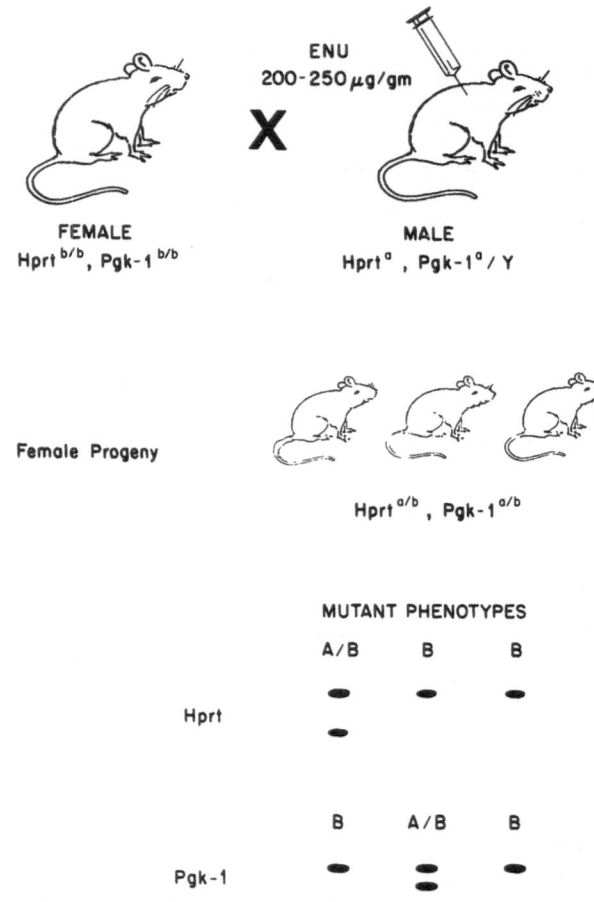

FIGURE 1: Screening protocol used to identify X-linked mutations.

MATERIALS AND METHODS

Mice: A recombinant X chromosome carrying both the M. castaneus Hprt^a allele and the M. musculus Pgk-1^a allele from the congenic strain C3H/HeHa Hprt^a, Pgk-1^a was transferred to the C57BL/6JRos inbred strain (Allelic transfer stock 29, AT29). Male mice from this stock were treated with ethyl nitrosourea (ENU/NEU) and mated after their return to fertility to mice from the C57BL/10.mdx (Hprt^b Pgk-1^b/Hprt^b Pgk-1^b) inbred strain. Backcross matings of F_1 females were performed to the C57BL/10.mdx strain.

Mutagen treatment: ENU (Sigma) at 10 mg/ml was prepared shortly before use by dissolving the solid in phosphate buffered saline at pH 6.8.(Russell et al., 1979). The males were exposed to a dose between 100-250 mg/kg body weight by a single intraperitoneal (i.p.) injection.

<u>Preparation of tissue samples for assay</u>: Blood was collected through heparinized capillary tubes from the orbital sinus. An equal volume of Johnson's buffer (Johnson <u>et al</u>., 1985) containing 10mM phosphate buffer pH 6.8, 0.25M sodium chloride, 0.01% Triton X-100, 15% Sucrose, 10mM dethioerythitol (DTE) and 1% bovine serum albumin (BSA) was added to each sample. The red blood cells were lysed in this buffer by incubating the suspension at 37°C for thirty minutes.

Tail samples were taken and chopped into small pieces with scissors in 100-200 ul of Johnson's buffer. Cells were lysed by a rapid freeze thawing cycle. Tissue debris was pelleted by centrifugation.

<u>HPRT analysis</u>: Resolution of the <u>Hprt</u> isozymes was performed on a horizontal polyacrylamide isoelectric focusing gel with a range in pH from 5-8 (Chasin and Urlaub, 1976) containing 5% acrylamide (32:1 acrylamide/bis-acrylamide ratio, BioRad), 5% Glycerol, 5% Pharmalyte pH 4-6.5 (Pharmacia), 0.8% Pharmalyte pH 3-10 (Pharmacia), 0.1 uM riboflavin-5'-phosphate (BioRad), 0.5% N,N,N'N'-tetramethylenediamine (BioRad) and 4.4 uM ammonium persulphate (BioRad). The cathode electrolyte contained 1M sodium hydroxide and the anode electrolyte contained 1M ortho-phosphoric acid. After the application of the samples at the anode end of the gel, the gels were pre-focused on constant current until the voltage reached 1,000V and then focused at a constant voltage of 1,000V for one hour. The gels were stained according to the protocol of Chasin and Urlaub (1976) using ^{14}C-labelled hypoxanthine (DuPont).

<u>PGK-1 analysis</u>: Electrophoresis condition and staining protocol were as described previously (Chapman <u>et al</u>., 1983). In principle, samples were run on cellulose acetate gels (Titan III, Helena) using a barbital/citrate buffer pH 8.8 at 200V for 1-1/2 hours. The gels were stained using a modification of the enzyme cascade reaction described by Bücher <u>et al</u>. (1980) and the isozymes visualized by the addition of 3-[4,5-dimethylthiazol-2-yl]-2,5-diphenyl tetrazolium (MTT, Sigma) and phenazine methosulphate (PMS, Sigma) at a final concentration of 1.5 mg/ml and 0.1 mg/ml, respectively.

RESULTS

A total of 1762 heterozygous G_1 female progeny from ENU-treated males were tested for mosaic expression of the indicator gene products HPRT and PGK-1. Of these offspring, nine displayed a non-mosaic pattern for both markers in the hemolysates (table 1). In every instance, only the maternally inherited allelic forms were expressed. Four of the nine were also non-mosaic in the tissues of the tail (table 1). The remaining five G_1 females expressed the paternal X-chrsomosome alleles in tissues from the tail in a normal mosaic pattern (table 1).

TABLE 1: Phenotypic deviants in the female progeny sired by ENU-treated males following their return to fertility.

| | BLOOD | | TAIL | | |
	HPRT	PGK-1	HPRT	PGK-1	Total
Normal mosaicism	A[*]	AB	-	-	1752
Non-mosaicism	B	B	B	B	4
Non-mosaicism (blood)	B	B	AB	AB	5

[*]Heterozygotes and homozygotes for the <u>Hprt</u>[a] allele cannot be distinguished on the basis of the blood phenotype.

Breeding tests were performed on all nine females to ascertain whether the marker alleles from the ENU-treated father would be transmitted and whether the pattern of non-mosaic expression was a heritable trait. The four G_1 females with non-mosaic expression in both tail and hemolysates did not transmit the marker alleles from the father and were therefore presumed to be XO genotypes. The five females that were non-mosaic in blood but mosaic in the tail produced heterozygous female progeny displaying the non-mosaic pattern of X chromosomal gene expression in the blood. These findings establish the heritability of the pattern observed in the original G_1 females and demonstrates that the non-mosaic pattern is not determined by the maternal or paternal origins of the gametes.

The HPRT and PGK-1 phenotypes observed in the hemolysate from two of the G_1 females (#556 and #704) were uniformly non-mosaic (figure 2). However, both females expressed the HPRT-A and PGK-1A allelic forms from the father in tissues from the tail (figure 2). The phenotype of #556 differed from that observed for other G_1 females and from the mutant #704 by having a marked decrease in the levels of HPRT-A and PGK-1A in the tissues from the tail and skeletal muscle.

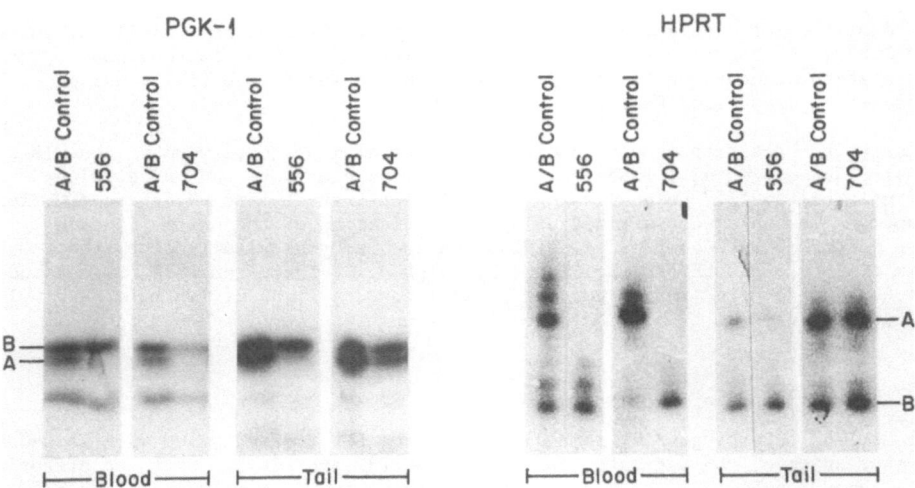

FIGURE 2: Electrophoretic separation of variant X-linked enzyme markers.

PROGENY ANALYSIS OF MUTANT FEMALE #556

The phenotypes in the offsprings produced by mating the 556 mutant female to a C57BL/10.mdx male are present in table 2. Nineteen female progeny were produced of which seven were homozygous (P_2 class) and another seven heterozygous for both indicator loci (P_1 class). Three of the P_1 class female progeny were non-mosaic in hemolysates indicating that the pattern observed in the 556 mother was heritable to at least half of her heterozygous daughters. These findings suggest that there is a mutation present on the Hprt^a, Pgk-1^a X chromosome from the ENU-treated male and that this mutation alters the mosaic expression of X chromosomes in females heterozygous for the mutation.

If the mutation were a cell-autonomous lethal condition we would predict that males receiving the mutant-bearing X chromosome would be absent in the progeny of female 556. A comparison of the relative frequency of male and female progeny, 21 males and 19 females, indicates that the sex ratio does not differ from the expected 1:1 ($x^2=0.1$). Moreover, the distribution of parental-type phenotypes among males indicates that there was no significant decrease in P_1 males (the mutant bearing X chromosome) compared with P_2 males ($x^2=0.529$). The lack of a demonstrable decrease in male progeny overall and in P_1 males in particular suggests that the mutation from 556, which alters mosaic X chromosome expression in blood, is not a cell-autonomous lethal nor is it behaving in a systemic lethal fashion in male progeny since P_1-type males are capable of transmitting the non-mosaic character to their daughters (data not shown).

TABLE 2: Phenotype of backcross progeny between phenotypic deviant 556 female and C57BL/10.mdx male

| | | Blood | | Tail | | Frequency |
		HPRT	PGK-1	HPRT	PGK-1	
Male offspring	P_1	A	A	-	-	7
	P_2	B	B	-	-	10
	R_1	A	B	-	-	1
	R_2	B	A	-	-	2
	Unclassified					1
					Total	21
Female offspring	P1	B	B	A<B	A<B	3
		A	AB	A<B	A<B	4
	P_2	B	B	B	B	7
	R_1	B	B	A<B	B	0
		A	B	A<B	B	3
	R_2	B	B	B	A<B	0
		B	AB	B	AB	1
	Unclassified					1
					Total	19

On the basis of the non-mosaic expression of the X chromosome in heterozygous female progeny from 556 we conclude that there is an X-linked mutation responsible for this phenotype and that this mutation has either variable penetrance in hemolysates or a map position distant to the Hprt and Pgk-1 marker genes. We have provisionally assigned this mutation the designated gene symbol $\underline{Xm}^{556}$ for X chromosome mutant 556.

PROGENY ANALYSIS OF MUTANT FEMALE #704

The phenotypes of offspring produced by female #704 mated with a C57BL/10.mdx male is shown in table 3. Twelve P_2 homozygous females were observed compared with 11 female progeny heterozygous for both indicator genes which is consistent with a 1:1 segregation of the two types of chromosomes from the 704 mother (χ^2=0.8). Eight out of the 11 heterozygous P_1 female progeny were non-mosaic for X chromosomal gene expression in blood suggesting the presence of a mutation on the Hprt^a, Pgk-1^a X chromosome from the original ENU-treated male. Examination of the sex-ratio in the progeny from 704 indicates that there is a significant deficit of males (χ^2=9.8, P<0.01) and in particular, a deficiency of the P_1 class. These findings indicate that the non-mosaic expression in blood of 704 and her heterozygous female progeny is a cell-autonomous lethal and that selective growth of the cells which express the non-mutant bearing X chromosome is sufficient to rescue the viability of mutant carriers.

TABLE 3: Phenotype of backcross progeny between phenotypic deviant 704 female and C57BL/10.mdx male

		Blood		Tail		Frequency
		HPRT	PGK-1	HPRT	PGK-1	
Male offspring	P_1	A	A	-	-	0
	P_2	B	B	-	-	10
	R_1	A	B	-	-	2
	R_2	B	A	-	-	0
					Total	12
Female offspring	P_1	B	B	AB	AB	8
		A	AB	AB	AB	3
	P_2	B	B	B	B	12
	R_1	B	B	AB	B	4
		A	B	AB	B	4
	R_2	B	B	B	AB	1
		B	AB	B	AB	1
					Total	33

If we assume that the mutation from 704 is fully penetrant then the mosaic expression for 3/11 heterozygous P_1 progeny suggests that the mutant locus lies outside of the Hprt-Pgk-1 region of the mouse X chromosome at an estimated distance of 27.3 ± 13.4 centiMorgans. The lack of R_2 male progeny which would involve a recombination between Hprt and Pgk-1 but retaining the distal portion of the X chromosome from the original mutagen-treated male suggests that the mutant locus may be distal to Pgk-1 on the mouse X chromosome.

Taken together, the transmission of the non-mosaic phenotype in heterozygous females and a deficit of males in the offspring from the G_1 female 704, indicates the presence of an X-linked mutation that acts as a cell-autonomous lethal. We have provisionally assigned this mutation the designated symbol Xm^{704} for X chromosome mutant 704. Preliminary data suggests that the mutant is fully penetrant in heterozygous carriers and that the locus maps distal to Pgk-1.

DISCUSSION

We initially asked whether we could use ENU to produce non-mosaic expression of X chromosomes in heterozygous females. Our screening methodology has identified at least 5 interesting phenodeviants in the G_1 female progeny of ENU-treated males. Two of these are described which illustrate different kinds of mutant phenotypes. One, Xm^{704}, behaves like a cell-autonomous lethal while the second, Xm^{556}, is more difficult to characterize. The Xm^{556} mutation is transmissible, but the apparent lack of full penetrance and the viability of males bearing the $Hprt^a$, $Pgk-1^a$ alleles associated with the Xm^{556} make it difficult to define the cell lineages most affected and the impact of the mutation on presumptive mutant bearing males. Preliminary work further suggests that Xm^{556} can be transmitted through a male which offers opportunities for following the mutant phenotype in a hemizygous X-chromosome background (data not shown). The phenotypic effects of Xm^{556} will be more comprehensively addressed in the accompanying manuscript (Ansell et al., this publication).

The phenotypic analysis of both mutants suggests that neither of them affect the process of X inactivation directly and that they act by cell selection from a mosaic population of cells which express both X chromosomes. From that standpoint, these mutations are similar to the phenotypes observed with at least one mouse mutant, xid and several X-linked human syndromes. Some appear to be specific to certain cell lineages (B cells - agammaglobulinemia; T cells and platelets - Wiskott-Aldrich syndrome), others, on the other hand, are less specific and significantly more variable in their phenotype (adrenoleukodystrophy, PGK-deficiency and Lesch-Nyhan syndrome). The mouse mutant X-linked immunodeficiency (xid) is one of a few examples that displays non-mosaic expression of other sex-linked enzymes specific to the B cell lineage (Forrester et al., 1987; Nahm et al., 1983). It is possible that the xid mutation in the mouse is homologous to the human agammaglobulinemia syndrome (Buckle et al., 1985). The X chromosomal controlling element (Xce) is another locus on the mouse X chromosome that influences the randomness of inactivation (Cattanach and Williams, 1972; West and Chapman, 1978). With at least three alleles, the Xce locus modifies the probability of X inactivation such that expression of sex-linked loci display a skewed phenotype depending upon which alleles are present in heterozygous females (Cattanach, 1970; Cattanach and Williams, 1972). It is not clear whether the new mutants we have described in the present study are analogous to known sex-linked loci in both mouse and man or whether they represent new and novel mutations. Further characterization is needed before any definitive conclusions can be made. Nonetheless, it would appear that at least one mutant has a specific effect on blood cell lineages. Whether this is a consequence of a mutation at a locus involved in blood cell production or at some other locus that has an indirect effect remains to be established.

In the case of Xm^{704}, we have preliminary evidence that the mutation may have been recovered in at least two other G_1 females from the same ENU-treated male. It will be important to ask whether other components of the hematopoietic lineage are affected by the mutation and whether prenatal hematopoiesis is affected. These determinations will help establish when mutant-bearing males die. In the final analysis, Xm^{704} may be a specific metabolic component of hematopoiesis. The apparent full penetrance of the mutant effects on mosaic expression and the lethality of mutant-bearing males will help in the localization of the Xm^{704} locus on the X chromosome relative to $Hprt$ and $Pgk-1$. At that point, we can construct additional crosses which will localize the gene on the X chromosome in multipoint linkage analysis (Mullins et al., in press).

This work was supported in part by NIH grants GM33160 and GM24125.

REFERENCES

Bode, V.C. (1984) Ethylnitrosourea mutagenesis and the isolation of mutant alleles for specific genes located in the t region of mouse chromosome 17. Genetics 108: 457-470.
Bücher, T., W. Bender, R. Fundele, H. Hofner and I. Linke (1980) Quantitative evaluation of electrophoretic allo- and isozyme patterns. FEBS Lett. 115: 319-324.

190

Buckle, V.J., J.H. Edwards, E.P. Evans, J.A. Jonasson, M.F. Lyon, J. Peters and A.G.
Searle (1985) Comparative maps of human and mouse X chromosome. Cytogenet. Cell
Genet. 40: 594-595.
Cattanach, B.M. (1970) Controlling elements in the mouse X-chromosome. III. Influence
upon both parts of an X divided by rearrangement. Genet. Res. 16: 293-301.
Cattanach, B.M., J.N. Perez and C.E. Pollard (1970) Controlling elements in the mouse
X-chromosome. II. Location in the linkage map. Genet. Res. 15: 183-195.
Cattanach, B.M. and C.E. Williams (1972) Evidence of non-random X chromosome
activity in the mouse. Genet. Res. 19: 291-316.
Chapman, V.M. (1987) X-chromosome regulation in oogenesis and early mammalian
development. In: Experimental Approaches to Mammalian Embryonic Development, eds.
J. Rossant & R.A. Pedersen, Cambridge University Press, pp.365-398.
Chapman, V.M., P.G. Kratzer and B.A. Quarantillo (1983) Electrophoretic variation
for X chromosome-linked hypoxanthine phosphoribosyl transferase (HPRT) in
wild-derived mice. Genetics 103: 785-795.
Chasin, L.A. and G. Urlaub (1976) Mutant alleles for hypoxanthine phosphoribosyl
transferase: Co-dominant expression, complementation and segregation in hybrid
Chinese hamster cells. Somat. Cell Genet. 2: 453-467.
Conley, M.E., P. Brown, A.R. Pickard, R.H. Buckley, D.S. Miller, W.H. Raskind, J.W.
Singer and P.J. Fialkow (1986) Expression of the gene defect in X-linked
agammaglobulinemia. New Engl. J. Med. 315: 564-567.
Dancis, J., P.H. Berman, V. Jansen and M.E. Balis (1968) Absence of mosaicism in the
lymphocyte of X-linked congenital hyperuricosuria. Life Sci. 7: 587-591.
Forrester, L.M., J.D. Ansell and H.S. Micklem (1987) Development of B lymphocytes in
mice heterozygous for the X-linked immunodeficiency (xid) mutation. J. Exp. Med.
165: 949-958.
Gartler, S.M. and A.D. Riggs (1983) Mammalian X-chromosome inactivation. Ann. Rev.
Genet. 17: 155-190.
Gealy, W.J., J.M. Dwyer and J.B. Harley (1980) Allelic exclusion of
glucose-6-phosphate dehydrogenase in platelets and T lymphocytes from a
Wiskott-Aldrich Syndrome carrier. Lancet I: 63-65.
Johnson, F.M. and S.E. Lewis (1981) Electrophoretically detected germinal mutations
induced in the mouse by ethylnitrosourea. Proc. Natl. Acad. Sci. (USA) 97:
3238-3141.
Johnson, G.G., T.A. Larsen, P. Blakley and V.M. Chapman (1985) Elevated levels of
erythrocyte hypoxanthine phosphoribosyltransferase associated with allelic
variation of murine Hprt. Biochem. 24: 5083-5089.
Krietsch, W.K.G., M. Dunnwald, I.M. Linke and T. Bücher (1985) Preferential
expression of the maternally inherited X-linked phosphoglycerate kinase allele in
human erythrocytes. Mol. Gen. Genet. 200: 497-499.
Lyon, M.F. (1961) Gene action in the X-chromosome of the mouse (Mus musculus L).
Nature 190: 372-373.
Nahm, M.H., J.W. Paslay and J.M. Davie (1983) Unbalanced X chromosome mosaicism in B
cells of mice with X-linked immunodeficiency. J. Exp. Med. 158: 920-931.
Nielsen, J.T. and V.M. Chapman (1977) Electrophoretic variation for
X-chromosome-linked phosphoglycerate kinase (PGK-1) in the mouse. Genetics 87:
319-325.
Nyhan, W.L., B. Bakay, J.D. Connor, J.F. Marks and D.K. Keele (1970) Hemizygous
expression of glucose-6-phosphate dehydrogenase in erythrocytes of heterozygotes
for the Lesch-Nyhan Syndrome. Proc. Natl. Acad. Sci. (USA) 65: 214-218.
Russell, L.B. (1961) Genetics of mammalian sex chromosomes. Science 133: 1795-1803.
Russell, W.L., P.R. Hunsicker, G.D. Raymer, M.H. Steele, K.F. Stelzner and H.M.
Thompson (1979) Dose-response curve for ethylnitrosourea-induced specific-locus
mutations in mouse spermatogonia. Proc. Natl. Acad. Sci. (USA) 79: 3589-3591.
West, J.D. (1982) X-chromosome expression during mouse embryogenesis. In: Genetic
Control of Gamete Production and Function, eds. P.G. Crosignani & B. L. Rubin,
Academic Press, New York, pp.49-91.
West, J.D. and V.M. Chapman (1978) Variation for X chromosome expression in mice
detected by electrophoresis of phosphoglycerate kinase. Genet. Res. 32: 91-102.

Mosaic Analysis of the Effects of a Novel X-Chromosome Mutation of the Haematopoietic System

J.D. Ansell, V.M. Chapman*, L.M. Forrester, D.J. Fowlis, C. MacKenzie, and H.S. Micklem

SUMMARY

Mutations specific to the X chromosome were identified in female offspring, sired by mice treated with the mutagen ethyl nitrosourea (ENU), by alterations in the mosaic patterns of X chromosome-linked enzyme polymorphisms in blood and other somatic tissues. Flow cytometric analyses were performed on haematopoietic and lymphoid cells of mice homozygous for one such mutation. Similar studies were made on heterozygotes that were, in addition, mosaic for electrophoretic variants of the enzyme phosphoglycerate kinase (PGK-1). The PGK-1 mosaic patterns in cells of different haematopoietic lineages were used to investigate the nature of the primary lesion induced by the mutation. Preliminary results indicate that one of the ENU mutations has effects on differentiation of T lymphocytes and possibly some other haematopoietic cells.

INTRODUCTION

X chromosome-linked genes in man code for a variety of immuno-deficiency syndromes and haematopoietic disorders. Three of the major categories of immunodeficiency diseases are inherited through the X chromosome: Bruton-type agammaglobulinaemia is characterised by an absence of plasma cells, which renders patients susceptible to bacterial infections (Geha et al. 1973); in Wiskott-Aldrich syndrome (eczema-thrombocytopenia-immunodeficiency syndrome) T lymphocytes and platelets are lacking and there are defects in the afferent limb of the immune response at the level of antigen processing (Blaese et al. 1968); Swiss-type agammaglobulinaemia (thymic epithelial hypoplasia, X-linked severe combined immuno-deficiency disease) patients are vulnerable to viral and fungal, as well as bacterial, infections and suffer from lymphocytopenia and atrophy of the thymus. A profound immunodeficiency is seen in some cases despite high levels of circulating B lymphocytes, which are however incapable of terminal differentiation into plasma cells (Yount et al. 1978).

Several other less common X-linked haematopoietic disorders have been recorded. These include; immunodeficiency with increased IgM (dysgammaglobulinaemia Type 1), granulomatous disease, X-linked thrombo-cytopenia, malignant reticuloendotheliosis, acute X-linked leukaemia and Duncan disease (X-linked progressive combined immuno-deficiency, X-linked lymphoproliferative disease, familial fatal Epstein-Barr infection). X-linkage has also been noted for a rare form of hypochromic anaemia and a proliferation defect in haematopoietic cells (McKusick 1986).

In summary, there may be a number of genes on the X chromosome that play important roles in the differentiation of immune function and

Department of Zoology, University of Edinburgh, West Mains Road, Edinburgh EH9 3JT, United Kingdom

* Roswell Park Memorial Institute, Buffalo, N.Y.

influence susceptibility to tumour development. These genes may also affect the differentiation of other haematopoietic elements. Few comparable disorders have been identified in mice or other experimental animals. The CBA/N mouse is homo- (or hemi-) zygous for the xid mutation and shows some similarity to the Bruton-type immunodeficiency syndrome (Scher 1982). However, the effect of the mutation is relatively mild. The mice do not respond to a class of 'T-independent' (TI-2) antigens and at least one population of B lymphocytes, characterised by high concentrations of membrane IgD (mIgD) and low concentrations of mIgM, is missing from the adult. Other X-linked loci in mice code for high, low or absent responses to specific antigens (Green 1981).

STRATEGIES FOR ANALYSIS OF X CHROMOSOME MUTATIONS IN MICE

Our own work in this laboratory has concentrated on the differentiation of B lymphocytes carrying the xid mutation in a heterozygous environment. The experimental strategy makes use of the phenomenon of X chromosome inactivation, an event which occurs shortly after implantation in female mammals and results in one or other of the X chromosomes in all somatic cells being functionally inactive. This is a random process, and results in an individual being a mosaic for any allelic differences on the X chromosome. Mosaicism for xid is not, in itself, detectable. However, we have been able to make use of another X-chromosome gene, Pgk-1, which has a detectable product; this is used as a marker for the presence of xid. The two alleles of Pgk-1 code for different electrophoretic forms of the enzyme phosphoglycerate kinase (PGK-1), A and B. These alloenzymes can be separated and quantified by simple electrophoretic techniques (Ansell and Micklem 1986). All somatic cells in female mice heterozygous for xid and Pgk-1 will be either PGK-1B with the xid mutant allele active or PGK-1A with the normal allelic counterpart of xid active. Any selection against cells carrying the xid mutant can be measured by looking at the relative expression of the Pgk alleles in that cell population. By separating subsets of B cells and other haematopoietic populations on a fluorescence activated cell sorter (FACS) we have been able to determine the cell types on which xid acts and the developmental stage at which it acts

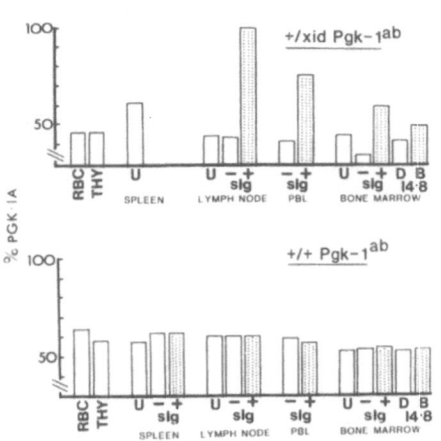

Fig. 1. Values of PGK-1A in cell lysates from a xid-heterozygous (+/xid Pgk-1ab) and a normal female (+/+ Pgk-1ab) mouse. Abbreviations : RBC, erythrocytes; THY, thymus; PBL, peripheral blood leucocytes; sIg, membrane immunoglobulin; + -, FACS-sorted cells positive or negative for sIg; 14.8, monoclonal antibody 14.8 against B220 antigen; B D, FACS-sorted cells staining brightly (B cells) or dully (pre-B cells) for B220. In the +/xid heterozygote, unbalanced mosaicism (stippled columns) is seen in peripheral B cells, but not in the bone marrow pre-B population.

(Witkowski et al. 1985, Forrester et al. 1987). An example of the data acquired by this approach is shown in Fig. 1. These and other data have shown that although the homozygous mutant is deficient only in certain classes of B lymphocyte, in the heterozygote virtually all mature B cells carrying an active mutant X chromosome are selected against. Further, this selection only operates on B cells after the stage at which membrane Ig (mIg) is expressed: earlier B-lineage cells in the bone marrow are unaffected.

This strategy can be used to analyse the effects of any X chromosome mutation at the cellular level. It has the additional advantage that genetic effects of single mutations can be analysed in a relatively normal heterozygous environment, thus enabling the nature of the primary lesion to be distinguished from other secondary effects which may constitute major parts of the syndrome associated with the homozygous (hemizygous) mutant.

ANALYSIS OF AN ENU-DERIVED MUTATION

The approach described above has been used in the analysis of an X chromosome mutation derived by ENU mutagenesis. The techniques of mutagenesis and the initial identification of mutants are described by Chapman (this volume). A female mouse was selected which showed random X chromosome expression in most somatic tissues, but selective expression of the non-mutagenised X chromosome in erythrocytes. This implied that during the course of erythropoietic differentiation, cells in which the mutant gene was active were at a selective disadvantage. In addition a preliminary experiment showed that lymph node cells had a non-mosaic phenotype. This suggested that the mutation may have been inimical to T lymphocyte differentiation, since most peripheral lymph node cells are T cells.

A number of homozygous mice derived from this original female have been analysed by flow cytofluorometry to investigate the effects of the mutation on various haematopoietic cell lineages. Female mice heterozygous for the mutant and for the A and B electrophoretic variants of PGK-1 have also been analysed and the mosaic phenotypes of sorted and unsorted haematopoietic cells investigated.

Single-cell suspensions of peripheral blood lymphocytes and from lymph node, spleen, thymus and bone marrow were prepared for FACS analysis and sorting. They were stained with monoclonal antibodies against Thy-1, Ly-3, L3T4 and B220 (Micklem 1986), a fluoresceinated goat anti-rat Ig serum being used as the second step. In addition cells of these organs as well as erythrocytes, brain and skeletal muscle, were prepared from heterozygous mice for alloenzyme analysis.

A series of dot plots taken from the FACS are shown in Figs. 2, 3 and 4, which illustrate some effects of this mutation on the haemato-poietic system. Fig. 2 shows the staining of bone marrow suspensions from a normal 3 month old CBA/Ca female (A), a homozygous mutant female (B) and a heterozygous female (C), with a monoclonal antibody against the B220 antigen. Dully staining (pre-B) and brightly stain-ing (mIg-expressing) cells usually comprise about 20% and 10% of the nucleated marrow cells respectively. In the mutant, these were reduced to 10% and 1% (mean of 5 animals). Although an approximately 1.5x increase in cellularity was seen in some mutant marrows, there appears to be some absolute reduction of B lymphopoiesis. Fig. 3 shows B220 staining in subcutaneous lymph node cells from the three types of animals. In a normal individual 14% of lymph node cells would be B cells (B220+ve). In the mutant this proportion was 47% with a proportionate decrease in the number of Thy-1+ve T cells

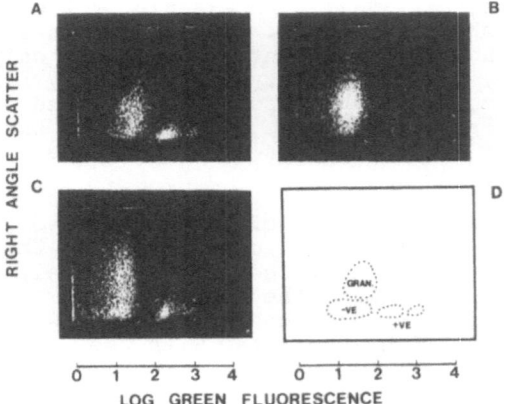

Fig. 2. FACS dot plots of bone marrow cells stained with a monoclonal antibody against B220 from a normal CBA/Ca control (A), an ENU homozygous mutant (B) and an ENU heterozygote (C). The diagram is of the cell populations in the control: the high-scattering granulopoietic and other cells (GRAN), a B220-negative population and two populations of B220-positive cells, the duller being pre-B cells and the brighter mIg-expressing B cells.

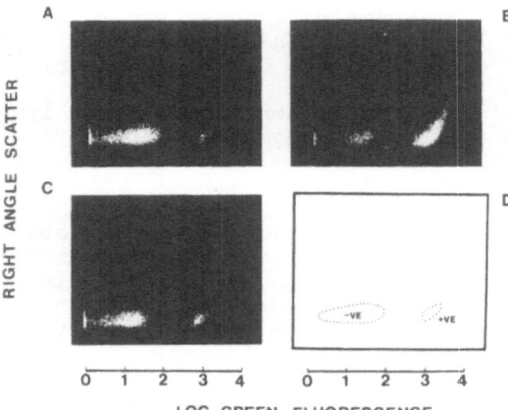

Fig. 3. Dot plots of lymph node cells stained for B220 as in Fig. 2. A, B and C are from the control, homozygous mutant and heterozygous mutant respectively. The homozygous mutant has a higher proportion of B220 +ve cells.

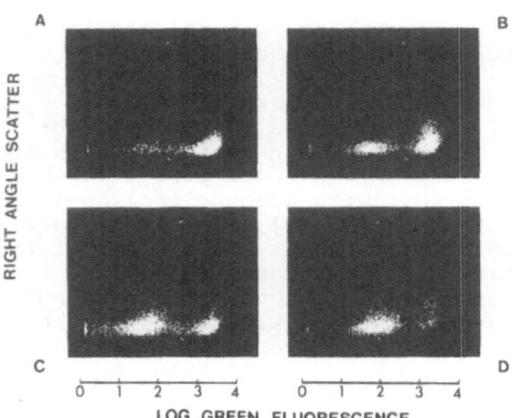

Fig. 4. Dot plots of lymph node cells (A and B) and spleen cells (C and D) stained with a monoclonal antibody against Thy-1. Thy-1 +ve cells are under-represented in the mutant (B and D) compared with the control (A and C) cell suspensions.

(Fig. 4, A and B). Similarly in the spleen (Fig. 4 C and D) the proportions of T cells in the mutant (4,D) are approximately half the normal value of 40%. Cells which stain for neither Thy-1 nor B220 usually account for 10% of splenocytes; in the mutant up to 55% of splenocytes are in this non-B, non-T category. It is apparent that one of the effects of this mutation was to alter the ratio of T to B lymphocyte numbers in the peripheral lymphoid organs. This was associated with increased granulopoiesis in the bone marrow (and a proportionate decrease in B lymphopoiesis), an increase in the numbers of granulocytes in the peripheral circulation (data not shown) and relative increases in the numbers of B lymphocytes in the peripheral lymphoid organs. Other preliminary observations on the homozygous mutant included decreased thymus size, decreased haematocrit and white blood cell count, increased bone marrow cellularity and increased size and cellularity of peripheral lymph nodes. Platelet counts were normal.

The heterozygotes appeared virtually normal. However analysis of the patterns of mosaicism for PGK-1 alloenzymes revealed defects at the cellular level in a number of organs. In normal heterozygotes all tissues would be expected to have a similar PGK-1 phenotype (McMahon et al. 1983, Micklem et al. 1987). The PGK-1 data for 5 ENU heterozygotes are summarised in Table 1. The data for skeletal muscle (SM) suggest that in these stocks two mutations may be segregating one of which has effects on the viability of muscle cells in the heterozygous environment. Since the original selection of these mutant stocks was on the basis of mosaic imbalance in blood, a double mutation would not have been detected. The mean ratio of PGK-1A:B in brain (BR) was 49:51). Against this yardstick PGK mosaicism in spleen (SPL) and bone marrow (BM) was slightly imbalanced in favour of the non-mutant X chromosome (PGK-1B in this case). This would suggest that there is no strong selection operating against B cells, or the bulk of differentiating haematopoietic cells, that carry an active mutant X chromosome. Platelets (PL) are relatively unaffected but circulating erythrocytes (E) have a greater imbalance. Selection against the mutant X is most apparent in cell suspensions from lymph node (LN) and thymus (THY). In lymph nodes of heterozygotes upwards of 80% of cells are T-cells. In thymus most cells are of T-lineage although in the preparation of cell suspensions it is possible to include varying proportions of stromal tissue. In two thymi, PGK-1A was less than 10%; in another, in which thymic lobes were analysed separately, one lobe was PGK-1B. In the one individual for which data are available so far FACS-sorted Thy-1+ve cells (T cells) from spleen and lymph node were shown to be entirely PGK-1B, i.e. devoid of cells carrying an active mutant X chromosome.

The data reviewed above indicate that the ENU mutation on the X chromosome has effects on T cell differentiation and may also have other effects on the haematopoietic system. Allozyme analysis of

Table 1.   Percent PGK-1A in cells from ENU heterozygotes.

Mouse	Age (wks)	E	PBL	LN	SPL	BM	THY	PL	BR	SM	THY1+VE SPL	THY1+VE LN
2261-1	7	16	–	18	35	–	20	–	51	0	–	–
2261-2	9	28	–	16	32	–	17	–	32	18	–	–
2115-1	7	28	–	–	–	–	–	–	–	–	0	0
2261-3	12	14	9	10	20	33	14,0	–	50	–	–	–
2261-4	16	43	38	14	31	40	0	27	50	40	–	–
2115-2	7	31	–	18	46	–	8	37	60	0	–	–

FACS-sorted cell lineages as described above, coupled with functional studies of the immune system, will enable us to determine the more precise effects of the lesion on haematopoietic differentiation and immune function.

We are indebted to Kay Samuel, Andrew Sanderson and Helen Taylor for technical assistance and to Dr. Paul Kincade for a gift of 14.8 antibody. LMF, DJF and CM were supported by Medical Research Council Postgraduate Studentships.

REFERENCES

Ansell JD and Micklem HS (1986) Genetic markers for following cell populations. In: Handbook of Experimental Immunology vol 2, 4th edn Ed DM Weir chap 56 Blackwells Scientific Publications

Blaese RM, Strober W, Brown RS and Waldmann TA (1968) The Wiskott-Aldrich syndrome. A disorder with a possible defect in antigen processing or recognition. Lancet 1:1056-1060

Forrester LM, Ansell JD and Micklem HS (1987) Development of B lymphocytes in mice heterozygous for the X-linked immuno-deficiency (XID) mutation. J exp Med 165:949-958

Geha RS, Rosen FS and Merler E (1973) Identification and character-isation of subpopulations of lymphocytes in human peripheral blood after fractionation on discontinuous gradients of albumin. The cellular defect in X-linked agammaglobulinemia. J Clin Invest 52:1726-1734

Green MC (1981) Catalog of mutant genes and polymorphic loci. In: Genetic Variants and Strains of the Laboratory Mouse. Ed MC Green pp 273-274. Gustav Fischer Verlag, Stuttgart, New York

McKusick VA (1986) X-linked phenotypes. In: Mendelian Inheritance in Man; Catalogs of Autosomal Dominant, Autosomal Recessive, and X-linked phenotypes. Seventh edition pp 981-1109 The John Hopkins University Press

McMahon A, Fosten M and Monk M (1983) X-chromosome inactivation mosaicism in the three germ layers and the germ line of the mouse embryo. J Embryol exp Morph 74:207-220

Micklem HS (1986) Monoclonal antibodies to murine haematopoietic cells. Methods in Hematology 13:182-206

Micklem HS, Lennon JE, Ansell JD and Gray RA (1987) Numbers and dispersion of repopulating hematopoietic cell clones in radiation chimeras as functions of injected cell dose. Exp Hematol 15: 251-257

Scher I (1982) The CBA/N mouse strain: an experimental model illustrating the influence of the X chromosome on immunity. Adv Immunol 33:1-71

Witkowski J, Forrester LM, Ansell JD and Micklem, HS (1985) Influence of the Xid mutation on B lymphocyte development in adult mice. In: Microenvironments in the Lymphoid System. Ed G Klaus Advances in Experimental Biology and Medicine 186:47-56 Plenum, New York

Yount WJ, Utsinger PD, Whisnant J and Folds JD (1978) Lymphocyte subpopulations in X-linked severe combined immunodeficiency (SCID): evidence against a stem cell defect; transformation response to calcium ionophore A23187. Am J Med 65:847-854

The *scid* Mouse Mutant

M. Bosma, W. Schuler, and G. Bosma

Occurrence of the scid Mutation

The scid mutation occurred in the C.B-17Icr (C.B-17) inbred strain, an immunoglobulin heavy chain (Igh) congenic partner strain of BALB/cAnIcr (BALB/c). The C.B-17 strain was derived from the 13th backcross generation of the original C.B stock of M. Potter. C.B-17 mice are not known to differ from BALB/c mice except that a portion of their chromosome 12 comes from the C57BL/Ka strain and includes the C57BL/Ka Igh locus and other closely-linked genes.

Mutant C.B-17scid mice were discovered in 1980 and reported in 1983 (Bosma et al. 1983). In the course of quantitating serum Ig levels in specific-pathogen-free mice, several C.B-17 mice were unexpectedly found to lack all of the major Ig classes (IgM, IgG3, IgG1, IgG2b, IgG2a and IgA). The ancestry of these mice was traced back to a single breeder pair; the male was agamma-globulinemic while the female appeared normal. Pedigree analysis revealed that the defect was recessively inherited. Selective genetic breeding led to the establishment of a colony of mutant mice and subsequent cellular analyses of these mice showed that they not only lacked functional B cells but also functional T cells. As this condition resembled that of severe combined immune deficiency (SCID), a syndrome first described in humans in the mid-50's (reviewed by Rosen et al. 1985), the mutant mice were called scid mice.

To ascertain the chromosomal location of the scid locus, scid mice were crossed with different linkage testing mouse stocks each of which expresses distinct genetic markers for one or more genes of known chromosomal location (in collaboration with M. Davisson, H. Sweet and L. Shultz of the Jackson Laboratory, Bar Harbor, ME). The F1 offspring were subsequently intercrossed with each other or backcrossed to scid mice as dictated by the recessive or dominant expression of the test markers. Only after the segregation analysis of more than 25 test markers in over 1800 offspring, was evidence obtained that scid is closely linked to mahoganoid (md), a recessive coat color marker on the centro-meric end of chromosome 16. The segregation of md and scid in 188 tested offspring of an F1 intercross agreed with expectation in that 25% and 22% of the mice typed homozygous for md and scid, respectively. However, none of the offspring typed homozygous for both md and scid; one would have expected ∿12 such mice (1/4 x 1/4 x 188) if both markers were unlinked.

To confirm the linkage of scid and md and to more precisely map scid on chromosome 16, a three-point cross was made involving md, scid and the lambda immunoglobulin light chain locus (Igl-1)

Institute for Cancer Research, Fox Chase Cancer Center, Philadelphia, PA 19111

which is also closely linked to md and is polymorphic (Epstein
et al. 1986). scid mice (scid, Igl-1^a, md$^+$) were crossed with a
recently derived recombinant mouse line (scid$^+$, Igl-1^b, md)
(described by Epstein et al. 1986) and then the F1 offspring were
intercrossed. The segregation of the three markers in the F2
generation is presently being analyzed (N. Ruetsch and G. Bosma
in collaboration with M. Davisson, H. Sweet and L. Shultz of the
Jackson Laboratory).

Effect of the scid Mutation on Lymphocyte Development

One of the earliest identifiable events in early B and T cell
development is the transcriptional activation of unrearranged Ig
and TCR genes (Kemp et al. 1980; Van Ness et al. 1981; Alt et al.
1982; Lennon and Perry 1985; Yancopoulos and Alt 1985). This
presumably reflects the early commitment of lymphocytes to the B
or T cell lineages; this may also reflect that certain Ig and TCR
genes are now accessible to the recombinase system. (Van Ness
et al. 1981; Yancopoulos and Alt 1985). Interestingly, transcriptional activation of Ig and TCR genes is clearly evident in
scid mice; Igh-V558, (Igh-Cμ) and (Igl-Cκ) transcripts are
readily detected in fetal liver and adult bone marrow and TCRγ
and TCRβ transcripts are present in adult thymus (W. Schuler,
A. Schuler, G. Bosma, G. Lennon and M. Bosma, unpublished
results). Nonetheless, all of these transcripts appear to derive
from unrearranged genes and thus cannot code for functional proteins, consistent with our inability to detect cells with Ig and
TCR rearrangements in freshly harvested lymphoid tissue of scid
mice (Schuler et al. 1986).

The above findings suggest that scid may impair Ig and TCR
rearrangements in developing B and T cells. Possibly, such
rearrangements are greatly reduced in frequency and/or are grossly abnormal. Evidence for the latter comes from the analysis of
transformed scid lymphocytes. Early B cells with Igh rearrangements can be recovered from scid bone marrow by transformation
with Abelson murine leukemia virus (A-MuLV). Strikingly, the
majority (>80%) of rearranged Igh alleles in A-MuLV transformed B
cells were shown to incur abnormal deletions (Schuler et al.
1986). The deletions extended varying distances into the Jh-Cμ
intron and spanned at least 3.5 kb from the most 3' Jh element.
This is illustrated in Figure 1. The detection of 5' flanking
regions of Dh elements juxtaposed to Cμ indicated that the deletions resulted from attempted Dh-to-Jh recombination. This is
confirmed in the accompanying report (Kim et al. 1987).

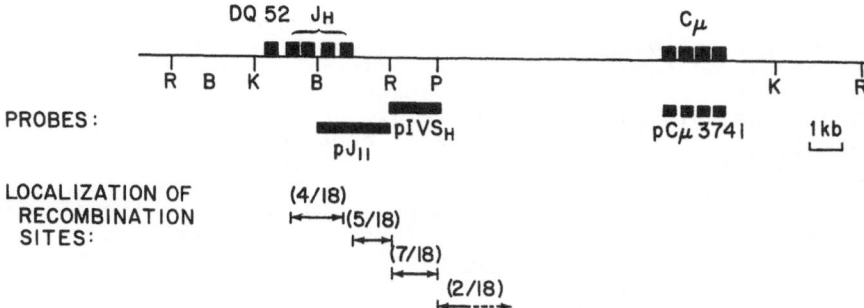

<u>Figure 1.</u> Partial restriction map of the <u>Igh</u> locus. The extent
of the abnormal J-associated deletions into the Jh-Cµ intron is
indicated for 14 of 18 alleles. Four of 18 rearrangements could
not be distinguished from normal rearrangements.

Abnormal rearrangements of antigen receptor genes also have been
seen in early <u>scid</u> T cells (Schuler <u>et al.</u> 1986) that appear as
spontaneous T cell lymphomas in ∿15% of <u>scid</u> mice (Custer <u>et al.</u>
1985). About 60% of the TCRβ rearrangements in these cells incur
deletions of the entire Jβ2 region, again as an apparent result
of attempted D-to-J recombination. However, defective rearrangements are not limited to D-to-J recombination, because in the
TCRγ locus, which lacks known D elements (rev. by Allison and
Lanier, 1987), abnormal deletions are also seen. The TCRγ deletions extend into the Vγ genes and flanking regions of Cγ genes
indicating faulty V-to-J recombination (Schuler <u>et al.</u> 1987 and
W. Schuler, A. Schuler and M. Bosma, unpublished results).

To explain the abnormal J-associated deletions and how they may
account for the <u>scid</u> phenotype, we proposed earlier (Schuler
<u>et al.</u> 1986) that the <u>scid</u> mutation causes highly error-prone Ig
and TCR rearrangements. Most developing <u>scid</u> lymphocytes would
accordingly lack an antigen receptor due to aberrant gene
rearrangements at both alleles of a critical antigen receptor
locus. The apparent absence of these nonfunctional cells in <u>scid</u>
lymphoid tissues might reflect their rapid turnover and elimination by macrophages, granulocytes and/or natural killer cells.
The latter cell types appear to function normally in <u>scid</u> mice
(Dorshkind <u>et al.</u> 1984; Custer <u>et al.</u> 1985; Dorshkind <u>et al.</u>
1985; Czitrom <u>et al.</u> 1985; Hackett <u>et al.</u> 1986; Bancroft <u>et al.</u>
1986). One way of detecting <u>scid</u> cells with aberrant gene
rearrangements would be to immortalize these cells before they
die. Transformation of early <u>scid</u> B and T cells presumably
serves this role.

To test further whether scid impairs the rearrangement of antigen
receptor genes, functionally rearranged Ig genes (Ig transgenes)
are being introduced into the scid mouse genome. This is being
done by selectively crossing the Ig transgenes of recently
established transgenic mouse strains (e.g., see Grosschedl et al.
1984; Storb et al. 1986) onto the genetic background of scid
mice. The expectation is that Ig transgenic scid mice will
develop B cells that express Ig proteins. Preliminary work (M.
Fried, K. Hayakawa, R. Hardy, G. Bosma and M. Bosma, unpublished
data) indicates that introduction of a functionally rearranged
Igh-Cμ gene alone (μ transgenic scid mice) results in near normal
numbers of Ly-5(B220)$^+$ IgM B cells in the bone marrow. Few such
cells are detected in the bone marrow of control, nontransgenic
scid mice. Whether these early scid B cells contain cytoplasmic
μ chains and abnormal Igl rearrangements remains to be ascertained.

Leaky scid Mice

A variable percentage (∿10-20%) of scid mice between the ages of
3-9 months appear "leaky" in that they produce detectable levels
of serum Ig (Bosma et al. 1983). Extensive characterization of
these scid(Ig$^+$) mice shows them to be oligoclonal for Ig-producing B cells and to contain a limited number of functional T cells
(Bosma et al. 1987; A. Carroll and M. Bosma, unpublished
results). In other respects, scid(Ig$^+$) mice resemble scid(Ig$^-$)
mice. Cells expressing common lymphocyte markers [e.g.,
Ly-5(B220), Ly-1] are virtually absent as are LPS and CON-A
responsive lymphocytes. Histologically, their lymphoid tissues
show the same general pattern of severe lymphocytic deficiency as
scid(Ig$^-$) mice.

The events responsible for scid(Ig$^+$) mice appear to be of somatic
origin as mice cannot be selectively bred for this condition;
also, the events seem to occur infrequently and may result in
unregulated terminal differentiation of the affected cells
because resting lymphocytes, responsive to lymphocyte mitogens
and/or expressing common lymphocyte surface antigens, are undetectable. The appearance of scid(Ig$^+$) mice might simply reflect
a low probability that a developing scid lymphocyte will make two
productive gene rearrangements at the appropriate Ig or TCR loci
(e.g., Igh and Igl or TCRβ and TCRα). Alternatively, an
occasional developing scid lymphocyte might revert to normal and
give rise to functional progeny. Genetic reversion at either
scid allele would presumably suffice to normalize a given cell.
Resolution of this issue awaits the results of further
experiments.

ACKNOWLEDGEMENTS

This research was supported by NIH grants AI-13323, CA-04946 and
CA-06927 and by an appropriation from the Commonwealth of
Pennsylvania. We thank M. Piatek for typing this manuscript.

REFERENCES

Allison JP, Lanier LL (1987) The T cell antigen receptor gamma gene: rearrangement and cell lineages. Immunol. Today 8: 293-296.

Alt FW, Rosenberg N, Enea V, Siden E, Baltimore D (1982) Multiple immunoglobulin heavy-chain gene transcripts in Abelson murine leukemia virus-transformed lymphoid cell lines. Molec. Cell. Biol. 2: 386-400.

Bancroft GJ, Bosma MJ, Bosma GC, Unanue ER (1986) Regulation of macrophage Ia expression in mice with severe combined immuno-deficiency: induction of Ia expression by a T cell-indepen-dent mechanism. J. Immunol. 137: 4-9.

Bosma GC, Custer RP, Bosma MJ (1983) A severe combined immuno-deficiency mutation in the mouse. Nature 301: 527-530.

Bosma GC, Fried M, Custer RP, Carroll A, Gibson D, Bosma MJ (1987) Evidence of functional lymphocytes in some (leaky) scid mice. J. Exp. Med. (in press).

Custer RP, Bosma GC, Bosma MJ (1985) Severe combined immuno-deficiency (SCID) in the mouse: pathology, reconstitution, neoplasms. J. Amer. J. Pathol. 120: 464-477.

Czitrom AA, Edwards S, Phillips RA, Bosma MJ, Marrack P, Kappler JW (1985) The function of antigen-presenting cells in mice with severe combined immunodeficiency. J. Immunol. 134: 2276-2280.

Dorshkind K, Keller GM, Phillips RA, Miller RG, Bosma GC, O'Toole M, Bosma MJ (1984) Functional status of cells from lymphoid and myeloid tissues in mice with severe combined immuno-deficiency disease. J. Immunol. 132: 1804-1808.

Dorshkind K, Pollack SB, Bosma MJ, Phillips RA (1985) Natural killer (NK) cells are present in mice with severe combined immunodeficiency (scid). J. Immunol. 134: 3798-3801.

Epstein R, Davisson M, Lehmann K, Akeson EC, Cohn M (1986) Position of Igl-1, md, and Bst loci on chromosome 16 of the mouse. Immunogenetics 23: 78-83.

Grosschedl R, Weaver D, Baltimore D, Constantini F (1984) Intro-duction of a μ immunoglobulin gene into the mouse germ line: specific expression in lymphoid cells and synthesis of functional antibody. Cell 38: 647-658.

Hackett J, Bosma GC, Bosma MJ, Bennett M, Kumar V (1986) Trans-plantable progenitors of natural killer cells are distinct from those of T and B lymphocytes. Proc. Natl. Acad. Sci. (USA) 83: 3427-3431.

Kemp DJ, Harris AW, Adams JM (1980) Transcripts of the immuno-globulin Cμ gene vary in structure and splicing during lymphoid development. Proc. Natl. Acad. Sci. (USA) 77: 7400-7404.

Kim MG, Schuler W, Bosma MJ, Marcu KB (1988) Aberrant Igh locus rearrangements in A-MuLV pre-B lines of scid mice: evidence for deregulated D-J recombination. Curr. Top. Microbiol. and Immunol. (in press).

Lennon GC, Perry RP (1985) Cμ-containing transcripts initiate heterogeneously within the IgH enhancer region and contain a novel 5'-nontranslatable exon. Nature 318: 475-478.

Rosen FS, Cooper MD, Wedgwood RJ (1984) The primary immuno-deficiencies. N. Engl. J. Med. 311: 235-242 and 300-310.

Schuler W, Schuler A, Bosma MJ (1987) Evidence for defective rearrangement of TCRγ genes in a mouse mutant (scid) with severe combined immune deficiency. J. Cell. Biochem. suppl. 11D p 216 (Abstract).

Schuler W, Weiler IJ, Schuler A, Phillips RA, Rosenberg N, Mak
    TW, Kearney JF, Perry RP, Bosma MJ (1986) Rearrangement of
    antigen receptor genes is defective in mice with severe
    combined immune deficiency. Cell 46: 963-972.
Storb U, Pinkert C, Arp B, Engler P, Gollahon K, Manz J, Brady W,
    Brinster RL (1986) Transgenic mice with μ and κ genes encoding
    antiphosphorylcholine antibodies. J. Exp. Med. 164: 627-641.
Van Ness GG, Weigert M, Coleclough C, Mather EL, Kelley DE, Perry
    RP (1981) Transcription of the unrearranged mouse Cκ locus.
    Sequence of the initiation region and comparison of activity
    with a rearranged Vκ-Cκ gene. Cell 27: 593-602.
Yancopoulos G, Alt FW (1985) Developmentally controlled and
    tissue-specific expression of unrearranged V_H gene segments.
    Cell 40: 271-281.

Aberrant Igh Locus Rearrangements in A-MuLV pre B Lines of *scid* Mice: Evidence for Deregulated D-J Recombination

M. G. Kim[1], W. Schuler[3], M. J. Bosma[3], and K. B. Marcu[1,2]

INTRODUCTION

Severe combined immune deficiency (scid) in mice is a recessive mutation (Bosma et al., 1983). Mice with this defect contain myeloid cells but no functional B and T cells indicating that their early lymphoid differentiation is defective. A-MuLV transformed, bone marrow derived pre B cells and spontaneous thymic lymphomas from scid animals displayed abnormal immunoglobulin and T cell receptor gene rearrangements with deletions around the J regions which may be a consequence of faulty D-J joining (Schuler et at., 1986). We have analysed the rearranged Igh loci in nine A-MuLV transformed scid pre B lines in some detail by Southern blotting and have determined the nucleotide sequences in the vicinity of two such aberrant Igh recombinations. We find that Igh locus deletions in scid pre B cells can involve up to all the D_H segments but do not extend to the V_H gene families. D_H and J_H coding sequences are both deleted at the site of recombination: Normal heptamer-nonamer recombination signal sequences separated by proper spacer lengths are not present but "heptamer like" sequences are found 5' of the recombination sites. These findings lend support to the idea that a deregulated, error prone D-J recombination contributes to the scid defect early in B and T cell development.

Deletions Involving D_H And J_H Regions in scid Pre B Lines

The locations of recombination sites within the J_H-C_μ intron of nine A-MuLV transformed scid pre B lines are shown in Figure 1. Breakpoints span over 10 Kb from amongst the J_H regions to the downstream S_μ repeats. They do not exhibit a clustered pattern though the majority reside around the Igh enhancer region. A-MuLV pre B lines established from normal mice show DJ or VDJ joins on both alleles (Alt et al., 1984). All nine scid pre B lines examined here displayed rearranged D_H bands upon either EcoRI or HindIII digestion. However germ line sized D_H segments are retained by all cell lines except for the S29 line which deleted all the D_H segments on one chromosome and only retained one on the other (Kim et al., submitted). The deletion of all the D_H segments could be due to VDJ joining. However, probes specific for the most D_H proximal V_H families (V_H81X and V_HQ52) revealed no deletions or rearrangements indicating that no V-D joins had occurred (Kim et al. submitted). There are three alleles with potentially functional D-J joinings (S11a1, S11a2, S33a) but these cell lines also still contain aberrantly rearranged alleles. One pre B line, S11, retains a germ line context J_H region which is highly atypical for A-MuLV transformed pre B cells (Alt et al., 1984). S11 is also unusual in containing four rearranged J_H segments and may be undergoing progressive recombinations which culminate in aberrant D-J deletions. However, it is also conceiveable that S11 is oligoclonal. Southern hybridization performed with a v-abl probe indicated that the majority of the scid lines possess one A-MuLV provirus, several have two, but S11 contains three A-MuLV genomes of equivalent intensity (data not shown). Limiting dilution cloning experiments will be necessary to assess the clonality of the S11 line.

[1] Genetics Graduate Program and [2] Depts.of Biochemistry, Microbiology & Pathology SUNY at Stony Brook, Stony Brook, NY 11784-5215;
[3] Institute for Cancer Research, Fox Chase Cancer Center, 7701 Burholme Avenue, Philadelphia, PA 19111

Current Topics in Microbiology and Immunology, Vol. 137
© Springer-Verlag Berlin · Heidelberg 1988

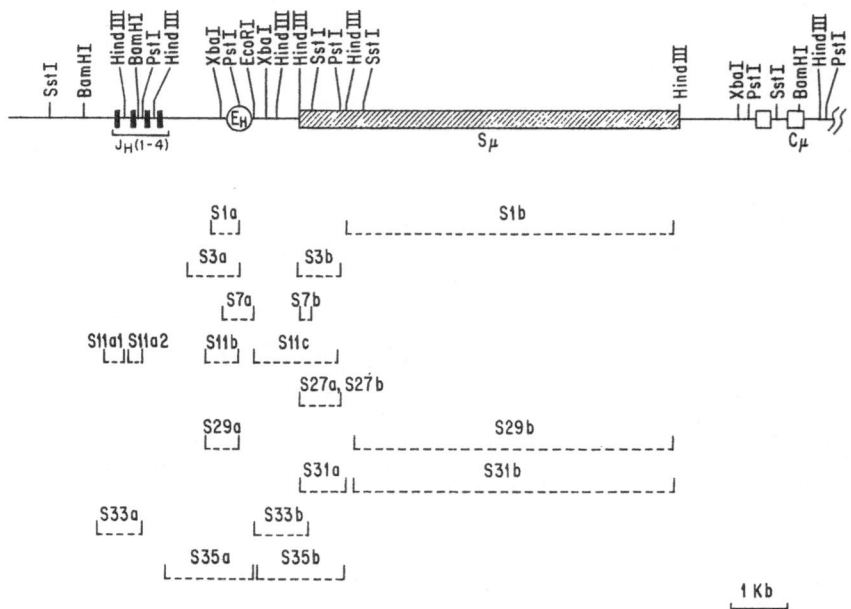

Figure 1. Locations of recombination sites within the J-C$_\mu$ intron of the Igh alleles of nine SCID pre B lines.

Features of the Nucleotide Sequences at Two _scid_ Igh Recombination Sites

We chose the S7 _scid_ pre B line for cloning and nucleotide sequence analysis since its Igh rearrangements are representative of the most common deletions in _scid_ pre B lines: one resides in the Igh enhancer region and the other nearby the S$_\mu$ tandem repeats. Comparative maps and structural features of the two S7 Igh alleles are shown in Figure 2. Genomic clones for each allele (a and b) were isolated and are denoted SE1(a) and SE3(b). Homologous regions were found 5' of their recombination sites. In addition, sequences upstream of the pSE3(b) recombination site hybridized with a 5' D$_{FL16.1}$ probe, but SE1(a) did not hybridize to either 5' D$_{FL}$ or 5'D$_{SP2}$ probes. Nucleotide sequence analysis of the recombination sites revealed that D$_H$ coding sequences and correct heptamer and nonamer recognition sequences separated by appropriate length spacer segments were absent (Figure 3). However, "heptamer like" sequences are found 5' of both breakpoints. Allele (a) contains a perfect heptamer (TACTGTG) in its 5' flanking D$_H$ sequences, 2 bp 5' of its rearrangement site, and allele (b) has a "heptamer like" sequence (TAGTGTA) in the analogous position. "Heptamer like" sequences are also found in the deleted DNA sequences within the IgH enhancer and the S$_\mu$ region, 10 and 15 bp 5' of the allele (a) and (b) breakpoint respectively. We also note that the sequences TG or TGG are positioned at the recombination sites of both alleles. Analogous sequences have been found at the recombination sites of Igh enhancer deletions, c-myc translocations (Aquilera et al., 1985) and retroviral insertions (reviewed in Panaganilova, 1985, Skalka and Leis, 1984) and an endonuclease activity specific for TG/AC sequences has been identified in chicken bursa and mouse liver extracts (Aquilera et al., 1985, Hope et al., 1986).

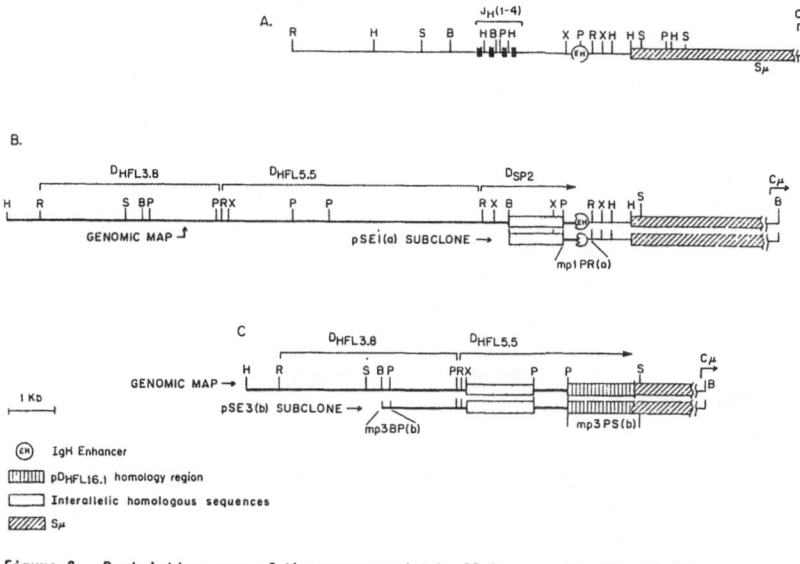

Figure 2. Restriction maps of the rearranged Igh alleles in the S7 cell line.
A: germ line configuration of J_H-$C_\mu$region, B: S7 allele (a), C: S7 allele (b).
R=EcoRI, H=HindIII, B=BamHI, S=SstI, P=PstI, X=XbaI.

Significance of "Heptamer Like" Sequences at scid Igh Recombination Sites

There are numerous examples where VDJ heptamer (but not nonamer) recognition
sequences reside nearby unusual Ig gene recombinations such as V_H-V_H gene
replacements (Kleinfield et al., 1986, Reth et al., 1986), chromosome
translocations in murine and human lymphoid malignancies (Showe et al., 1987,
Otsu et al., 1987), and abnormal light chain gene rearrangements (Siminovitch
et al., 1985, Durdik et al., 1984, Seidman and Leder, 1980). A number of
these rearrangements also contain "heptamer like" sequences and their distance
from the recombination sites varies from 0-12 bp (see Table I).

The presence of "heptamer like" sequences near the recombination sites of the
two sequenced Igh alleles may be fortuitous or may indicate the involvement of
these sequences in the abnormal deletions of D_H and J_H coding segments. The
later possibility is consistant with the absence of symmetrical deletions in
these loci. Nuclear factors which specifically bind to the D-J heptamer-
nonamer sequences (Aquilera et al., 1987) and their flanking DNA (Weaver and
Baltimore, 1987) have been recently identified and sequence specific
endonuclease activities unique to B cells have also been detected (Desiderio
et al., 1984, Kataoka et al., 1984). Whether any of these factors are absent
or defective in scid pre B cells remain to be determined.

A.

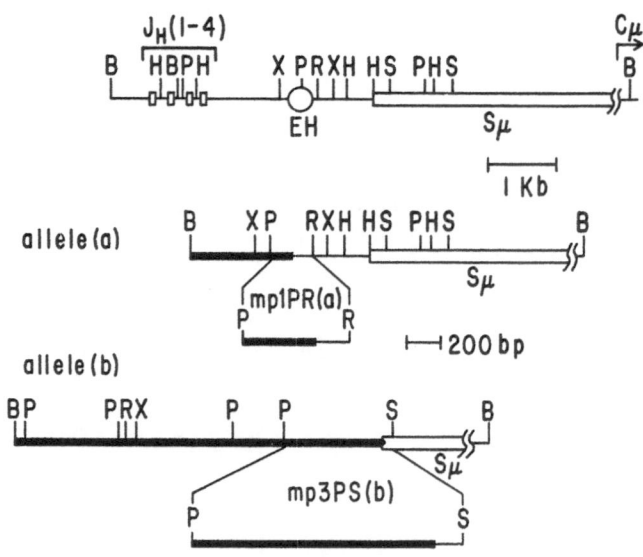

B.

| 1PR (a) | ACGATCCCAG ACCACCCACA CCATCCAGAG TCAGAGACTA TGAGCTAGCC |
| IGH-ENH | GTCATGTGGC AAGGCTATTT GGGGAAGGGA AAATAAAACC ACTAGGTAAA |

| 1PR (a) | TAGCATCTGC ATCATTCTAA GTTTCAGACC CAATAPCCTA TC[TACTGTG]G |
| IGH-ENH | CTTGTAGCTG TGGTTTGAAG AAGTGGTTTT GAAA[CACTCT_G]TCCAGCCCC |

| 1PR (a) | GCCAAACCGA AAGTCCAGGC TGAGCAAAAC ACCACCTGGG TAATTTGCAT |
| IGH-ENH | A--------- ---------- ---------- ---------- ---------- |

C.

| 3PS (b) | CATTGAGTCC TGGGGGCATG AGTGTGCCCA GGTAAATTCC TTACCCACTC |
| IGH-5'Sμ | AAACCAGGCA CCGCAAATGG TAAGCCAGAG GCAGCCACAG CTGTGGCTGC |

| 3PS (b) | AGCATAAATT TCCAGTCCCA CAGACTACAT CACCTTTGAG TAGGAATGTT |
| IGH-5'Sμ | TCTTAAAGCT TGTAAACTGT TTCTGCTTAA GAGGGACTGA GTCTT[CAGTC] |

| 3PS (b) | AAAAGT[TAGT GTA]GATGAAG AGACATTTGT GTCTTTGAGT ACCGTTGTCT |
| IGH-5'Sμ | [AT]TGCTTTAG GGGGAGA--- ---------- ---------- ---------- |

Figure 3. Nucleotide sequences of the recombination sites of the rearranged Igh alleles in S7 cells. Nucleotide sequences of the corresponding regions within the BA1B/c Igh enhancer and Sμ are shown for comparison. The arrows indicate breakpoints and heptemer like sequences are boxed.

Table **I**. Heptamer-like sequences found nearby aberrant Igh gene recombinations[a]

Aberrant Phenomenon	Cell line	Location	Heptamer like Sequence	Reference
SCID deletion	S7 (allele a)	5' DH	T A C T G T G	this paper
		IgH Enh	C A C T c T G	
"	S7 (allele b)	5' DH	T A g T G T a	this paper
		5' S_μ	c a G T C A t	
Enhancer deletion	MOPC 195	3' JH4	T A C T G g G	Aquilera et al
		S_μ	a g G A C A C	(1985)
"	MOPC 467	5' JH4	(C A C T G T G)[b]	"
		S_μ	T A g T c T G	
"	9.2.2.1 (MPC11 variant)	JH	(C A g A G T t)[b]	Eckhardt & Birshstein
		5' $C_{\gamma 2a}$	(C c a T G T G)[b]	(1985)
Switch variant	9.7.1 (MPC11 variant)	$C_{\gamma 2a}$	a g C T G T G	"
		$C_{\gamma 2b}$	c T G T C c t	
			(C A C A G T G)[b]	
Etn	P3.26Bu4	$S_{\gamma 2b}$	(C A C T G g G)[b]	Shell et al. (1987)
Line 1	PD31(300-18)	Line 1	C A C c a T G	Yancopoulos et al. (1986)
t(12:15)	MPC11	myc	c a G A C A C	Stanton et al.
		$S_{\gamma 2a}$	a c C A G a G	(1984)
"	ABPC45	5' myc	(C g C A G T c)[b]	Fahrlander et al. (1985)
"	ABPC33	5' myc	T A t T G T G	Kim & Marcu
		5'$S_{\gamma 2a}$	(t g a T G T G)[b]	unpublished
"	J558	S_α	a g C T G T G	Gerondakis et al. (1984)
"	W267	myc	T c C a G T c	"
		S_α	(g A C T G T G)[b]	
"	HOPC1	myc	C c C T G T G	"
		S_α	(C A g T G T G)[b]	
"	P3	myc	C c C T G c G	"
		S_μ	g A C T G a c	
t(6:15)	ABPC4	C_κ	g A C T G c t	Webb et al.
		pvt-1	C A g A G T t	(1984)

D-J heptamer consensus   T/C A C T/A G T G

Aberrant Rearrangement Frequencies % = 63 60 70 93 87 77 70
Normal Rearrangement Frequencies % =   76 72 72 96 98 100 96   Akira et al. (1987)

a. Heptamer sequences were found 0~12bp from the breakpoints. Capital letters are conserved sequences, small letters are nonconserved sequences.
b. Sequences are found on the antisense strand.

REFERENCES

Aquilera R, Hope TJ, Sakano H. (1985) Characterization if immunoglobulin enhancer deletions in murine plasmacytomas. EMBO J 4:3689-3693.

Aquilera RJ, Pikora S, Okazaki K , Sakano H. (1987) A pre-B cell nuclear protein which specifically interacts with immunoglobulin V-J recombination sequences. Cell in press.

Alt FW, Rosenberg N, Casanova RJ, Thomas E, Baltimore D. (1982) Immunoglobulin heavy chain expression and class switching in a murine leukemia cell line. Nature 296:325-331.

Alt FW, Yancopoulos GD, Blackwell TK, Wood C, Thomas E, Boss M, Coffman R, Rosenberg N, Tonegawa S, Baltimore D, (1982) Ordered rearrangement of immunoglobulin heavy chain variable region segment. EMBO J 3:1209-1219.

Akira S, Okazaki K, Sakano H. (1987) Two pairs of Recombination Signals CACTGTG and GGTTTTGT are sufficient to cause Immunoglobulin V-J Joining. Science in press.

Borzillo GV, Cooper MD, Kubagawa H, Landay A, Burrows PD. (1987) Isotype switching in human B lymphocyte malignancies occurs DNA deletion: Evidence for nonspecific switch recombination. J Immunol 139:1326-1335.

Bosma GC, Custer RP, Bosma MJ. (1983) A severe combined immunodeficiency mutation in the mouse. Nature 301:527-530.

Desiderio S, Baltimore D. (1984) Double stranded cleavage by cell extract near recombinational signal sequences of immunoglobulin genes. Nature 308:860-862.

Durdik J, Moore MW, Selsing E. (1984) Novel light-chain gene rearrangements in mouse light chain-producing B lymphocytes. Nature 307:746-752.

Eckhardt LA, Birshtein BK. (1985) Independent immunoglobulin class switch events occurring in a single myeloma cell line. Mol Cell Biol 5:856-868.

Fahrlander FD, Sumegi J, Yang J-Q, Wiener F, Marcu KB, Klein G. (1985) Activation of the c-myc oncogene by the immunoglobulin heavy-chain gene enhancer after multiple switch region-mediated chromosome rearrangements in a murine plasmacytoma. Proc Natl Acad Sci USA 82:3746-3750.

Gerondakis S, Cory S, Adams JM. (1984) Translocation of the myc cellular oncogene to the immunoglobulin heavy chain locus in murine plasmacytomas is an imprecise reciprocal exchange. Cell 36:973-982.

Hope TJ, Aquilera RJ, Minie ME, Sakano H. (1986) Endonucleolytic activity that cleaves immunoglobulin recombination sequences. Science 231:1141-1145.

Kataoka T, Kondo S, Nishi M, Kodaira M, Honjo T. (1984) Isolation and characterization of endonuclease J: a sequence specific endonuclease cleaving immunoglobulin genes. Nucleic Acids Res 12:5995-6010.

Klein S, Sablitzky F, Radbruch A. (1984) Deletion of the IgH enhancer does not reduce immunoglobulin heavy chain production of a hybridoma IgD class switch variant. EMBO J 3:2473-9476.

Kleinfield R, Hardy RR, Tarlinton D, Dangl J, Herzenberg LA, Weigert M. (1986) Recombination between an expressed immunoglobulin heavy-chain gene and a germline variable gene segment in a Lyl[+] B-cell lymphoma. Nature 322:843-846.

Otsu M, Katamine S, Uno M, Yamaki M, Ono Y, Klein G, Sasaki M, Yopita Y, Honjo T. (1987) Molecular characterization of novel reciprocal translocation t(6:14) in an Epstein-Barr virus transformed B cell precursor. Mol Cell Biol 7:708-717.

Panganiban AT. (1985) Retroviral DNA integration. Cell 42:5-6.

Reth M, Gehrmann P, Petrac E, Wiese P. (1986) A novel V_H to $V_H DJ_H$ joining mechanism in heavy-chain-negative (null) pre B cells results in heavy-chain production. Nature 322:840-842.

Schuler W, Weiler IJ, Schuler A, Phillips RA, Rosenberg N, Mak TW, Kearney JF, Perry RP, Bosma M. (1986) Rearrangement of antigen receptor genes is defective in mice with severe combined immune deficiency. Cell 46:963-972.

Seidman JG, Leder P. (1980) A mutant immunoglobulin light chain is formed by a aberrant DNA and RNA splicing events. Nature 286:779-783.

Shell B, Szurek P, Dunnick W. (1987) Interruption of two immunoglobulin heavy chain switch regions in murine plasmacytoma P3.2bBu4 by insertion of retrovirus-like element Etn. Mol Cell Biol 7:1364-1370.

Showe LC, Moore RCA, Erikson J, Croce CM. (1987) Myc oncogene involved in a t(8:22) chromosome translocation is not altered in its putative regulatory regions. Proc Natl Acad Sci USA 84:2824-2828.

Siminovitch KA, Bakhshi A, Goldman P, Korsmeyer SK. (1985) A uniform deleting element mediates the loss of genes in humans B cells. Nature 316:260-262.

Skalka AM, Leis J. (1984) Retroviral DNA integration. BioEssay 1:206-210.

Stanton LW, Yang J-Q, Eckhardt LA, Harris LJ, Birshtein BK, Marcu KB. (1984) Product of a reciprocal chromosomal translocation involving the c-myc gene in a murine plasmacytoma. Proc Natl Acad Sci USA 81:829-833.

Yancopoulos GD, DePinho PA, Zimmerman KA, Lutzker SA, Rosenberg N, Alt FW. (1986) Secondary genomic rearrangement events in pre B cells $V_H DJ_H$ replacement by a LINE-1 sequence and directed class switching. EMBO J 5:3259-3266.

Weaver D, Baltimore D. (1987) B lymphocyte-specific protein binding near an immunoglobulin-chain gene J segment. Proc Natl Acad Sci USA 84:1516-1520.

Webb E, Adams JM, Cory S. (1984) Variant (6:15) translocation in a murine plasmacytoma occurs near an immunoglobulin gene but far from the myc oncogene. Nature 312:777-779.

ACKNOWLEDGEMENTS

We thank Hitoshi Sakano for providing data on normal V-D-J heptamer consensus matches and for preprints of manuscripts. This research was supported by NIH grants GM26939 (awarded to KBM), AI13323 and CA04946 (awarded to MJB) and an appropriation from the Commonwealth of Pennsylvania. WS is a recipient of a research fellowship from the Deutsche Forschungsgemeinschaft and KBM is a Catacosinos Cancer Research Professor.

V$_H$ Family Usage and Binding Analyses of Polyreactive Monoclonal Autoantibodies Derived from Nonimmunized Adult BALB/c Mice

A. B. Hartman[1,3], C. P. Mallett[2], J. Srinivasappa[3], B. S. Prabhakar[3], A. L. Notkins[3], and S. J. Smith-Gill[2]

INTRODUCTION

The presence of natural autoantibodies in the B-cell repertoire of normal healthy mice has been well established and suggests that some autoreactive B cells could be activated by the internal environment, i.e., naturally activated (Dighiero et al. 1983; Prabhakar et al. 1984; Steele and Cunningham 1978). In order to better understand the naturally activated repertoire, we have examined the reactivity patterns of a panel of BALB/c hybridomas from unmanipulated adult spleen cells. This panel of natural antibody hybridomas (NAbs), selected first for organ binding by indirect immunofluorescence microscopy, was used to examine the following questions:

1. Are organ-reactive NAbs polyreactive?

2. Is there preferential V$_H$ usage in NAbs?

GENERATION OF NAb PANEL

Fusion of pooled spleen cells derived from two normal 12-week-old non-immunized BALB/cAn mice was carried out as previously described (Prabhakar et al. 1984). Hybridomas were first screened against frozen BALB/cAn tissue sections by using indirect immunofluorescence microscopy (Srinivasappa et al. 1986). As summarized in Table 1, 22 of 103 antibodies screened were positive for organ binding. Thirteen of these 22 antibodies were reactive to tissues in more than one organ, while nine displayed single organ specificity. Eighty-five hybridomas were then screened for antigen binding (Table 1). Eleven antibodies were positive for antigen binding against an initial test panel of four antigens (bovine serum albumin, galactan, cytochrome c, and chicken hen egg white lysozyme); all but one of these antibodies also exhibited organ reactivity. From these antibodies, a panel composed of three mono-organ-reactive antibodies, six multi-organ-reactive antibodies, and one non-organ-reactive antibody was selected for further study. All but one of these antibodies were of the IgM heavy chain class; the other antibody, NAb1, was identified as an IgG2b. These 10 NAbs were examined for V$_H$ family usage and for reactivity against a larger panel of antigens. Figure 1 shows organ-binding patterns for three of the NAbs.

[1]Department of Biologics Research, Walter Reed Army Institute of Research, Washington, DC
[2]Laboratory of Genetics, National Cancer Institute, and the
[3]Laboratory of Oral Medicine, National Institute of Dental Research, National Institutes of Health, Bethesda, MD

Current Topics in Microbiology and Immunology, Vol. 137
© Springer-Verlag Berlin · Heidelberg 1988

Table 1. Primary screening of NAbs

	Organ binding			Antigen binding		
	Isotype			Isotype		
	IgM	IgG	Total	IgM	IgG	Total
Antibodies Tested	-	-	103	-	-	85
Antibodies Positive	18	4	22	11	-	11
Monoreactive NAbs	6(2[a])	3(1[a])	9	2	-	2
Multireactive NAbs	12(6[a])	1	13	9(1[a])	-	9

[a]NAbs selected for detailed characterization in this study.

V$_H$ FAMILY USAGE OF THE TEN NAbs

V$_H$ family usage of the 10 NAbs was determined by slot blot analysis (Bellon et al. 1987), utilizing V$_H$ gene probes V$_H$J558, V$_H$3609, V$_H$S107, V$_H$36-60, and V$_H$QUPC52 obtained from Peter Brodeur (Brodeur and Riblet 1984), and V$_H$X24, V$_H$37.1 (7183 family), and V$_H$22.1 (J606 family), described previously (Hartman and Rudikoff 1984). V$_H$ family usage was then confirmed by sequencing of the heavy chain from the VDJ join back through the FR3 region. Sequencing was performed by primer extension of poly(A)$^+$-selected mRNA from each hybridoma and subsequent sequencing of the cDNA transcripts utilizing Maxam-Gilbert techniques (Clarke et al. 1985; Maxam and Gilbert 1980). Sequencing results (Table 2, Hartman et al. 1988) revealed that four V$_H$ families were expressed by the 10 NAbs: V$_H$J558, V$_H$Q52, V$_H$3609, and V$_H$7183. When V$_H$ family usage in the 10 NAbs was compared to estimates of potential (germline) and available repertoires (Holmberg et al. 1986), we found an apparent random V$_H$ usage in the NAbs of the adult mouse. In fact, the NAbs in our study were found to be encoded by the four most abundant families (V$_H$J558, V$_H$Q52, V$_H$7183, and V$_H$3609), which together account for an estimated 80% of the germline V$_H$ genes (Riblet and Brodeur 1986).

ANTIGEN REACTIVITY OF THE TEN NAbs

The 10 NAbs were screened against a larger panel of haptens and both self and non-self antigens by using particle concentration immunofluorescence (Jolley et al. 1984) with an automated system (Screen Machine, Pandex Laboratories, Mundelein, IL). The results of this screening (Table 2, Hartman et al. 1988) confirmed the patterns shown by the initial screen against four antigens. Two antibodies, NAb1 and NAb8, did not bind any antigen in the panel, while the other eight antibodies exhibited polyreactive binding profiles. Each of the polyreactive NAbs showed a unique pattern of antigen binding, indicating that the polyreactivity exhibited by these antibodies is not indiscriminate. Since all but one of the organ-reactive IgM NAbs were also polyreactive, these results confirm the conclusions of Holmberg et al. (1986) that self-reactivity is likely a consequence of polyreactivity or antibody "degeneracy." We also found a striking

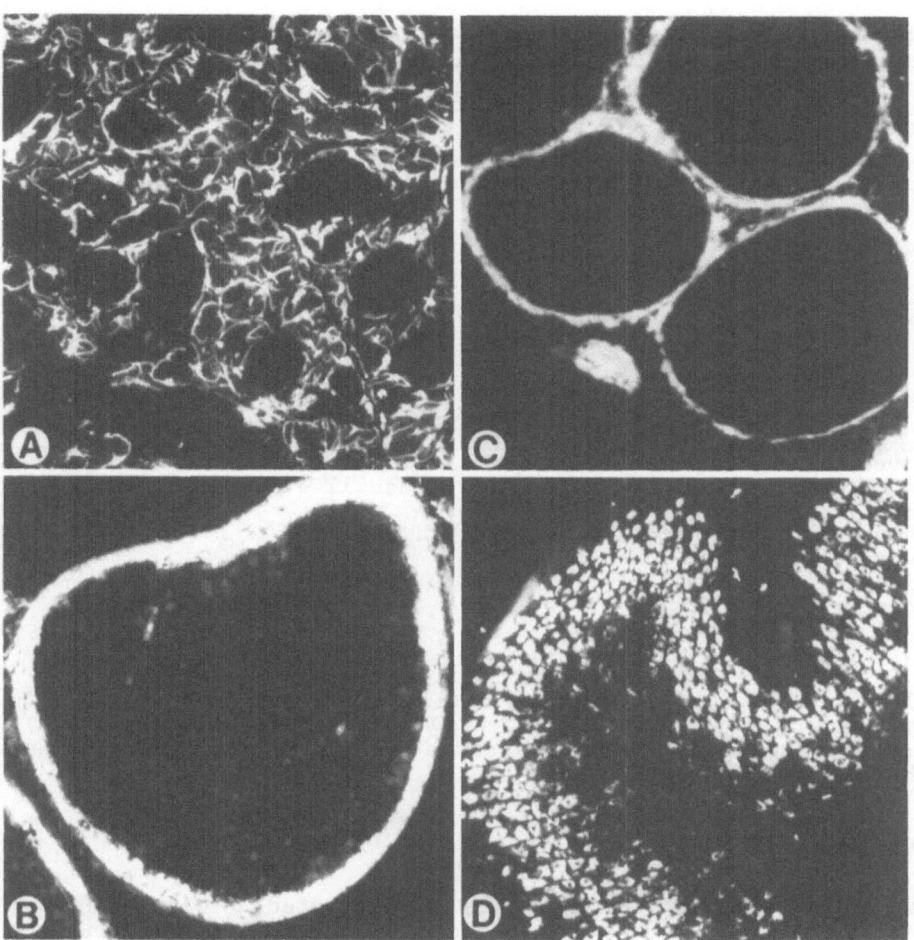

Fig. 1. Reactivity of NAbs with BALB/c organs. Indirect immunofluorescence reactivity of NAb2 with tissue in salivary gland (A),
NAb7 with smooth muscle in oviduct (B) and testis (C), and NAb8 with
parietal cells in stomach (D). Original magnifications: A, x125;
B, x125; C, x80; and D, x125.

214

Table 2. Summary of NAbs derived from adult BALB/c mice[a]

Antibody	Organ reactivity	Antigen reactivity	V_H family	Ig heavy chain class[b]
NAb1	+[c]	none	7183	γ_{2b}
NAb2	++[d]	poly	3609	μ
NAb3	++	poly	3609	μ
NAb4	++	poly	Q52	μ
NAb5	+	poly	Q52	μ
NAb6	++	poly	Q52	μ
NAb7	++	poly	J558	μ
NAb8	+	none	J558	μ
NAb9	++	poly	J558	μ
NAb10	0[e]	poly	J558	μ

[a]Sequence and binding data described in detail elsewhere (Hartman et al. 1988).
[b]All NAbs described here have κ light chains.
[c]Mono-organ reactive.
[d]Multi-organ reactive.
[e]No reactivity.

correlation between apparent affinities of the antibodies and V_H family usage in the order $V_H3609 > V_HQ52 > V_HJ558$ (data not shown). In general, the V_HJ558 antibodies were less reactive, in agreement with Holmberg (1987).

CONCLUSIONS

1. The majority (8/9) of IgM NAbs demonstrated a wide range of reactivities for both self and non-self antigens that were unique for a given antibody. This is consistent with the hypothesis that self-reactivity may reflect general polyreactivity.

2. NAb V_H usage is diverse and appears to be representative of the germline repertoire.

3. We did see a correlation between V_H family usage and apparent affinity for a broad spectrum of antigens. This suggests that different V_H families may vary in their natural "germline" affinities for complex antigens.

4. We propose that possible functions for polyreactive natural antibodies are to act as a first line of defense and offer protection for the host against a variety of foreign agents.

ACKNOWLEDGMENT

CPM was supported by American Cancer Society Postdoctoral Fellowship PF-2699.

REFERENCES

Bellon B, Manheimer-Lory A, Monestier M, Moran T, Dimitriu-Bona A, Alt F, Bona C (1987) High frequency of autoantibodies bearing cross-reactive idiotopes among hybridomas using V_H7183 genes prepared from normal and autoimmune strains. J Clin Invest 79: 1044-1053

Brodeur PH, Riblet R (1984) The immunoglobulin heavy chain region (Igh-V) locus in the mouse. I. 100 Igh-V genes comprise seven families of homologous genes. Eur J Immunol 14: 922-930

Clarke SH, Huppi K, Ruezinsky D, Staudt L, Gerhard W, Weigert M (1985) Inter- and intraclonal diversity in the antibody response to influenza hemagglutinin. J Exp Med 161: 687-704

Dighiero G, Lymberi P, Mazie JC, Rouyre S, Butler-Browne GS, Whalen RG, Avrameas S (1983) Murine hybridomas secreting natural monoclonal antibodies reacting with self antigens. J Immunol 131: 2267-2272

Hartman AB, Mallett CP, Srinivasappa J, Prabhakar BS, Notkins AL, Smith-Gill SJ (1988) Organ-reactive autoantibodies from nonimmunized adult BALB/c mice are polyreactive and exhibit a random pattern of V_H gene usage. Submitted for publication

Hartman AB, Rudikoff S (1984) V_H genes encoding the immune response to β-(1,6)-galactan: somatic mutation in IgM molecules. EMBO J 3: 3023-3030

Holmberg D (1987) High connectivity, natural antibodies preferentially use 7183 and QUPC52 V_H families. Eur J Immunol 17: 399-403

Holmberg D, Freitas AA, Portnoi D, Jacquemart F, Avrameas S, Coutinho A (1986) Antibody repertoires of normal BALB/c mice: B lymphocyte population defined by state of activation. Immunol Rev 93: 147-169

Jolley ME, Wang CJ, Ekenberg SJ, Zvelke MS, Kelso DM (1984) Particle concentration fluorescence immunoassay (PCFIA): a new, rapid immunoassay technique with high sensitivity. J Immunol Methods 67: 21-35

Maxam AM, Gilbert W (1977) A new method for sequencing DNA. Proc Natl Acad Sci USA 74: 560-564

Prabhakar BS, Saegusa J, Onodera T, Notkins AL (1984) Lymphocytes capable of making monoclonal antibodies that react with multiple organs are a common feature of the normal B cell repertoire. J Immunol 133: 2815-2817

Riblet R, Brodeur PH (1986) The Igh-V repertoire of the mouse. Mt Sinai J Med 53: 170-174

Srinivasappa J, Saegusa J, Prabhakar BS, Gentry MK, Buchmeier MJ, Wiktor TJ, Koprowski H, Oldstone MBA, Norkins AL (1986) Molecular mimicry: frequency of reactivity of monoclonal antiviral antibodies with normal tissues. J Virol 57: 397-401

Steele EJ, Cunningham AJ (1978) High proportion of Ig-producing cells making autoantibody in normal mice. Nature 274: 483-484

Pleiotropic Effects of Deleterious Alleles at the "Motheaten" Locus

L. D. Shultz

INTRODUCTION

Our understanding of basic immunologic mechanisms has been advanced through the study of mutations that cause defects in the development or regulation of the immune system. We have recently reviewed more than 30 genes known to cause abnormalities in this system (Shultz and Sidman 1987). Although certain immunological mutations have served as models for specific human diseases, their chief value is as tools with which to dissect complex processes and thus increase our understanding of the immune system in normal and pathologic states. Among these mutations, deleterious alleles at the motheaten locus cause the most severe immunological changes known to be caused by a single locus. Mice homozygous for the recessive allelic genes "motheaten" (me) or "viable motheaten" (me^V) on Chromosome 6 are severely immunodeficient and develop autoimmune disease early in life. The first recorded mutation at the motheaten locus occurred in 1965 in the C57BL/6J strain of mice at the Jackson Laboratory (Green and Shultz 1975). In 1966, an independent mutation named me^{2J}, was found in an inbred stock carrying the mutation hydrocephalus. Although the mutation me^{2J} was used to carry out linkage tests, propagation of this stock has been discontinued. In 1980, the me^V mutation occured on the C57BL/6J strain background. Homozygotes (me/me) and (me^V/me^V) have a mean lifespan of 3 and 9 weeks respectively (Shultz et al. 1984). Early experimentation with me/me mice indicated multiple immunologic abnormalities. However, the short lifespan of these mice made it difficult to distinguish basic defects in the immune system from those defects associated with incomplete maturation and with poor health. The three-fold increase in longevity of me^V/me^V mice has stimulated recent additional experimentation. This report focuses on the phenotypic effects of mutations at the motheaten locus and discusses recent findings suggesting that these deleterious alleles cause microenviromental defects demonstrable at the level of hematopoietic progenitors.

HISTOPATHOLOGIC ABNORMALITIES

While me/me mice can usually be recognized by the second postnatal day, when small abscesses appear on the surface of the skin, me^V/me^V mice cannot be identified by the presence of skin lesions until 4-5 days of age (Green and Shultz 1975; Shultz et al. 1984). In both me/me and me^V/me^V mice, neutrophils accumulate in the dermis and penetrate as far as the panniculus muscle. These subepidermal lesions displace hair follicles and result in patchy absence of pigment, giving the animals their characteristic "motheaten" appearance. The cutaneous abnormalities are not prevented under germ-free conditions in offspring derived by hysterectomy (Lutzner and Hansen, 1976) and therefore appear to be associated with autoimmune disease rather than with infection. The finding that doubly homozygous nu/nu me^V/me^V mice develop focal skin lesions similar to those in intact me^V/me^V mice (Shultz et al. 1984)) indicates that differentiated T cells are not required for development of these lesions. In addition to cutaneous abnormalities appearing early in life, me^V/me^V mice have a significant reduction in numbers of Ia^+ epidermal Langerhans cells after 5 weeks of age. By 8 weeks, the mutant mice show a three-fold reduction in numbers of Langerhans cells compared with littermate control animals. This age-associated reduction in Langerhans cells might

The Jackson Laboratory , Bar Harbor, ME 04609

reflect a general abnormality in Ia[+] dendritic cell populations since recent evidence suggests that Langerhans cells serve as precursors of Ia[+] dendritic cells in lymphoid organs (Schuler and Steinman 1985). Because cutaneous lesions are the first phenotypic abnormalities seen in *me/me* and *me^V/me^V* mice, they may herald immunopathologic changes that appear later in life.

Histopathological abnormalities in lymphoid tissues of *me/me* and *me^V/me^V* mice are similar in appearance (Green and Shultz 1975; Shultz et al. 1984). The thymus appears histologically normal until 4 weeks of age when cortical depletion becomes evident. Involution progresses in *me^V/me^V* mice until 16 weeks of age when nothing grossly recognizable as a thymus can be found in the mediastinal area. In contrast to thymic atrophy, the spleens of *me/me* and *me^V/me^V* mice show marked hypercellularity from birth onwards. Splenomegaly in these mice results from increased erythropoiesis and myelopoiesis and is accompanied by depletion of lymphoid cells from the periarteriolar regions. In contrast to the increased erythropoiesis in the spleen, the bone marrow shows decreased erythropoiesis and increased myelopoiesis. As in the spleen, lymph nodes from *me/me* and *me^V/me^V* mice lack well-defined lymphoid follicles. While lymph nodes from the mutant mice show increased size, there is a decreased incidence of lymphocytes and increased numbers of neutrophils, plasma cells, and multinucleated giant cells. In both the spleen and lymph nodes, atypical plasmacytoid cells containing discrete immunoglobulin inclusions appear by 4 weeks of age. These inclusions have been termed Russell bodies, and the cells containing them have been termed Mott cells (Russell 1890). Mott cells have been reported previously to be present following hyperimmunization (Zlotnick et al. 1959) as well as in association with chronic inflammatory diseases and lymphoid malignancy in man and experimental animals (Gebbers and Otto 1976; Hsu et al. 1972; Blom et al. 1976). Experimentation with *me^V/me^V* mice has shown Mott cells to be thymic-dependent plasmacytoid cells that are defective in Ig secretion (Shultz et al. 1987). Mott cells appear to result from host responses to polyclonal B cell activation and they may be indicative of a mechanism by which spontaneous autoantibody secretion is reduced following chronic antigenic stimulation.

In both *me/me* and *me^V/me^V* mice, the immediate cause of death depends on focal intra-alveolar hemorrhages with accumulation of macrophages and neutrophils in pulmonary alveoli (Green and Shultz, 1976; Shultz et al. 1984)). Such macrophage accumulation may be due to an increased multiplication rate since these cells show increased proliferative capacity in vitro (McCoy et al. 1982; McCoy et al. 1983). Since cultured splenocytes from *me/me* mice spontaneously produce high levels of colony-stimulating activity (CSA) in vitro, it has been suggested that the elevation in macrophage proliferation may result from defective regulation of CSA (McCoy et al 1984). The development of pneumonitis in *me/me* mice has been described in detail by Rossi et al (1985) who suggest that the pulmonary lesion in these mice may be a valuable model for following the natural progression of interstitial lung disease associated with autoimmunity. The increased lifespan of *me^V/me^V* mice is associated with a more chronic lung disease than the acute pulmonary lesions commonly observed in *me/me* mice. Pulmonary as well as renal lesions in these mice accompany the autoimmune changes. Immune complex and complement deposition are evident in the lungs and kidneys of *me^V/me^V* mice by 10 weeks of age (Shultz et al. 1984). Elevated blood urea nitrogen levels are seen in mutant mice surviving to 15 weeks.

Despite their increased lifespan, both female and male *me^V/me^V* mice are sterile. Thus, maintenance of *me^V/me^V* as well as *me/me* mice is accomplished by transplanting ovaries of females to histocompatible hosts. Breeding of such ovary recipients to pedigreed C57BL/6J +/+ males provides the heterozygotes needed to produce mutant offspring and also reduces the possibility of subline divergence. Sterility in male me^V/me^V mice is associated with Leydig cell depletion and low testosterone levels. Although there is no direct evidence that the decrease in Leydig cell numbers is due to autoimmune disease, the role of inflammatory processes in sterility is suggested by neutrophil aggregation between the testicular tubules at 1-2 weeks of age (Shultz et al. 1984). While testosterone implants result in production of normal appearing spermatids in me^V/me^V mice, attempts to restore fertility with such implants have been unsuccessful.

PERIPHERAL BLOOD CHANGES

In *me/me* mice, the elevated white cell count which becomes evident by 2 weeks of age is attributable to increased numbers of neutrophils and monocytes (Green and Shultz 1975). The high number and incomplete maturation of peripheral granulocytes is consistent with the presence of chronic inflammatory lesions in the skin and lung. In contrast, while me^V/me^V mice show a high percentage of circulating neutrophils at an early age, peripheral white blood cell counts remain normal until 7 weeks of age. By 10 weeks, these mice develop a two-fold increase in total white blood cells and a five-fold increase in the percentage of neutrophils (Shultz et al. 1984). Although *me/me* mice have normal red cell counts, me^V/me^V mice develop severe macrocytic hypochromic anemia by 9 weeks of age. The presence of hemagglutinating antibodies in sera from these mice suggests that anemia may be secondary to autoimmune disease.

ABNORMALITIES IN LYMPHOID CELLS AND IN IMMUNE FUNCTION

While the incidence of splenic B cells is markedly reduced in *me/me* and me^V/me^V mice, there are increased numbers of plasma cells. Almost all the B cells present in these mice show low levels of IgD and express the Ly-1 surface glycoprotein, which marks a minor population of B cells in normal mice and the IgM autoantibody-producing B cells in NZB mice (Sidman et al. 1986). Such Ly-1[+] B cells are thought be responsible for producing natural autoantibodies (Hayakawa et al 1984) and anti-idiotypic antibodies (Kearney and Vakil 1986) in normal animals. The levels of IgM in *me/me* and me^V/me^V mice are 25 to 50 times greater than those in littermate control mice, and sera from the mutant mice contain multiple autoantibodies (Shultz and Green 1976; Shultz and Zurier 1978; Sidman et al. 1986). Hyperimmunoglobulinemia is not due to increased production of B cells (McCoy et al 1985), but to a dramatic overproduction of two B cell maturation-promoting lymphokines that appear to underlie the observed polyclonal B cell activation (Sidman et al. 1984; Sidman et al 1985). The role of lymphoid cells in the morbidity of me^V/me^V mice is indicated by the observation that animals simultaneously homozygous for the mutation "severe combined immunodeficiency" *(scid)* and me^V show a significant increase in longevity compared with me^V/me^V mice (Shultz and Sidman 1987). While Ly-1[+] B cells contribute to certain pathologic changes in *me/me* mice, recent work by Scribner et al (1987) suggests that development of such cells and expression of autoantibodies do not underlie the "motheaten" phenotype. These investigators examined the interaction of the *me* mutation with the mutation "X-linked immunodeficiency" *(xid)* . The *xid* gene prevents the marked expansion of Ly-1[+] B cells (Hayakawa et al. 1983). Although the *xid* gene prevented development of Ly-1[+] B cells and markedly diminished autoantibody levels, combination of *me* with *xid* on the NSF strain background did not increase longevity nor reduce the severity of granulocytic lesions compared with NSF-*me/me* mice.

Motheaten mice show severely impaired responses to thymic-dependent and thymic-independent antigens, have reduced proliferative responses to B cell and T cell mitogens, and lack cytotoxic T cell as well as natural killer (NK) cell activity (Shultz and Green, 1976; Sidman et al. 1978b; Kincade 1978; Davidson et al. 1979; Clark et al. 1981). Immunodeficiency in these mice is believed not to be due to any primary defect in IL-1 or IL-2 production or utilization (Stanton et al. 1985). A recent investigation of me^V/me^V mice has shown severe defects in immunologic function similar to those reported in me/me mice. However, while splenic T cells from me^V/me^V mice are defective in proliferative responses to Con A and lack cytotoxic T cell activity, lymph node cells from these mice show normal Con A blastogenic and cytotoxic T cell responses (Shultz et al., unpublished data)

HEMATOPOIETIC PROGENITOR CELL ABNORMALITIES

The transfer of hematopoietic progenitor cells from mice with heritable immunologic dysfunction into normal irradiated recipients has been used to evaluate experimentally the role of intrinsic stem cell defects in the disease process. Despite the normal ontogeny, tissue distribution and differentiative capacity of hematopoietic stem cells, intravenous transfer of bone marrow or spleen cells from me/me mice into 1000 R gamma-irradiated congenic +/+ recipients results in death from severe pulmonary hemorrhage and inflammation at 2-3-weeks after injection (Shultz et al. 1983). Thus, determination of pathologic changes in irradiated recipients of bone marrow or spleen cells from me/me mice has been limited to short term experiments. The longer lifespan of me^V/me^V mice is evidently determined at the level of hematopoietic progenitors. Lethally-irradiated +/+ recipients of me^V/me^V bone marrow cells survive three-fold longer than recipients of me/me marrow cells (Shultz 1987). Pathologic changes in me^V/me^V marrow recipients are similar to those seen in me^V/me^V mice and include splenomegaly, pneumonitis, granulocytic skin lesions and hyperimmunoglobulinemia. Death from acute pulmonary injury prevents assessment of the ability of me/me bone marrow cells to repopulate the lymphoid system of irradiated recipients. However, as discussed below, the increased survival time of me^V/me^V bone marrow recipients enables such studies.

The loss of cells from the thymus of me/me and me^V/me^V mice after 4 weeks of age was initially thought to be associated with the occurrence of thymocytotoxic autoantibodies. However, based on recent studies, it is more likely that thymic involution in these mice is caused by a defect at the level of hematopoietic progenitor cells. Bone marrow cells from me^V/me^V mice are unable to repopulate the thymus of irradiated congenic recipients after intravenous (I.V.) injection. Using a newly developed intrathymic (I.T.) transfer system, Greiner et al (1986) showed that prothymocytes are present in normal numbers in these mutant mice. Thus, the defective thymic repopulation following I.V. injection appeared to be associated with a prothymocyte homing defect rather than with a decrease in prothymocyte numbers. The intriguing finding that the apparent defect in the thymus homing capacity can be corrected by mixing normal congenic +/+ bone marrow cells with those from me^V/me^V mice before I.V. injection into irradiated recipients indicates that the impaired thymic repopulation function may be due in part to a defect in a radiosensitive accessory cell population (Komschlies et al 1987).

Results using three different types of bone marrow culture systems have indicated that deleterious alleles at the me locus cause microenvironmental abnormalities that may affect multiple hematopoietic lineages. Medlock et al (1987) utilized a newly developed in vitro culture system that selectively supports the generation in vitro of terminal deoxynucleotidyl transferase positive (TdT+) cells. This system has been used to investigate the pathogenesis of abnormal lymphopoiesis in me/me and me^V/me^V mice. These results demonstrated that bone marrow cell feeder layers derived from *me/me* and *me^V/me^V* mice did not support the generation of rat TdT^+ cells in vitro, whereas stromal cell feeder layers derived from littermate normal mice do so. Since composite feeder layers formed from mixing mutant and normal bone marrow cells likewise failed to support the generation of TdT^+ cells in vitro, defective lymphopoiesis in the mutant bone marrow cultures appeared to be secondary to inhibitory factors. Although the stromal microenvironment of *me/me* and *me^V/me^V* mice did not support the growth of TdT^+ cells, mutant mouse bone marrow cultured on littermate control feeder layers generated normal numbers of TdT^+ cells. These data suggested that a microenvironmental defect in the bone marrow of these mutant mice played an important role in the impaired development of functional lymphoid cells. Early lineage B cells identified by the B220 antigen, as well as numbers of TdT positive cells, were found to be markedly depleted in the bone marrow of *me/me* and *me^V/me^V* mice. Although the mutant mice showed a severe decrease in numbers of TdT^+ bone marrow cells at all ages tested, frequency of TdT^+ cells in the thymus and levels of TdT enzymatic activity in thymuses from *me/me* and *me^V/me^V* mice were normal.

More recently, Hayashi et al (1988) analyzed hematopoietic cells from *me^V/me^V* mice using Whitlock-Witte cultures for lymphocytes and Dexter cultures for myeloid cells. Neither lymphocytes nor granulocytes were formed in *me^V/me^V* bone marrow cultures. Moreover, co-cultures of bone marrow from normal and mutant mice were defective. These data further indicate that dysregulation of the bone marrow microenvironment in *me^V/me^V* mice underlies abnormal lymphopoiesis and myelopoiesis. Although the mechanism whereby *me^V/me^V* bone marrow cells inhibited normal hematopoietic cell development remains unknow, inhibition was not due to soluble factors but instead appeared to be dependent on direct cellular interactions.

CONCLUSIONS

Homozygosity for deleterious alleles at the motheaten locus results in marked abnormalities in multiple hematopoietic lineages. Defects in lymphoid cell populations in *me/me* and *me^V/me^V* mice result in severe immunodeficiency and autoimmune disease. Although the underlying mechanism by which the mutant alleles affect the immune system is not well understood, it appears that defects in lymphoid cell and myeloid development and function might be secondary to abnormalities in the hematopoietic microenvironment. As the products of the alleles at the *me* locus become known, additional insight will be gained into mechanisms underlying normal immune function and immunologic disease processes.

ACKNOWLEDGEMENTS

This work was supported by NIH grant CA 20408. Its contents are soley the responsibility of the Jackson Laboratory. I am grateful to Dale Rex Coman, Robert Evans, and Derry Roopenian for critical reading of this manuscript.

REFERENCES

Blom J, Mansa B, Wiik A (1976) A study of Russell bodies in human monoclonal plasma cells by means of immunofluorescence and electron microscopy. Acta Pathol Microbiol Scand [A] 84:335-349

Clark E A, Shultz L D, Pollack S B (1981) Mutations in mice that influence natural killer (NK) cell activity. Immunogenetics 12:601-613

Davidson W F, MorseH C III, Sharrow S O, Chused T M (1979) Phenotypic and functional effects of the motheaten gene on murine B and T lymphocytes. J Immunol 122:884-891

Gebbers J O, Otto H F (1976) Plasma cell alterations in ulcerative colitis. An electron microscopic study. Path Eur 11:271-279

Green M C, Shultz L D (1975) Motheaten, an immunodeficient mutant of the mouse. I. Genetics and Pathology. J Hered 66:250-258

Greiner D L, Goldschneider I, Komschlies K L, Medlock E S, Bollum F J, Shultz L D (1986) Defective lymphopoiesis in bone marrow of motheaten (*me/me*) and viable motheaten (*me^V/me^V*) mice. I. Analysis of development of prothymocytes, early lineage B cells, and terminal deoxynucleotidyl transferase-positive cells. J Exp Med 164:1129-1144

Hayakawa K, Hardy R R, Parks D R, Herzenberg L A (1983) The " Ly-1 B "cell population in normal, immunodefective, and autoimmune mice. J. Exp. Med. 157:202-218

Hayakawa K, Hardy R R, Honda M, Herzenberg L A, Steinberg A D Herzenberg L A (1984) Ly-1 B cells: Functionally distinct lymphocytes that secrete IgM autoantibodies. Proc Natl Acad Sci (USA) 81:2494-2498

Hayashi Shin-Ichi, Witte P L, Shultz L D , Stanley E R, Kincade P W (1988) Lymphopoiesis in culture is prevented by interaction with adherant bone marrow cells from mutant motheaten mice. J. Immunol In Press

Hsu SM, Hsu LP, McMillan P N, Fanger H. (1972) Russell bodies. A light and electron microscopic immunoperoxidase study. Am J Clin Pathol 77:26-31

Kearny J, Vakil M (1986) Functional idiotype networks during B cell ontogeny. Ann Immunol (Inst Pasteur) 137C:77

Kincade P (1978) Incidence and characteristics of functional B lymphocytes in motheaten mice. In Genetic control of autoimmune disease , ed. N R Rose, P E Bigazzi, N L Warner, pp. 241-249, Amsterdam: Elsevier North Holland

Komschlies K L , Greiner D L, Shultz, L D, Goldschneider I (1987) Defective lymphopoiesis in bone marrow of motheaten (*me/me*) and viable motheaten (*me^V/me^V*) mice. III. Normal mouse bone marrow cells enable *me^V/me^V* prothymocytes to generate thymocytes after intravenous transfer. J Exp Med 166:1162-1167

Lutzner M A, Hansen C T (1976) Motheaten: An immunodeficient mouse with markedly less ability to survive than the nude mouse in a germfree environment. J Immunol 116:1496-1497

McCoy K, Chi E, Engel D, Rosse C, Clagget J (1982) Abnormal in vitro proliferation of splenic mononuclear phagocytes from motheaten mice. J Immunol 128:1797-1804

McCoy K L, Chi E, Engel D, Clagett J (1983) Accelerated rate of mononuclear phagocyte production in vitro by splenocytes from autoimmune motheaten mice. Am J. Pathol. 112:18-26

McCoy K L, Nielson K , Clagett J (1984) Spontaneous production of colony-stimulating activity by splenic Mac-1 antigen-positive cells from autoimmune motheaten mice. J Immunol 132:272-276

McCoy K L, Clagget J, Rosse C (1985) Effects of the motheaten gene on murine B cell production. Exp Hematol 13:554-559

Medlock E S, Goldschneider I, Greiner D L, Shultz, L D (1987) Defective lymphopoiesis in bone marrow of motheaten *(me/me)* and viable motheaten *(me^V/me^V)* mice. II. Description of a microenvironmental defect for the generation of terminal deoxynucleotidyl transferase-positive bone marrow cells in vitro. J Immunol 138:3590-3597

Rossi G A, Hunninghake G W, Kawanami O, Ferrans V J Hansen C T, Crystal R G (1985) Motheaten mice - an animal model with an inherited form of interstitial lung disease. Am. Rev. Respir. Dis. 131:150-158

Russell, W (1890): An address on a characteristic organism of cancer. B Med J 2:1356-1360

Scribner C L, Hansen C T, Klinman D M, Steinberg A D (1987) The interaction of the *xid* and *me* genes. J Immunol 138:3611-3617

Schuler G, Steinman R M (1985) Murine epidermal Langerhans cells mature into potent immunostimulatory dendritic cells in vitro. J Exp Med 161:526-546

Shultz L D, Green M C (1976) Motheaten, an immunodeficient mutant of the mouse. II. Depressed immune competence and elevated serum immunoglobulins. J Immunol 116:936-943

Shultz L D, Zurier R B (1978) Motheaten, a single gene model for stem cell dysfunction and early onset autoimmunity. In Genetic control of autoimmune disease , ed. N. R. Rose, P. E. Bigazzi, N. L. Warner, pp. 229-240, Amsterdam: Elsevier North Holland

Shultz L D, Bailey C L, Coman D R (1983) Hematopoietic stem cell function in motheaten mice. Exp Hematol 11:667-680

Shultz L D, Coman D R, Bailey C L, Beamer W G, Sidman C L (1984) "Viable motheaten", a new allele at the motheaten locus. I. Pathology. Am JPathol 116:179-192

Shultz L D, Sidman C L (1987) Genetically determined murine models of immunodeficiency. Ann Rev Immunol 5:367-403

Shultz L D, Coman D R, Sidman C L, Lyons B (1987) Development of plasmacytoid cells with Russell bodies in autoimmune viable motheaten mice. Am J Pathol 127:38-50

Shultz, L D (1987) Hematopoietic stem cell defect in viable motheaten mutant mice. Fed Proc 46:1032

Sidman C L, Shultz L D, Unanue E R (1978a) The mouse mutant "motheaten" I. Development of lymphocyte populations. J Immunol 121:2392-2398

Sidman C L, Shultz L D, Unanue E R (1978b) The mouse mutant motheaten. II. Functional studies of the immune system. J Immunol 121:2399-2404

Sidman C L , Marshall J D , Masiello N C, Roths J B, Shultz, L D (1984) Novel B-cell maturation factor from spontaneously autoimmune viable motheaten mice. Proc Soc Natl Acad Sci. USA 81:7199-7202

Sidman C L, Shultz L D, Evans R (1985) A serum-derived molecule from autoimmune viable motheaten mice potentiates the action of a B cell maturation factor. J Immunol 135:870-872

Sidman C L, Shultz L D, Hardy R R, Hayakawa K, Herzenberg L A(1986) Production of immunoglobulin isotypes by Ly-1$^+$ B cells in viable motheaten and normal mice. Science 232:1423-1425

Stanton T H, Tubbs C, Clagett J (1985) Cytokine production and utilization by the motheaten mouse. J Immunol 135:4021-4026

Ward J M (1978) Pulmonary pathology of the motheaten mouse. Vet Path 15:170-178

Zlotnick A, Gertichter B, Nir I (1959) Experimental production of "grape cells" and their relationship to the serum gamma globulin and seromucoids. Blood 14:564-570

Characterization of Mott Cell Hybridomas from Autoimmune "Viable Motheaten" Mutant Mice

P. A. Schweitzer and L. D. Shultz

INTRODUCTION

Mott cells are abnormal plasma cells with discrete glycoprotein inclusions termed Russell bodies. These inclusions can be detected by their intense staining with periodic acid-Schiff's reagent (PAS). While Mott cells are present in low numbers in normal tissues (Lisco 1942), they are abundant in certain patients with multiple myeloma (Maldonado et al. 1966), trypanosomiasis (Mott 1905), and AIDS (Armstrong et al 1985). Mott cells can be found in experimental animals after hyperimmunization (White 1954) and in association with autoimmune disease of genetic origin (Alanen et al. 1985; Shultz et al. 1987). Although Mott cells have been recognized since 1890 (Russell 1890), neither the factors required for their development nor the role of these cells in normal and in diseased states have been determined. Mott cells are commonly found in lymphatic tissues from autoimmune, "viable motheaten" (me^V) mutant mice after 5 weeks of age (Shultz et al 1987). In order to analyze the defect(s) associated with development of Mott cells, permanent cell lines (hybridomas) were established that retain the Mott cell phenotype; i.e., plasmacytoid cells containing large amounts of immunoglobulin (Ig) within Russell bodies.

METHODOLOGY AND RESULTS

Cells from cervical lymph nodes of me^V/me^V mice were fused to the non-secreting myeloma parent, SP2/0. Aminopterin-resistant hybrids were then screened for the presence of cells containing discrete PAS-positive cytoplasmic inclusions. Mott cell hybridomas appeared at an unexpectedly high frequency. Approximately one-third of hybridomas from me^V/me^V mice contained Russell bodies. Staining of the Mott cell hybridomas with isotype-specific affinity-purified fluorescein-conjugated antisera revealed that although the majority produced mk Ig, a small percentage produced ml Ig. Globular, medusoid, or crystalline Russell bodies were observed by transmission electron microscopy (Fig. 1). After cloning, the Mott cell hybridomas retained their individual morphologic characteristics. However, the hybridomas were often unstable, losing detectable Russell bodies after extended culture.

In order to investigate the defect that causes abnormal Ig secretion from Mott cell hybridomas, additional hybridomas were made between me^V/me^V lymph node cells and the P3X63 myeloma fusion partner, which secretes IgG1 (MOPC21). Hybridomas with the Mott cell phenotype were observed at the same frequency as obtained in a parallel fusion with the non-secretor, SP2/0. In addition, by immunofluorescence microscopy, both IgG1 (presumably MOPC21) and IgM (from the me^V/me^V lymph node cells) were found in the Russell bodies.

Although these Mott cell hybridomas clearly retain Ig in intracellular rough endoplasmic reticulum (RER)-bound vesicles, Ig in supernatants was readily detectable by ELISA. We are currently trying to determine whether this Ig was secreted from Mott cell hybridomas or released from ruptured cells. IgM from the supernatant of Mott cell hybridomas eluted from a gel filtration column at a molecular size corresponding to pentameric IgM, approximately 10^6 daltons. This is the expected molecular weight for secreted IgM.

The Jackson Laboratory, Bar Harbor, ME 04609.

IgM-dependent plaque-forming cells (PFC) are sensitive to the inhibitor of protein synthesis, cycloheximide (Paige and Skarvall 1982). This sensitivity been used to determine whether Mott cells from NZB mice secrete Ig (Alanen et al. 1985). PFC from certain me^V/me^V Mott cell hybridomas were not inhibited by cycloheximide; these PFC were presumably caused by ruptured cells. However, the PFC from other Mott hybridomas were prevented by treatment with cycloheximide. These preliminary experiments indicate that some Mott cell hybridomas are able to secrete Ig in addition to retaining the Ig intracellularly.

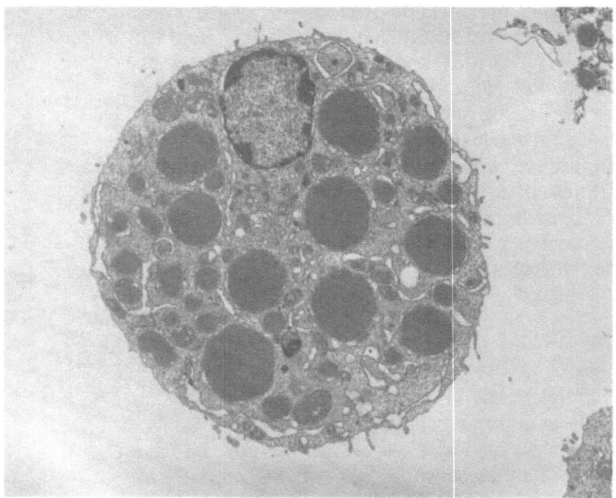

Fig. 1 Transmission electron micrograph of a Mott cell hybridoma. Numerous osmophilic, globular Russell bodies are evident (x4800).

DISCUSSION

Mott cells may represent a stage of B cell development in which the secretion of Ig is regulated after maturation to the plasma cell stage. Mott cell development requires functional T cells and can be antigen specific. The development of Mott cells in me^V/me^V mice is dependent upon the presence of functional T cells because in mice doubly homozygous for the nude and viable motheaten genes or in me^V/me^V mice thymectomized at birth, Mott cells do not develop (Shultz et al. 1987). White (1954) demonstrated that many Russell bodies in Mott cells were antigen binding (i.e. had anti-bacterial antibodies) following hyperimmunization of mice and rabbits with crude bacterial antigens. Identifying the epitopes to which the immunoglobulins from Mott cell hybridomas react would be informative for understanding the mechanisms underlying the development of Mott cells. However, the highly cross reactive nature of autoantibodies (Satoh et al. 1983) might make a definitive identification of the antigen difficult.

Several characteristics differentiate the me^V/me^V Mott cell hybridomas from previously described Mott cell hybridomas (Alanen et al. 1985; Weiss et al. 1984). The Ig produced by Mott cell hybridomas from me^V/me^V mice was IgM, whereas the hybridomas described by

Alanen et al. (1985) produced either IgG1 or IgG3 and that described by Weiss et al. (1984) produced only light chains. Also, Mott cell hybridomas from me^V/me^V mice arise at a thirty-fold higher frequency than from NZB mice (Alanen et al. 1985).

Although the P3X63 myeloma parent had the enzymes/proteins required for Ig secretion (P3X63 secretes IgG1), Mott cell hybridomas were obtained at a similar frequency to fusions with the non-secretor, SP2/0. The Russell bodies in these hybridomas contained both IgM and IgG1. This indicates that abnormal Ig secretion is not a result of an alteration in the primary amino acid sequence of the Ig heavy chain. However, the possibility of a defective light chain gene has not been ruled out. Since neither the SP2/0 nor the P3X63 myeloma parent rescues the defective Ig secretion, Mott cell hybridomas may represent a stage of B cell development frozen by fusion. Therefore, the development of Mott cells may not be directly caused by the action of defective me^V/me^V genes.

If Mott cells synthesize normal Ig chains and have no defects in the secretory organelles and/or proteins required for intracellular transport, yet are defective Ig secretors (judged by the buildup of Ig intracellularly), the possibility exists that Mott cells are not "down-regulated" plasma cells but rather synthesize Ig at a rate that overloads the protein secretory apparatus. Overproduction of Ig might explain not only the secretion of some Ig by Mott cell hybridomas but also the abundance of intracellular Ig in Russell bodies. Although it appears that these Mott cell hybridomas can secrete Ig, secreted Ig has not yet been detected from Mott cells from me^V/me^V mice, in vivo (Shultz et al. 1987). The release of high molecular weight IgM is not inconsistent with Ig sequestered in the RER and an inability to secrete IgM (Tartakoff and Vassalli 1979). However, the inhibition of PFC by cycloheximide indicates that some plaques are not a consequence of ruptured cells but are the result of active Ig secretion. This issue is being investigated further at the biochemical level.

ACKNOWLEDGEMENTS

This study was supported by NIH grants CA 20408 and DK 07449. Its contents are solely the responsibility of the Jackson Laboratory. We thank Ed Leiter and Derry Roopenian for critical review of this manuscript.

REFERENCES

Alanen A, Pira U, Lassila O, Roth J, Franklin, RM (1985) Mott cells are plasma cells defective in immunoglobulin secretion. Eur. J. Immunol. 15: 235-242

Armstrong JA, Dawkins RL, Horne R (1985) Retroviral infection of accessory cells and the immunological paradox in AIDS. Immunol Today 6: 121-122

Lisco H (1942) Russell bodies occurring in the lymph follicles of the intestinal tract of pigs. Anat Rec 82:59-66

Maldonado JE, Brown AL, Bayrd ED, Pease GL (1966) Cytoplasmic and intranuclear electron-dense bodies in the myeloma cell. Arch Path 81: 484-500

Mott FW (1905) Observations on the brains of men and animals infected with various forms of trypanosomes. Proc Roy Soc 76: 235-242

Paige CJ, Skarvall H (1982) Plaque formation by B cell clones. J. Immunol. Meth. 52:51-61

Russell W (1890) An address on a characteristic organism of cancer. Brit. Med J. 2:1356-1360

Satoh J, Prabhakar BS, Haspel MV, Ginsberg-Fellner F, Notkins A (1983) Human monoclonal autoantibodies that react with multiple endocrine organs. N. Engl. J. Med. 309: 217-220

Shultz LD, Coman DR, Lyons BL, Sidman CL, Taylor S (1987) Development of plasmacytoid cells with Russell bodies in autoimmune "viable motheaten" mice. Amer. J. Path. 127: 38-50

Tartakoff A, Vassalli P (1979) Plasma cell immunoglobulin M molecules: their biosynthesis, assembly, and intracellular transport. J. Cell Biol. 83: 284-299

Weiss S, Burrows PD, Meyer J, Wabl MR (1984) A Mott cell hybridoma. Eur. J. Immunol. 14: 744-748

White RG (1954) Observations on the formation and nature of Russell bodies. Brit. J. Exp. Path. 35: 365-376

A Molecular Genetic Approach to *gld* "Autoimmune" Disease

M. F. Seldin[1], H. C. Morse III[2], and A. D. Steinberg[1]

INTRODUCTION

A number of inbred strains, various crosses, and recombinant inbred lines of mice spontaneously develop autoimmune manifestations of which resemble those of patients with systemic lupus erythematosus and to some extent, Sjogren's syndrome and rheumatoid arthritis. Although several laboratories have characterized many of the immune abnormalities that occur secondary to genetic traits that segregate as Mendelian units, the primary defects have been elusive. Single gene defects which lead to or accelerate autoimmune disease include lpr, an unmapped autosomal recessive mutation (Murphy and Roths, 1978; Andrews et al, 1978) Yaa, the Y-chromosome-linked accelerator factor in BXSB mice (Murphy and Roths, 1979) and gld (generalized lymphoproliferative disease), a spontaeous autosomal mutation mapped to distal mouse chromosome 1 (Roths et al, 1984).

The gld mutation results in profound lymphadenopathy with expansion of an unusual T cell population and autoantibody production in C3H/HeJ mice (Roths et al, 1984; Davidson et al, 1985; Davidson et al, 1986; Mountz et al, 1986; Seldin et al, 1987a). By 16 weeks of age C3H-gld/gld mice of both sexes develop peripheral and mesenteric lymphadenopathy, splenomegaly, antinuclear antibodies including anti-dsDNA and hypergammaglobulinemia. The lymph nodes of these mice are heavily populated with dull Thy-1+, dull Ly-1, Ly-4⁻ (L3T4⁻), Ly-2⁻ cells These cells have high expression of cell surface antigens Ly-5(B220), Ly-6, Ly-22, Ly-24 and PC-1 and absence of sIg, ThB and Ia (Davidson et al, 1986; Seldin et al, 1987a). These lymphocytes exhibit polyclonal rearrangement of TCR-beta but not Ig heavy chain genes and express full length TCR-alpha and TCR-beta mRNA (Mountz et al, 1986; Davidson et al, 1986). Lymph node cells of these mice also express large amounts of the myb proto-oncogene which is ordinarily only expressed at high levels in the thymus or after mitogenic stimulation of T cells (Mountz et al, 1986; Seldin et al, 1987a). The phenotypic expression of the gld mutation is very similar to that of the nonallelic lpr mutation but unlike the lpr mutation the gld mutation occurred in a stable inbred strain of mouse and has been successfully mapped utilizing a 3 point cross analysis (Roths et al, 1984).

Our group has undertaken a molecular genetic approach to the understanding of the pathophysiology of this genetically determined disease in which the mutant or deficient normal gene product(s) remains undefined. The "gene first" approach has successfully been employed with the use of cDNA-mRNA subtraction hybridization to uncover the alpha and beta chains of the T cell receptor for antigen (Hedrick et al, 1984; Saito et al, 1984), and the use of DNA mediated gene transfer induction of fibroblast transformation in the cloning of certain oncogenes (Kontriris and Cooper, 1981; Perucho et al, 1981; Murray et al, 1981). It is more difficult to

[1]Cellular Immunology Section, National Institute of Arthritis, Muskuloskelatal and Skin Diseases, and [2]Laboratory of Immunopathology, National Insitute of Allergy and Infectious Disease, National Institutes of Health, Bethesda, MD.

approach those genes for which there is less certainty about the organs in which they are expressed and for which there are no available in vitro functional assays. Newly developed techniques allowing rapid cloning of genes large distances from available markers are dependent only on gene location and the type of mutation (Collins et al, 1987; Poustka et al, 1987). These techniques involving "chromosome jumping" depend on precise mapping and subsequent molecular characterization of the region containing the genetic defect. We have initiated a large breeding study to obtain mice with chromosome recombination events close to the gld gene which should allow the precise localization of this gene.

RESULTS and DISCUSSION

In order to detect chromosome recombination events by the use of restriction fragment length polymorphisms (RFLPs) and identify crossover events near the gld locus, we are breeding [(C3H-gld/gld x Mus spretus)F1 x C3H-gld/gld] backcross mice. Mus spretus was chosen because of the increased likelihood of being able to detect unique bands at any locus (Potter et al, 1986). Thus far over 1200 backcross mice have been generated. The general strategy is outlined in Fig. 1.

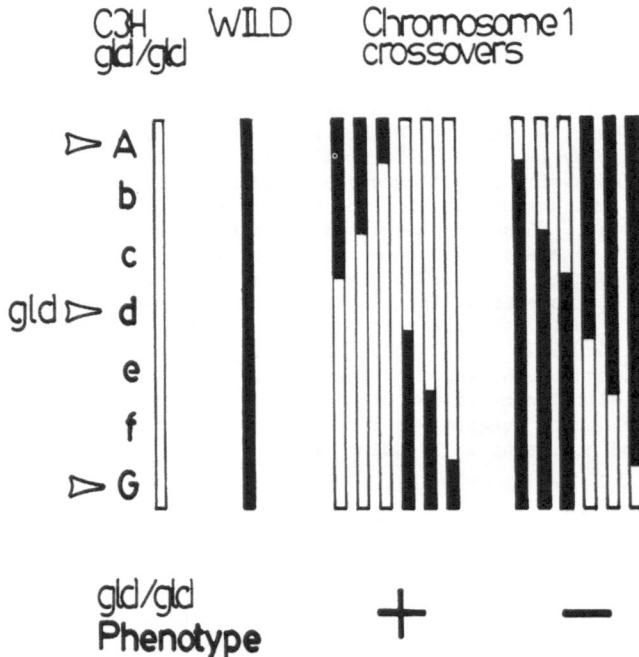

Figure 1. Mapping gld by RFLPs using [(C3H-gld/gld x wild) x C3H-gld/gld] backcross DNAs. Only the relevant chr.1 crossover events are depicted. Using typed markers, crossovers at A or G can be detected. This will limit the number of DNA samples to those potentially informative. After RFLPs with a given probe (B-F) have been identified between C3H-gld/gld and wild (M.spret), the backcross DNA can be characterized as illustrated. This will determine gene order and map distances. Only those probes that are closer to gld than the nearest crossover event (D), will yield a pattern directly corresponding to the phenotype.

Initial studies have centered on establishing a molecular genetic map of distal mouse chromosome 1 including the gld gene. We utilized clones of genes either previously localized to distal mouse chromosome 1, or likely to be located in this region based on the possibility of a large conserved linkage group between distal mouse chromosome 1 and human chromosome 1q. To clarify gene positions we examined backcross mice (currently 95 studied) and 7 sets of recombinant inbred RI strains. Potentially informative RFLPs in backcross mice were determined by hybridizing candidate genetic probes on Southern blots containing genomic DNA from C3H/HeJ-gld/gld parental mice and (C3H-gld/gld x M. spretus)F1 mice digested with various restriction endonucleases. Allelic variants were similarly identified in RI parental strains. Figure 2 shows the results of these studies which indicated the positions of 8 genes (Cfh, C4bp, Ren-1,2, Ly-5, At-3/gld, Apo-A2, Ly-17, and Spna-1) spanning over 25 centi-Morgans on distal chromosome 1.

Mouse Chromosome 1

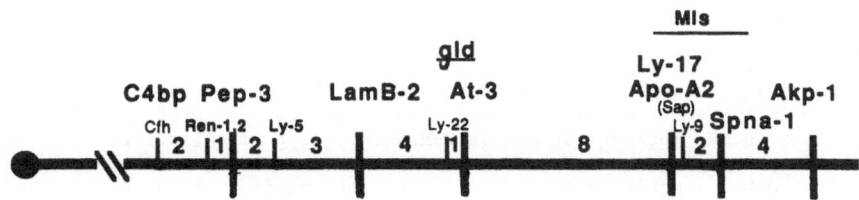

Figure 2. Distal mouse chromosome 1. The map distances and confidence intervals were established based on a Bayesian analysis of data obtained from both recombinant inbred lines and backcross mice. The placement of Cfh, C4bp, Ren-1,2, Ly-5, At-3, Ly-17, Apo-A2, and Spna-1 are based on Southern blot analysis of RFLPs. Cfh was detected utilizing a 4.4 kb Hpa I fragment from the mouse cDNA probe pMH8 (D'Eustachio et al, 1986). C4bp was detected using a 1.8 kb Pst I fragment from the mouse cDNA clone pMBP.15 (Kristensen et al, 1987). Ren-1,2 was detected with a 1.4 kb Pst I insert from the mouse cDNA clone Id-2 (Field et al, 1984). Ly-5 polymorphisms were detected using a 2400 bp Bam HI fragment isolated from the cDNA clone pLy-5-68 (Seldin et al, 1987b). At-3 associated RFLPs were detected with a 1.3 Pst I insert from the human cDNA clone pAt3 (Bock et al, 1985). The Ly-17 probe was a 1.3 kb Eco RI insert from the Ly-17 alpha chain cDNA clone J774 (Ravetch et al, 1986). The Apo-A2 probe was a 600 bp Eco RI insert from a mouse cDNA clone (A. Lusis, R.C. LeBoeuf, and M. Lucero - unpublished clone). The Spna-1 probe was a 750 bp Pst I insert from the mouse cDNA clone pMaSpl (Seldin et al, 1987c).

The gld gene was mapped with respect to these genes in the 95 backcross mice. Each was phenotypically typed on the basis of 1. obvious lymphadenopathy including the presence of enlarged mesenteric lymph nodes, 2. elevated IgM or IgG anti-DNA antibodies, and 3. the increased ratio ofspleen cell Ly-5(B220) vs. Kappa expression. The data indicated that there were no recombinants between an At-3 associated RFLP and gld. All 33 phenotype + mice were homozygous C3H at this locus and all 45 mice that had the heterozygous genotype were phenotype negative.

These data also indicate that the gld phenotype has variable penetrance in [(C3H-gld/gld x M. spretus)F1 x C3H-gld/gld] backcross mice. That is some mice that are homozygous for the C3H alleles throughout the region in which the gld locus must be located do not manifest the gld/gld phenotype. This must be due to other genetic factors since the variability in penetrance occurred even in litter mates housed in the same cage and was not present in C3H-gld/gld parental mice. Thus epistatic effects of genes not linked to gld are implicated. Epistatic effects of background genes have previously been noted upon the introduction of lpr/lpr a similar but nonallelic mutation, into various inbred domestic strains of mice (Kemp et al, 1982; Davidson et al, 1984, Izui et al, 1984; Morse et al, 1985; Samuelson et al, 1986).

The [(C3H-gld/gld x M.spretus)F1 x C3H-gld/gld] backcross mice may thus prove useful in characterizing additional genes involved in the pathogenesis of autoimmune disease. In addition to the variable penetrance of gld in current studies a small number of phenotype[+] backcross mice had profound glomerulonephritis which does not occur in the parental mice. This autoimmune manifestation is likely to be dependent on M.spretus genes in addition to gld/gld (M.F.Seldin and H.Austin unpublished results). These results are consistent with the observation that lpr, a similar but nonallelic mutation, results in profound glomerulonephritis in MRL-lpr/lpr but not in C3H/HeJ-lpr/lpr mice (Izui et al, 1984).Future genotyping of large numbers of backcross mice may allow identification of other genetic loci involved in the manifestations of autoimmune disease.

Evolving molecular technology should allow eventual characterization of genes such as gld. The ability to clone large segments of eukaryotic genes up to 500 kb has recently been reported (Burke et al, 1987). Analytical tools such as pulse and alternating field gel electrophoreses and the ability to clone segments of DNA large distances away from a well mapped initial cloned sequence promise to yield insights into the molecular mechanisms that lead to disease (Collins et al, 1987; Poustka et al, 1987). The identification of an RFLP closely linked to the gld gene identifies a starting point for an approach to understanding a genetic defect that results in abnormal T cells and autoimmune disease.

SUMMARY

A spontaneous autosomal recessive mutation (gld) on distal chromosome 1 results in profound lymphadenopathy with expansion of an unusual T cell population and auto-antibody production in C3H/HeJ mice. Our group has undertaken a molecular genetic approach to the understanding of the pathophysiology of this genetically determined disease in which the mutant or deficient normal gene product(s) remains undefined. [(C3H-gld/gld x Mus spretus)F1 x C3H-gld/gld] backcross mice are being utilized to allow precise mapping and eventual cloning of this gene.

Initial studies have centered on clarification of gene positions on telomeric mouse chromosome 1. DNA from both backcross mice (95 studied) and multiple recombinant inbred lines have been studied utilizing genetic probes for 7 gemes on chromosome 1 genes. The gene order was determined

to be (centromere) - C4bp, Ren-1,2, Ly-5, [At-3/gld], Apo-A2/Ly-17, Spna-1
- (telomere).   No crossovers between an At-3 associated restriction
fragment length polymorphism and gld were observed.

The [(C3H-gld/gld x Mus spretus)F1 x C3H-gld/gld] backcross mice may also
prove valuable in characterizing additional genes.   Some backcross mice
with the gld/gld genotype have variable penetrance of the gld/gld
phenotype; others exhibit autoimmune pathology not present in C3H-gld/gld
mice.   Thus detailed mapping of these backcross mice may result in the
identification of genes contributing to or inhibiting autoimmune disease.

Acknowledgment

We wish to thank Dr. M. Potter for providing Mus spretus mice and allowing
the use of the Hazleton Animal Facility under NCI contract No1-CB94326, Dr
L.A. D'Hoostelaire for valuable discussions, Drs. B. Tack, J. Ravetch, K.
Gross, P. Curtis, F.-W. Shen, R.C. LeBoeuf, and A. Lusis for their kind
gift of clones and Marena Mattson for her excellent care of our mice.

REFERENCES

Andrews, B.B., Eisenberg, R.A., Theofilopoulos, A.N., Izui, S., Wilson,
    C.B., McConahey, P.J., Murphy, E.D., Roths, J.B., Dixon, F. (1978)
    Spontaneous murine lupus-like syndromes.   Clinial and immunological
    manifestations in several strains. J. Exp. Med. 148:1198-1215.
Bock,S.C., Harris, J.F., Balazs, I., Trent, J.M. (1985) Assignment
    of the human antithrombin III structural gene to 1q 23-25. Cytogenet.
    Cell. Genet. 39:67-69.
Burke, D.T., Carle, G.F., Olsen, M.V. (1987) Cloning of large exogenous
    DNA into yeast by means of artificial chromosome vectors. Science.
    236:806-812.
Collins, F.S., Drum, M.L., Cole, J.C., Lockwood, W.K., Vande Woude, G.F.,
    Iannuzzi, M.C. (1987) Construction of a general human chromosome
    jumping library, with application to cystic fibrosis. Science.
    235:1046-1049.
Davidson, W.F., Roths, J.B., Holmes, K.L., Rudikoff, E., Morse, H.C.III.
    (1984) Dissociation of severe lupus-like disease from polyclonal B
    cell activation and IL-2 deficiency in C3H-lpr/lpr mice. J. Immunol.
    133:1048-1056.
Davidson, W.F., Holmes, K.L., Roths, J.B., Morse, H.C.III. (1985)
    Immunologic abnormalities of mice bearing the gld mutation suggest a
    common pathway for murine non-malignant lymphoprokiferative disorders
    with autoimmunity. Proc. Natl. Acad. Sci. (USA) 82:1219-1223.
Davidson, W.F., Dumont, F.J., Bedigian, H.G., Fowlkes, B.J., Morse,
    H.C.III. (1986)   Phenotypic, functional and molecular genetic
    comparisons of the abnormal lymphoid cells of C3H-lpr/lpr and C3H-
    gld/gld mice. J. Immunol. 136:4075-4084.
D'Eustachio, P., Kristensen, T., Wetsel, R.A., Riblet, R., Taylor, B.A.,
    Tack, B.F. (1986) Chromosomal location of the genes encoding complement
    components C5 and factor H in the mouse. J. Immunol. 137:3990-3995.
Field, L.J., McGowan, R.A., Dickinson, D.P., Gross, K.W. (1984) Tissue
    and gene specificity of mouse renin expresssion. Hypertension. 6:597-
    603.
Hedrick, S.M., Cohen, D.I., Nielson, E.A., Davis, M.M. (1984)   Nature
    308:149-153.
Izui, S., Kelly, V.E., Masuda, K., Yoshida, H., Roths, J.B., Murphy, E.D.
    (1984) Induction of various autoantibodies by mutant gene lpr in
    several strains of mice. J. Immunol. 133:227-233.

Kemp, J.D., Cowdery, J.S., Steinberg, A.D., Gershon, R.K. (1982) Genetic control of autoimmune disease: interactions between xid and lpr. J. Immunol. 128:388-392.

Krontiris, T.G., Cooper, G.M. (1981) Proc. Natl. Acad. Sci.,U.S.A. 78:1181-1184.

Mountz, J.D., Huppi, K.E., Seldin, M.F., Mushinski, J.F., Steinberg, A.D. (1986) T cell receptor gene expression in autoimmune mice. J. Immunol. 137:1029-1036.

Morse, H.C.III, Roths, J.B., Davidson, W.F., Longdon, W.Y., Fredrickson, T.N., Hartley, J.W. (1985) Abnormalities induced by the mutant gene, lpr: Patterns of disease and expression of murine leukemia viruses in SJL/J mice homozygous and heterozygous for lpr. J. Exp. Med. 161:602-616.

Murray, M.J., Shilo,B., Shih, C., Cowing, D., Hsu, H.W., Weinberg, R.A. (1981) Three different human tumor cell lines contain different oncogeness. Cell. 25:355-361.

Murphy, E.D., Roths, J.B. (1977) A single gene model for massive lymphoproliferation with autoimmunity in new mouse strain MRL. Fed. Pro.36:1246.

Murphy, E.D., Roths, J.B. (1979) A Y chromosome-associated factor producing accelerated autoimmunity and lymphoproliferation in strain BXSB. Arthritis Rheum. 22:1188-1194.

Perucho, M., Goldfarb, M., Shinzer, K., Lama, C., Fogh, J., Wigler, M. (1981) Human tumor derived cell lines contain common and different transforming genes. Cell. 27:467-476.

Poustka, A., Pohl, T.M., Barlow, D.P., Frischauf, A., Lehrach, H. (1987) Construction and use of human chromosome jumping libraries from Not I digested DNA. Nature 325:353-355.

Ravetch, J.V., Luster,A.D., Weinshank, R., Kochan, J., Pavlovec, A., Portnoy, D.A., Hulmes, J., Pan, T.-C.E., Unkeless, J.C. (1986) Structural heterogeneity and functional domains of murine immunoglobulin G Fc receptors. Science 234:718-725.

Roths, J.B., Murphy, E.D., Eicher, E.M. (1984) A new mutation, gld, that produces lymphoproliferation and autoimmunity in C3H/HeJ mice. J. Exp. Med. 159:1-20.

Samuelson, L.E., Davidson, W.F., Morse, H.C.III., Klausner, R.D. (1986) Abnormal tyrosine phosphorylation on T-cell receptors in lymphoproliferative disorders. Nature 324:674-676.

Saito, H., Kranz, D.M., Takagaki, Y., Hayday, A.C., Eisen, H.N., Tonegawa, S. (1984) A third rearranged and expressed gene in a clone of cytotoxic T lymphocytes. Nature. 312:36-40.

Seldin, M.F., Reeves, J.P., Scribner, C.L., Roths, J.B., Davidson, W.F., Morse, H.C.III, Steinberg, A.D. (1987a) Effect of xid on autoimmune C3H-gld/gld mice. Cell Immunol. 107:249-255.

Seldin, M.F., D'Hoostelaere, L.A., Steinberg, A.D., Saga, Y., Morse, H.C.III. (1987b) Allelic variants of Ly-5 in inbred and natural populations of mice. Immunogenetics 26:74-78.

Seldin, M.F., Morse, H.C.III, D'Hoostelaere, L.A., Britten, J.L., Steinberg, A.D. (1987c) Mapping of alpha-spectrin on distal mouse chromosome 1. Cytogenet. Cell. Genet. 45:52-54.

Genetic Analysis of BALB/cJ Subline Resistance to Actively Induced Experimental Allergic Orchitis (EAO) and Experimental Allergic Encephalomyelitis (EAE)

C. Teuscher, E. P. Blankenhorn, and W. F. Hickey

INTRODUCTION

EAO and EAE are two organ-specific autoimmune diseases which can be readily induced in genetically susceptible strains of mice (Teuscher et al. 1985a; Arnon 1981). Murine EAO is manifest as inflammation of the testes (orchitis), aspermatogensis, epididymitis, and vasitis (Kohno et al. 1983), whereas acute EAE is manifest clinically by varying degrees of paraparesis and paralysis, accompanied by lymphocytic and mononuclear cell infiltration of the central nervous system (CNS) (Arnon 1981). It was previously demonstrated that significant differences in susceptibility to actively induced EAO and EAE exist among various sublines of BALB/c mice (Teuscher et al. 1985b; Teuscher et al. 1987a; Munoz and Mackay 1984; Hickey et al. 1986). Of the 13 substrains studied, BALB/cJ mice were consistantly resistant to the induction of both diseases. The BALB/cJ substain is unique within the BALB/c family since it differs from other BALB/c substrains by several characteristic phenotypes (Potter 1985). One such phenotype, which may be relevant to disease susceptibility, is the elevated levels of serum alpha-fetoprotein (AFP) in adult BALB/cJ mice. It has been suggested that AFP may be immunosuppressive and that it is capable of suppressing EAE (Murgita and Tomasi 1975; Abaramsky et al. 1982; Brenner et al. 1985), although these findings are not conclusive (Fujinami et al. 1976). The serum AFP level, which is under the control of the Afr-1 locus (Olsson et al. 1977), normally drops dramatically at birth, from several milligrams/ml to a few hundred nanograms/ml. However, the mutant $Afr-1^b$ allele in BALB/cJ mice results in elevated adult AFP levels (from 2 to 5 ug/ml). If AFP is responsible for suppressing disease susceptibility in BALB/cJ mice, this phenomenon would be expected to segregate in a genetic test-cross where resistance to EAO and EAE would be found in mice bearing two copies of the $Afr-1^b$ allele.

MATERIALS AND METHODS

Animals: BALB/cJ and BALB/cByJ male and female mice were purchased from Jackson Laboratory (Bar Harbor, ME). All substrain breeding stock as well as F_1 hybrid and backcross mice were generated and maintained under identical enviornmental and nutritional conditions in the animal facilities of the Division of Laboratory Animal Medicine, the University of Pennsylvania School of Medicine (Philadelphia, PA). Animals were housed in groups of five animals or less per cage (BALB/cJ male mice were housed individually) and fed Purina mouse pellets and acidified water ad libitum. All animals appeared to be in good health at the time of immunization and were between 8 and 10 weeks of age when studied.

Induction and evaluation of disease: For the induction of EAO, male mice were immunized under ether anesthesia with 10 mg dry weight mouse testicular homogenate (MTH) in 0.05 ml of phosphate buffered saline (PBS) emulsified

with an equal volume of complete Freund's adjuvant (Difco, Detroit, MI)
(CFA) supplemented with 0.45 mg M. tuberculosis (H37Ra). Each animal
received 0.1 ml of the emulsion distributred equally in both hind footpads.
Immediately thereafter, each aniamal received 10.0 ug of crude pertussigen
dissolved in 0.1 ml of 0.015 M Tris-HCl buffer containing 0.5 M NaCl and
0.017% Triton X-100 pH 7.6 by i.p. injection and 5.0 ug again 24 hours
later. All animals were killed 30 days after immunization. The testes were
fixed in Bouin's fixative, embedded in paraffin, and 5-um thick sections
were cut and stained with hematoxylin-eosin for histological examination. A
pathology index (PI) was determined on each testis by examing two to four
sections taken at four different levels. The four major lesions of EAO
(orchitis, aspermatogensis, epididymitis, and vasitis) were semiquantitated
in a double-blind fashion as previously descrived (Teuscher et al. 1985a;
Tung et al. 1985; Teuscher et al. 1987a; Adekunle et al. 1987). The PI for
each animal was calculated as the average PI for the histopathologic changes
in both testes. The overall PI for each substrain was calculated as the
average of the individual PI for all animals of a particular substrain.

For the induction of EAE, female mice received 0.1 ml of encephalitogenic
emulsion in each hind foot pad and scruff of the neck, distributed equally
among these three sites. The emulsion consisted of equal volumes of 0.9 N
saline containing 40.0 mg/ml lyophilized, homogenized pool of allogeneic
mouse CNS prepared from SWR mice and CFA supplemented with 4.0 mg/ml M.
tuberculosis (H37RA). Thus each animal received 2.0 mg of CNS tissue in
adjuvant. On the day of immunization or 3 days thereafter mice were given
10.0 ug of crude pertussigen i.v. and 5 ug i.p. as detailed above. The mice
were observed for daily signs of EAE from day 10 to day 30 postinjection.
All animals were sacrificed for histopathologic evaluation at the peak of
illness; on the 30th day all animals which had not exhibited EAE clinically
were killed and their CNS were studied for histological evidence of EAE in a
double-blind fashion. A PI of the degree of histologic EAE severity was
assigned: 0, no evidence of CNS inflammation; 1, small, primarily
meningeal, scattered inflammatory infiltrates; 2, large but scattered
infiltrates in meninges and parenchyma; and 3, large, numerous, occasionally
confluent inflammatory infiltrates (Teuscher et al. 1987b).

Determination of murine AFP levels: Serum was collected from the animals at
the time of sacrifice and stored at $-70°$ C. Murine AFP was quantitated
using a solid-phase radioimmunoassay as previously described (Blankenhorn et
al. 1985). Briefly, polyvinyl chloride 96-well plates were coated with
Protein A-Sepharose-purified monospecific rabbit anti-mouse AFP overnight at
$4°$ C, blocked with 1% bovine serum albumin in PBS and rinsed, and diluted
mouse serum (1/5, 1/10 and 1/20) was added in duplicate to the wells and
incubated for 2 hours at room temperature. Radioiodinated pourified murine
AFP was added to the plates at a concentration of 20,000 cpm/well and
binding to the antibodies was allowed to proceed at $4°$ C overnight. The
plates were washed, dried, sliced into individual wells, and counted.
Determination of the amounts of AFP was made using a computer-based
calculation of the percentage inhibition by mouse serum at each dilution
compared with a standard curve of inhibition afforded by dilutions of pure
AFP performed in parallel.

Statistical analysis: Statistical comparisons were carried out by the
Student T test, the Wilcoxon ranked sum test, or the X^2 test. All

comparisons in this study were considered statistically significant when P was less that 0.05.

RESULTS AND DISCUSSION

BALB/cByJ mice were susceptible to both EAO and EAE, whereas mice of the BALB/cJ subline were resistant to the induction of both diseases (Tables 1 and 2). Aspermatogensis and autoimmune vasitis were found to correlate with susceptibility to autoimmune orchitis, while only marginal autoimmune epididymitis was observed. With respect to EAE, as has been frequently demonstrated (Lando et al. 1979), mice of the BALB/cJ subline showed no clinical evidence and only very marginal histologic evidence of disease. However, the majority of BALB/cByJ mice showed clear clinical and histopathological susceptibility. Susceptibility to both diseases was inherited as a dominant trait in (BALB/cByJ X BALB/cJ)F_1 hybrid animals.

TABLE 1: Susceptibility of BALB/c Substrains to EAO

Substrain	n	Orchitis PI	% Aspermatogenesis	Epididymitis PI	Vasitis PI
BALB/cJ	10	0	0	0	0
BALB/cByJ	8	5.3	52.2	1.6	3.0
(BALb/cByJ X BALB/cJ)F_1	5	3.9(NS)[a]	39.7(NS)	1.3(NS)	2.6(NS)

[a] NS, not significantly different from susceptible parental subline (P>0.05).

TABLE 2: Susceptibility of BALB/c Substrains to EAE

Substrain	n	Clinical EAE			Histologic EAE	
		No-Symptoms	Flaccid tail and weakness	Hind Limb paralysis and/or moribund state	Infiltrate detected	Inflammatory PI
BALB/cJ	15	15	0	0	3	0.2
BALB/cByJ	29	12	3	14	21	1.5
(BALB/cByJ X BALB/cJ)F$_1$	7	4	0	3	6	1.4(NS)[a]

[a] NS, not significantly different from susceptible parental subline ($P > 0.05$).

Susceptibility and resistance to EAO and EAE were examined in male and female (BALB/cByJ X BALB/cJ)F$_1$ X BALB/cJ backcross animals, respectively, and the circulating AFP levels of all animals were determined. The classification of mice susceptible or resistant to EAO and EAE with respect to their circulating AFP levels in shown in Tables 3 and 4.

These data suggest that BALB/cJ substrain mice posess either a single difference in a common regulatory gene which controls susceptibility to both diseases or two differences, one in a regulatory gene affecting susceptibility to EAO and one in a regulatory gene controlling susceptibility to EAE (the ratio of disease resistant to disease susceptible animals is 13:15 or 0.9:1.0 for EAO amd 16:18 or 0.9:1.0 for EAE). The identity and location of this regulatory locus is currently unknown. The genetic mechanisms involved in the regulation of organ specific autoimmune disease are, for the most part, poorly understood. To elucidate such conditions and the genes controlling them, it would be useful to examine experimental animals which have a very high degree of genetic similarity, but differ in the phenotypic expression of certain traits, i.e., coinsogenic strains. We propose that such a model may exist among the BALB/c substrains for EAE and EAO, both of which involve T-lymphocyte-mediated, organ specific autoimmunity. In addition, the mutant Afr-1^b allele expressed by BALB/cJ mice did not segregate with disease resistance. Since very high circulating levels of AFP were found in both susceptible and resistant backcross mice, it would appear that resistance is not due to the purported immunosuppressive effects of AFP. Association of disease resistance with additional BALB/cJ substrain variations embodied in a set of differential phenotypes which include

TABLE 3: Distribution of High-AFP (Afr-1$^{b/b}$) and Low-AFP (Afr-1$^{a/b}$) Mice in the (BALB/cByJ X BALB/cJ)F$_1$ X BALB/cJ Backcross Generation According to Susceptibility to EAO

EAO	High-AFP(Afr-1$^{b/b}$)	Low-AFP(Afr-1$^{a/b}$)	Total
Susceptible	6	7	13
Resistant	6	9	15
Total	12	16	

TABLE 4: Distribution of High-AFP (Afr-1$^{b/b}$) and Low-AFP (Afr-1$^{a/b}$) Mice in the (BALB/cByJ X BALB/cJ)F$_1$ X BALB/cJ Backcross Generation According to Susceptibility to EAE

EAE	High-AFP(Afr-1$^{b/b}$)	Low-AFP(Afr-1$^{a/b}$)	Total
Susceptible	7	9	16
Resistant	6	12	18
Total	13	21	

aggressive fighting behavior, differences in the expression of the
lymphocyte associated Qa antigens, increased levels of three adrenal enzymes
involved in catecholamine biosynthesis (tyrosine hydroxylase, dopamine-beta-
dehydrogenase, and phenylethanolamine N-methyltransferase), or resistance to
plasmacytoma induction and susceptibility to pristane-induced arthritis
(Potter 1985), has not yet been examined in linkage studies. Thus, EAO and
EAE resistance is currently unassociated with any other known phenotypic
differences characterizing BALB/cJ mice. Nevertheless, the fact that
disease resistance is not linked to the mutant Afr-1[B] allele suggests that
multiple mutational events may have occured in several regulatory genes
rather than a single mutation in a pleitropic regulatory gene that affects
the expression of all of the differential phenotypes observed in BALB/cJ
subline mice.

REFERENCES

Abaramsky O, Brenner T, Mizrachi R, Soffer, D (1982) Alpha-fetoprotein
suppresses experimental allergic encephalomyelitis. J Neuroimmunol 2, 1-7
Adekunle AO, Hickey WF, Smith SM, Tung KSK, Teuscher, C (1987) Experimental
allergic orchitis in mice: IV. Preliminary characterization of the major
murine testis specific aspermatogenic autoantigen(s). J Reprod Immunol
12, 49-62
Arnon, R (1981) Experimental allergic encephalomyelitis-susceptibility and
suppression. Immunol Rev 55, 5-30
Blankenhorn EP, Wax JS, Matthai R, Potter, M (1985) Genetic analysis of
alpha-fetoprotein levels in BALB/c sublines. Curr Top Microbiol Immunol
122, 53-57
Brenner T, Evron S, Soffer D, Abramsky O, (1985) Treatment of
experimental allergic encephalomyelitis in rabbits with alpha-fetoprotein.
Israel J Med Sci 21, 945-949
Fujinami RS, Paterson PY, Parmely MJ, Thompson JS, Goeken NE (1976) Lack of
suppressive effects of alpha-fetoprotein on development of experimental
allergic encephalomyelitis in rats. Nature (London) 264, 782-783
Hickey WF, Kirby WM, Teuscher C (1986) BALB/c substrain differences in
susceptibility to experimental allergic encephalomyelitis (EAE). Ann NY
Acad Sci 475, 331-333
Kohno S, Munoz, JJ, Williams TM, Teuscher C, Bernard CCA, Tung KSK (1983)
Immunopathology of murine experimental allergic orchitis. J Immunol 130,
2675-2682
Lando Z, Teitlbaum D, Arnon R (1979) Genetic control of susceptibility to
experimental allergic encephalomyelitis in mice. Immunogenetics 9, 435-
442
Munoz JJ, Mackay IR (1984) Production of experimental allergic
encephalomyelitis with the aid of pertussigen in mouse strains considered
genetically resistant. J Neuroimmunol 7, 91-96
Murgita RA, Tomasi, TB (1975) Suppression of the immune response by
fetoprotein. J Exp Med 141, 440-452
Olsson M, Lindahl G, Ruoslahti E (1977) Genetic control of alpha-
fetoprotein synthesis in the mouse. J Exp Med 145, 819-827
Potter M (Ed) (1985) The BALB/c Mouse. Curr Top Microbiol Immunol 122

Teuscher C, Smith SM, Goldberg EH, Shearer GM, Tung KSK (1985a)
   Experimental allergic orchitis in mice: I. Genetic control of
   susceptibility and resistance to induction of autoimmune orchitis.
   Immunogenetics 22, 323-333
Teuscher C, Potter M, Tung KSK (1985b) Differential susceptibility to
   experimental autoimmune orchitis in BALB/c substrains. Curr Top Microbiol
   Immunol 122, 181-188
Teuscher C, Smith SM, Tung KSK (1987a) Experimental allergic orchitis in
   mice: III. Differential susceptibility and resistance among BALB/c
   sublines. J Reprod Immunol 10, 219-230
Teuscher C, Blankenhorn EP, Hickey WF (1987b) Differential susceptibility
   to actively induced experimental allergic encephalomyelitis and
   experimental allergic orchitis among BALB/c substrains. Cell Immunol (In
   press)
Tung, KSK, Teuscher C, Smith S, Ellis L, Dufau ML (1985) Factors that
   regulate the development of testicular autoimmune disease. Ann NY Acad
   Sci 438, 171-188

Genetic Control of Murine Susceptibility
to 3-Methylcholanthrene-Induced T Cell Lymphoma

S. T. Ishizaka and F. Lilly

INTRODUCTION

It has been known since the 1940's that genetic background has an effect on the susceptibility of mice to lymphoma induced by chemical carcinogens (Law 1941; Morton 1941). In most cases, however, the biochemical basis for this variation in susceptibility has yet to be elucidated. We describe here our work on a system in which T cell lymphoma is induced in mice by exposure to the coal tar-derived carcinogen 3-methylcholanthrene (MCA). One gene controlling the likelihood of developing lymphoma after exposure to MCA has been identified, and it appears that the remaining differences in susceptibility which cannot be attributed to this known locus may themselves stem from the action of a second single gene. This fact makes more feasible the mapping and identification of the biochemical entity involved.

AHH INDUCIBILITY: AN EPISTATIC EFFECT

Table 1 outlines the responses of various strains of inbred mice to skin painting with MCA in benzene. It can be seen that some strains respond with the generation of papillomas localized at the site of MCA application. Other strains develop thymic lymphoma, and some do not show any neoplastic effects at all. We have shown (Duran-Reynals 1978) in backcross studies that papilloma development segregates with inducibility at the Ah locus. This gene (Thomas 1972) controls the expression of an enzyme, aryl hydrocarbon hydroxylase (AHH), that metabolizes MCA to its reactive epoxide form. Presumably AHH-inducible strains respond to percutaneous MCA with the production of AHH, which metabolizes MCA resulting in its reaction with DNA and subsequent skin tumorigenesis (Thomas 1973). This reaction appears to effectively block MCA entry into the circulation of the animal, as AHH inducible strains do not manifest lymphoma after MCA exposure. The lymphoma response is limited to strains in which MCA does not evoke an increase in AHH production. It should be noted that noninducible strains are not devoid of AHH, but simply do not augment its level after polycyclic hydrocarbon exposure (Nebert 1969). The endogenous enzyme in noninducible strains may be responsible for the MCA processing presumed to be necessary for lymphomagenesis.

Table 1
Strain-specific patterns of tumorigenesis following MCA exposure

Mouse Strain	Incidence of Skin Tumors	Incidence of Thymic Lymphoma
CBA/J	high	none
BALB/c	high	none
A/J	high	none
RF/J	none	high
DBA/1J	none	high
DBA/2J	none	high
ST/bN	none	low
SWR/J	low	low

Department of Genetics, Albert Einstein College of Medicine,
Bronx, NY 10461

Current Topics in Microbiology and Immunology, Vol. 137
© Springer-Verlag Berlin · Heidelberg 1988

A SECOND LOCUS AFFECTING SUSCEPTIBILITY

It is clear from Table 1 that the <u>Ah</u> locus is not the only factor affecting a mouse strain's susceptibility to lymphoma: AHH noninducible strains exhibit MCA-induced lymphoma incidences which can be classified as either low (10-40%) or high (60-90%). The work to be discussed in this section focuses on these AHH noninducible strains; those which exhibit high incidences of lymphoma after MCA exposure are referred to as "susceptible", while those which have low incidences are termed "resistant". Crosses between MCA lymphoma susceptible and resistant strains indicate that resistance is a dominant trait, and four different backcrosses of (resistant x susceptible) F_1 to the susceptible strain give incidences halfway between those of the susceptible and resistant parental strains. This pattern is consistent with the determination of resistance by a single locus (Mayer 1980). This is confirmed by second generation backcross experiments (our unpublished data) in which half the (SWR/J x RF/J) x RF/J females backcrossed to RF/J males gave rise only to susceptible offspring, and half produced offspring with a lymphoma rate halfway between the RF/J and SWR/J rates. The fact that a single locus appears to be involved should facilitate the mapping and identification of the gene determining resistance, however we have not yet been successful in determining the linkage of this trait.

In order to determine where in a resistant animal this resistance is expressed we have constructed bone marrow chimeras in which marrow from a resistant strain is transferred to a lethally irradiated animal of a susceptible strain. Reciprocal transfers were also made, and animals were then treated with MCA after a 2 month engraftment period. The results indicated that resistance is an inherent characteristic of marrow-derived cells, and cannot be derived from stroma: susceptible RF/J marrow developing in resistant (ST/bN x RF/J) F_1 animals gave rise to a high incidence of RF/J lymphomas, while (ST/bN x RF/J) F_1 marrow in an RF/J recipient develops lymphoma only at a low rate (Ishizaka 1987).

This finding led us to examine some properties of marrow-derived cells which might influence an animal's susceptibility to induced thymic lymphoma. In unpublished studies no correlation was seen between the resistance of a strain and thymic levels of superoxide dismutase or DNA repair. The former is an enzyme that decreases the level of superoxide, a tumor promoting agent (Cerutti 1985); the latter is clearly of interest in a system where a mutagenic agent induces disease. Neither was any relation found between high levels of NK activity, a nonspecific immune cytytoxic function of marrow-derived cells, and resistance to MCA-induced lymphoma.

Unpublished experiments from our laboratory have also examined the susceptibility of various mouse strains to X-ray-induced lymphoma, using a fractionated dose regimen. In all AHH noninducible strains examined to date high rates of X-ray-induced lymphoma correlate with high MCA-induced lymphoma susceptibility. Similarly, all strains exhibiting MCA resistance also have low rates of X-ray induced lymphoma. This suggests that the two phenomena may derive from a single locus. We hope to clarify this point using recombinant inbred lines derived from one susceptible and one resistant parental strain.

It is interesting to consider the theoretical ramifications if it is found that resistance to X-ray-induced and MCA-induced lymphoma do in fact map to a single gene. Resistance can presumably stem from three possible mechanisms: an ability to avoid damage (perhaps through some protective system), a means of efficiently repairing mutagenic damage, or a surveillance system that can prevent the outgrowth of transformed cells. In this last case it is not difficult to envision a system that would deal equally well with both X-ray and chemically induced tumors. In the former two cases it is more challenging (and therefore more interesting) to define systems which would deal with both irradiation and a polycyclic hydrocarbon as mutagenic agents. In this connection it should also be noted that one possible scenario for lymphoma induction involves the activation and reinsertion of

242

endogenous viral genomes near some mouse gene controlling cell growth. Chinsky et al. (1985) have examined a number of primary RF/J MCA-induced thymic lymphomas and have found no evidence for such an event, nor have we found any alterations in the Pim-1 locus, a common insertion site in Moloney MuLV-induced tumors (unpublished data).

REFERENCES

Cerutti PA (1985) Prooxidant states and tumor promotion. Science 227:375-381
Chinsky J, Goodenow MM, Jackson M, Lilly F, Leinwand L, Childs G (1985) Comparison of endogenous murine leukemia virus proviral organization and RNA expression in 3-methylcholanthrene-induced and spontaneous thymic lymphomas in RF and AKR mice. J Virol 53:94-99
Duran-Reynals ML, Lilly F, Bosch A, Blank KJ (1978) The genetic basis of susceptibility to leukemia induction in mice by 3-methylcholanthrene applied percutaneously. J Exp Med 147:459-469
Ishizaka S, and Lilly F (1987) Genetically determined resistance to 3-methylcholanthrene-induced lymphoma is expressed at the level of bone marrow-derived cells. J Exp Med 166:565-570
Law LW (1941) The induction of leukemia in mice following percutaneous application of 9,10-dimethyl-1,2-benzanthracene. Canc Res 1:564-571
Mayer A, Lilly F, Duran-Reynals ML (1980) Genetically dominant resistance in mice to 3-methylcholanthrene-induced lymphoma. Proc Natl Acad Sci USA 77:2960-2963
Morton JJ, Mider GB (1941) Some effects of carcinogenic agents on mice subject to spontaneous leukoses. Canc Res 1:95-98
Nebert DWL, Gelboin HV (1969) The in vivo and in vitro induction of aryl hydrocarbon hydroxylase in mammalian cells of different species, tissues, strains, and developmental and hormonal states. Arch Biochem Biophys 134:76-89
Thomas PE, Kouri RE, Hutton JJ (1972) The genetics of aryl hydrocarbon hydroxylase induction in mice: A single gene difference between C57BL/6J and DBA/2J. Biochem Genet 6:157-168
Thomas PE, Hutton JJ, Taylor BA (1973) Genetic relationship between aryl hydrocarbon hydroxylase inducibility and chemical carcinogen induced skin ulceration in mice. Genetics 74:655-659

Multigenic Control of Colon Carcinogenesis in Mice Treated with 1,2-Dimethylhydrazine

D. Fleiszer*, J. Hilgers**, and E. Skamene*

INTRODUCTION

In spite of major research efforts, cancer of the colon remains the second commonest cancer killer in North America. Epidemiologic studies on large populations have implicated numerous dietary factors which encourage the appearance of these tumors but a clear cause - effect relationship for individuals has not been established (Armstrong and Dou, 1975; Kinlen, 1983; Review, 1982; Walker, 1976; Weisberger et al, 1982; Willett and MacMahou, 1984). The large majority of colon cancers are classified as idiopathic. There are notable exceptions, however, such as the "cancer families", familial polyposis, Gardner's syndrome and others where the genetic background of the host appears to play an important role (Lynch et al, 1973; Lynch and Lynch, 1980). In the majority of cases the problem remains of explaining why some individuals, given similar environments, develop colon cancer and others do not. One possibility is that subtle genetic factors are present, causing one individual to be susceptible and another resistant to developing colon cancer. Very little work appears to have been done, at an experimental level, to explore this possibility.

Previous work done in our laboratory and by others, has shown that the colon carcinogen dimethylhydrazine (DMH) induces tumors in animals that are very similar to human tumors, both in behavior and histology (Filipe 1975; Fleiszer et al. 1980; Maskens 1976; Newberne and Rogers, 1973; Sunter et al, 1978; Wiebecke et al, 1973). Since 1980 the popularity of this model has grown rapidly and with the use of many new species and strains it has become evident that there is wide variation in the sensitivity to the carcinogen from one strain to the next (Diwan and Blackman 1980; Diwan and Meier, 1976; Diwan et al, 1977; Evans et al, 1974; Evans et al., 1975; Fleiszer and Skamene, unpublished; Thurnherr et al, 1973; Table 1). To date there has been very little done to study this strain variation. Two studies based on a classical mendelian analysis, suggested the difference is due to a single autosomal dominant gene (Boffa et al, 1986; Evans et al, 1977). Some preliminary data from unreported work done in our own laboratory suggested this may not be the case and the current experiment, utilizing two recombinant inbred (RI) colonies with a well defined genetic background, was undertaken.

*Montreal General Hospital Research Institute, Montreal, Quebec H3G 1A4, Canada
**Netherlands Cancer Institute, Amsterdam, The Netherlands

Table 1. Strain variation in susceptibility to DMH-induced colon carcinogenesis in inbred mice

Susceptible	Relatively resistant	Resistant
CF1	C57BL/6J	AKR/J
SWR/J	BALB/cHeA	DBA
ICr/Ha		C57BL/Ha
P/J		
A/J		
STS/A		

MATERIALS AND METHODS

Three hundred and sixteen mice representing the two progenitor strains, A/J (A) and C57BL/6J (B), their F_1 progeny and 23 AXB/ BXA recombinant inbred strains were tested for relative resistance or sensitivity to the colon carcinogen dimethylhydrazine. One hundred and thirty-three mice representing the two progenitor strains, BALB/cHeA (C) and STS/A (S), and 14 CXS recombinant inbred strains were similarly tested. A and B mice were obtained from Jackson Laboratories. The F_1 and AXB/BXA RI strains were propagated at the Montreal General Hospital (ES) from breeding stock supplied by Dr. Muriel Nesbitt, University of Californa, La Jolla (Nesbitt and Skamene, 1984). The C and S mice and their RI counterparts were produced at the Netherlands Cancer Institute, Amsterdam (Hilgers and Arends, 1985). Animals were housed in identical cages with wood chip bedding in groups of 3-6 animals per cage and fed standard chow and water ad lib. After a minimum of two weeks acclimatization, at eight weeks of age, each animal was given DMH at a dose of 15 mg/kg, by subcutaneous injection. This was continued once a week for a total of twenty weeks. After a further six weeks, the animals were killed and the number of gross colon tumors counted. Means and standard errors were determined for each group. A weighted cluster analysis for 2, 3 and 4 segregating populations was performed. The "student t" test was used to determine the level of significance of differences between the A and B progenitors and the F_1 strain.

RESULTS

  The average number of tumors and standard errors for each strain are shown in Figure 1. A/J and STS/A mice were susceptible, with the mean number of tumor nodules 19.0 and 11.3, respectively. C57BL/6 and BALB/c mice typed as resistant with the mean number of tumor nodules 1.0 and 1.4, respectively. The F_1 hybrids (C57BL/6J x A/J) were susceptible with the mean number of tumor nodules being 11.7. Although this suggests that the susceptibility is dominant over resistance it should be noted that there was a significant difference (p = 0.07) between the susceptible (A/J) parent and F_1 hybrids suggesting either an incomplete penetrance or a gene dose effect.

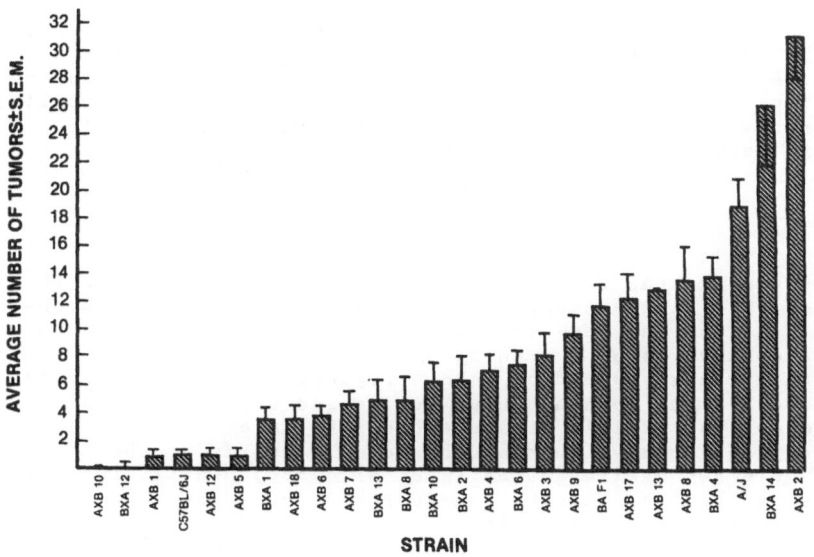

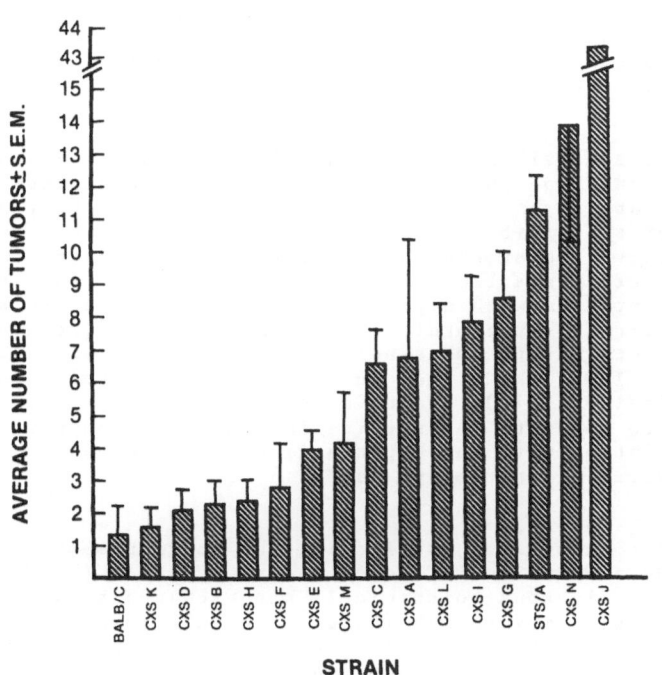

Figure 1. Colonic tumor load in DMH-treated recombinant inbred
mice of AXB/BXA (top) and CXS (bottom) series.

The 23 AXB/BXA RI strains had mean tumor loads ranging from 0 to 32 and the 14 CXS strains had mean tumor loads ranging from 1.6 to 43.3. A cluster analysis of the RI strain results, weighted by the standard deviation and the sample size within each strain, failed to reveal any convincing separation into identifiable phenotypic groups in either set of strains.

DISCUSSION

It has been suggested that sensitivity to dimethylhydrazine is determined by a single autosomal gene (Boffa et al, 1986; Evans et al, 1977). In one case (Evans et al, 1977) this conclusion was based on work using a grading system in which the colon tumor burden was given a score from 0 to 4 depending on its appearance. The A/J and F_1 mice both had high scores and were considered to carry the dominant allele of susceptibility in either homozygous or heterozygous forms. In the other case, details of the analysis were not available (Boffa et al, 1986). Utilizing this method we had similar results (unreported), but when we actually counted the number of tumors found in a given colon, there was, in fact, a statistical difference between F_1 and their A progenitor. It thus seems that we are dealing with a quantitative trait with a threshold expression. In such a situation, as pointed out by Wright (1934), the results of Mendelian analysis may lead to erroneous conclusion and the monogenic theory of inheritance needs to be proved by further breeding tests to ascertain that the single gene for dominant trait breeds true.

The RI strain analysis performed in this study clearly establish-ed that more than one gene was involved in the regulation of DMH-induced carcinogenesis. We have demonstrated that there was a spectrum of susceptibility ranging from the extremely resistant AXB-10 strain to the exquisitely susceptible AXB-2 strain. Similarly, there was a broad range of tumor burden from the CXS K to the CXS J strains with a gradually increasing average number of tumors among the intermediate strains. If a single gene was involved in determining DMH sensitivity each RI strain should statistically look like either the susceptible or resistant progenitor (Bailey 1971). Using a weighted cluster analysis we were unable to separate the strains into distinct phenotypic groups, consistent with the hypothesis that DMH sensitivity is based on several, if not many, genes.

This is hardly surprising considering the large number of factors which have been found to influence tumor formation (Table 2). For example, indigenous colonic cell kinetics can be used to predict susceptibility to DMH (Deschner et al, 1983; Glickman et al, 1987). The kinetics of colon mucosa is a complex process requiring the interaction of numerous cell systems each with its own complex set of controlling genes. Differences in drug metabolism have also been suggested as an underlying reason for the differential strain susceptibility. The degree of alkylation of DNA, by DMH, has been shown to correlate with susceptibility and resistance (Cooper et al, 1978). The metabolism of DMH to its proximate carcinogen is also a complex process requiring

several enzyme systems each with its own genetic background
(Evans 1982; Fiala 1977; Sohn et al, 1985). The degree of DNA
damage caused by DMH has also been found to correlate with strain
susceptibility to DMH - induced colon tumors (Bolognesi and
Boffa, 1986). There are many more examples of the complexity of
DMH carcinogenesis and it would be unrealistic to expect that all
of these phenotypic expressions are the result of a common
mechanism simple enough to be coded for by a single gene. It is
much more likely that there are several or many mechanisms, each
with its own rate - limiting step, and that the cell machinery
involved in each, requires several if not many genes for its
functioning.

Table 2. Some factors affecting or associated with induced tumors

---

 1) Dietary factors: Fat
                        Fiber
                        Protein
                        Cholesterol
 2) Bile acids
 3) Microflora
 4) Bacterial B-glucuronidase
 5) Mucosal B-glucuronidase
 6) Cellular kinetics
 7) Ornithine decarboxylase
 8) Mucin
 9) Age
10) Hormones
11) Immune system
12) Flagyl
13) Disulfiram

We now plan to search for various genes and combinations of genes
associated with susceptibility or resistance to the carcinogen in
recombinant congenic strains. Once these have been identified,
they can be studied individually and their relative contribution
to carcinogenesis determined. Similar associations might then be
searched for in man.

REFERENCES

Armstrong B, Dou R (1975) Environmental factors and cancer
    incidence and mortality in different countries with special
    reference to dietary practices. Int J Cancer 15:617-631
Bailey DW (1971) Recombinant - inbred strains. Transplantation
    1971 11(3):325-327
Boffa L, Bolognesi C, Muriani M (1986) Correlation between
    1,2-dimethylhydrazine (DMH) susceptibility and AH gene
    expression in mice (Abstract #476). Proc Am Assoc Cancer Res
    27:121
Bolognesi C, Boffa L (1986) Correlation between incidence of
    1,2-dimethylhydrazine-induced colon carcinomas and DNA damage
    in six genetically different mouse strains. Cancer Lett
    30:91-95

Cooper HK, Buecheler J, Kleihues P (1978) DNA alkylation in mice
  with different susceptibility to 1,2-dimethylhydrazine-induced
  colon carcinogenesis. Cancer Res 38:3063-3065
Deschner E, Long F, Hakissian M, Herrmann S (1983) Differential
  susceptibility of AKR, C57BL/6J and CF1 mice to
  1,2-dimethylhydrazine-induced colonic tumor formation predicted
  by proliferative characteristics of colonic epithelial cells.
  J Natl Cancer Inst 70(2):279-282
Diwan BA, Blackman KA (1980) Differential susceptibility of three
  sublines of C57BL/6 mice to the induction of colorectal tumors
  by 1,2-dimethylhydrazine. Cancer Lett 9:111-115
Diwan B, Meier H, Blackman KE (1977) Genetic differences in the
  induction of colorectal tumors by 1,2-dimethylhydrazine in
  inbred mice. J Natl Cancer Inst 59:455-458
Diwan B, Meier H (1976) Colo-rectal tumors in inbred mice treated
  with 1,2-dimethylhydrazine. Proc Am Assoc Cancer Res 17:106
Evans J (1982) Differential susceptibility of mouse strains to
  induction of multiple large bowel neoplasms by
  1,2-dimethylhydrazine. In: Malt RA, Williamson RE (eds)
  Colonic carcinogenesis: Falk symposium 31. MTP Press Ltd,
  Lancaster, p 177
Evans J, Hauschka T, Mittelman A (1974) Brief communication:
  Differential susceptibility of four mouse strains to induction
  of multiple large bowel neoplasms by 1,2-dimethylhydrazine.
  J Natl Cancer Inst 52:999-1000
Evans J, Mittelman A, Hauschka T (1975) Genetics of colon tumor
  induction in mice by 1,2-dimethylhydrazine. Proc Am Assoc
  Cancer Res 16:16
Evans JT, Shows TB, Sproul EE, Paolini NS, Mittelman A, Hamschka
  TS (1977) Genetics of colon carcinogenesis in mice treated with
  1,2-dimethylhydrazine. Cancer Res 37:134-136
Fiala E (1977) Investigations into the metabolism and mechanism
  of action of the colon carcinogen 1,2-dimethylhydrazine and
  azoxymethane. Cancer 40:2436-2445
Filipe MI (1975) Mucinous secretion in rat colonic mucosa d
  carcinogenesis induced by dimethylhydrazine. Br J Cancer
  32:60-77
Fleiszer D, MacFarlane J, Murray D, Brown RA (1980) Effects of
  diet on chemically induced bowel cancer. Can J Surg
  23(1):67-73
Fleiszer D, Skamene E. Unpublished observation.
Glickman LT, Suissa S, Fleiszer D (1987) Proliferative
  characteristics of colonic crypt cells in C57BL/6J and A/J mice
  as predictors of subsequent tumors formation. Cancer Res
  47:4766-4770
Hilgers J, Arends J (1985) A series of recombinant inbred strains
  between the BALB/c HeA and STS/A mouse strains. Curr Topics in
  Microbiol & Immunol 122:31-37.
Kinlen LJ (1983) Fat and cancer. Br Med J 286:1081-1082
Lynch HT, Guirgis HA, Swartz M (1973) Genetics and colon cancer.
  Arch Surg 106:669-675
Lynch HT, Lynch PM (1980) The cancer family syndrome: A pragmatic
  basis for syndrome identification. Dis Colon Rectum 22:106-110
Maskens AP (1976) Histogenesis and growth pattern of
  1,2-dimethylhydrazine-induced rat colon adenocarcinoma. Cancer
  Res 36:1585-1593
Nesbitt MN, Skamene E (1984) Recombinant inbred mouse strains
  derived from A/J and C57BL/6J: a tool for the study of genetic
  mechanisms in host resistance to infection and malignancy. J
  Leuk Biol 36:357-364

Newberne PM, Rogers AE (1973) Adenocarcinoma of the colon animal
  model of human disease. Am J Pathol 72:541-544
Review. Committee on diet, nutrition and cancer, National
  Research Council: Diet, Nutrition and Cancer (1982).
  Washington DC, National Academy Press
Sohn OS, Puz C, Caswell N, Fiala ES (1985) Differential
  susceptibility of rat and guinea pig colon mucosa DNA to
  methylation by methylazoxymethyl acetate in vivo. Cancer Lett
  29:293-300
Sunter JP, Appleton DR, Wright NA, Watson AJ (1978) Pathological
  features of the colonic tumors induced in rats by the
  administration of 1,2-dimethylhydrazine. Virchows Arch B
  29:211-223
Thurnherr N, Deschner E, Stonehill E (1973) Induction of
  adenocarcinomas of the colon in mice by weekly injection of
  1,2-dimethylhydrazine. Cancer Res 33:940-945
Walker ARP (1976) Cancer and diet, with special reference to
  intakes of fat and fiber. Am J Clin Nutr 29:1417-1426
Weisberger, IH, Wynder EL, Horne CL (1982) Nutritional factors in
  etiologic mechanisms in the carisation of gastrointestinal
  cancers. Cancer 50:2541-2549
Wiebecke B, Krey U, Lohrs U, Eder M (1973) Morphological and
  autoradiographical investigations on experimental
  carcinogenesis in polyp development in the intestinal tract of
  rats and mice. Virchows Arch A 360:179-193
Willett WC, MacMahou B (1984) Diet and cancer. New Engl J Med
  310:633-638, 697-703
Wright S. (1934) Results of crosses between inbred strain of
  guinea pigs, differing in number of digits. Genetics 19:537

Effect of the *Gv-1* Locus on Moloney Ecotropic Murine Leukemia Virus Induced Disease in Inbred Wild Mice

C.J. Villar[1], T.N. Fredrickson[2], and C.A. Kozak[1]

INTRODUCTION

The nonacute retroviruses induce neoplastic disease following a long latency period. During this latency period, the infectious ecotropic murine leukemia virus (MuLV) spreads throughout the mouse resulting in chronic viremia. As the virus spreads, it recombines with germline copies, or proviruses, of nonecotropic MuLVs to produce infectious mink cell focus-forming (MCF) viruses. These MCF viruses resemble their ecotropic MuLV progenitors but contain novel sequences in their envelope (env) genes which encode the major virion glycoprotein, and in the long terminal repeats (LTRs) which contain transcriptional control signals. These recombinant viruses have an expanded host range and are themselves leukemogenic. The mechanisms involved in the production of MCF viruses are unknown, although it has been established that multiple recombinations occur, and novel viruses have been isolated from preleukemic tissues which may represent intermediate recombinants in this process (Cloyd and Chattopadhyay 1986). Proviral sequences related to both the xenotropic and MCF host range classes of infectious MuLVs ultimately contribute to the altered env and LTR regions of the MCF virus (Holland et al. 1985; Quint et al. 1984). Although the specific proviruses involved in this process have not been identified, it has been suggested that the xenotropic provirus Bxv-1 contributes LTR sequences to the leukemogenic MCF MuLV (Hoggan et al. 1986).

Various studies have shown that numerous cellular genes are responsible for resistance to MuLV-induced leukemogenesis and that many of these genes significantly affect the disease process by suppressing MuLV replication. Thus, the resistance allele at Fv-4 prevents exogenous infection by ecotropic MuLVs (Kai et al. 1976). Fv-4 mediated resistance is absolute and the resistant mice are not at all susceptible to virus-induced neoplastic disease (Suzuki 1975). Other genes which serve to lower virus titers by 1–3 logs also have a dramatic effect on virus-induced disease (Rowe and Hartley 1983). Thus, the resistance allele of the Rmcf locus reduces cellular susceptibility in tissue culture to MCF MuLVs, and alleles at the Fv-1 locus restrict replication of N- or B-tropic MuLVs. These genes will alter the onset as well as the ultimate incidence of lymphomas.

In this study, we examined virus-induced leukemogenesis in mice in which expression of germline nonecotropic MuLVs is restricted: the inbred strain 129 GIX⁻ and the wild mouse M. spretus (Morocco). 129 GIX⁻ mice carry the recessive allele at the Gv-1 locus. Gv-1 was initially described as a locus that controls expression of the GIX antigen on thymocytes (Stockert et al. 1972). GIX is now known to be the major MuLV envelope glycoprotein (Tung et al. 1975; Obata et al. 1975). More recent studies have shown that Gv-1 acts by coordinately suppressing transcription of the different proviral genes found in 129 GIX⁻ mice.

[1]Laboratory of Molecular Microbiology, National Institute of Allergy and Infectious Diseases, National Institutes of Health, Bethesda, MD 20892
[2]Department of Pathology, University of Connecticut, Storrs, CT 06268

Table 1. Production of infectious MCF MuLV and induction of lymphomas in M. spretus and 129 GIX⁻ mice inoculated as neonates with ectropic MoMuLV

Mice	Age (mo)	No. With MCF MuLV/No. Tested	No. Lymphomas/ No. Total
129 GIX⁻	5	2/3	0/3
	8	1/1	0/1
	16	NT	2/3
M. spretus	5	2/2	1/8
	9	NT	1/3

We have now found that the wild mouse Mus spretus (Morocco) also shows a similar phenotype in that these animals contain multiple proviruses, but fail to express any detectable retroviral RNA. Therefore, we examined both of these mice following inoculation with ectropic Moloney MuLV (MoMuLV) for retrovirus-related message, the production of MCF MuLVs, and tumorigenesis to determine whether transcriptionally suppressed retroviral sequences can contribute to the generation of MCF MuLVs and ultimately to neoplastic disease.

EFFECT OF Gv-1 ON PROVIRUS EXPRESSION AND MoMuLV INDUCED LEUKEMOGENESIS

RNA was extracted from various tissues of uninoculated 129 GIX⁻ mice. Consistent with the results reported by Levy and his colleagues (1982, 1985), Northern blot analysis of these samples demonstrates that the amount of retrovirus-related message detected in these mice is dramatically reduced compared with that of 129 GIX⁺ mice (data not shown). Comparable results were obtained using different segments of the retroviral genome as hybridization probes.

129 GIX⁻ mice were inoculated intraperitoneally and in the region of the thymus with MoMuLV one to three days after birth. Mice were sacrificed at various time intervals. Spleen and thymus cells were plated as infectious centers on mink lung and mouse SC-1 cells, and examined for infectious MCF virus by serological methods (Cloyd and Evans 1987) or by focus formation on mink cells. Mice sacrificed for virus testing were examined for gross signs of neoplastic disease, and all mice were examined weekly for signs of sickness such as palpable lymph nodes or spleen or labored breathing. Mice sacrificed for virus testing were examined for abnormally enlarged lymphoid organs. Histological examinations were performed on tissue samples from selected mice.

As shown in Table 1, infectious MCF virus could be isolated from these mice by 5 weeks. Gross pathology as well as histological examination showed some evidence of lymphomas after 16 weeks. These results are comparable to those reported for MoMuLV infection in other inbred strains (Moloney 1960). Therefore, Gv-1 mediated reduction of retrovirus transcription does not appear to have a dramatic effect on MCF virus production in these mice.

MoMuLV INDUCED LEUKEMOGENESIS IN M. SPRETUS (MOROCCO)

While our results with 129 GIX⁻ mice suggest that the suppressive effects of Gv-1 do not alter production of infectious MCF MuLVs, it should be noted that Gv-1 mediated suppression is not total. In unin-

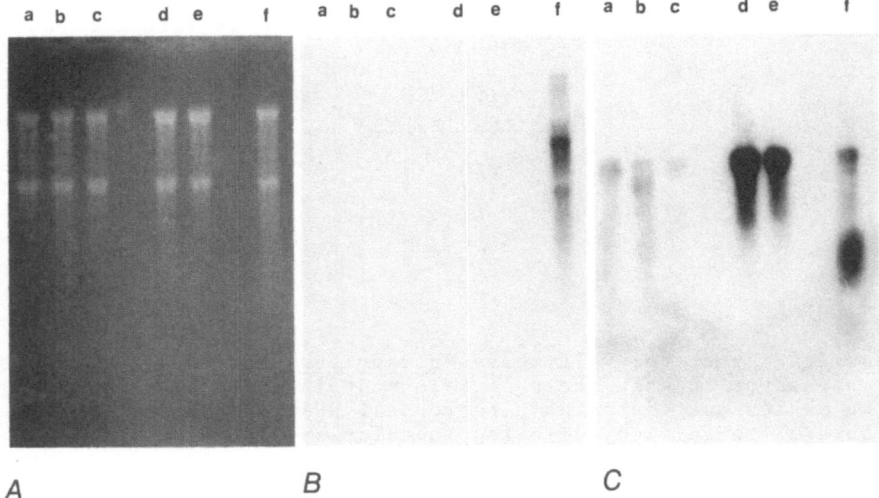

Fig. 1. Northern blot analysis of RNAs extracted from various tissues of M. spretus (Morocco). Panel A, Ethidium bromide stained gel; Panel B, Northern blot hybridized with pXenv, a 455 base pair fragment reactive with both xenotropic and MCF MuLVs; Panel C, Same membrane stripped and hybridized with an actin probe. Lane a, brain; b, heart; c, kidney; d, spleen; e, thymus; f, AKR mouse thymoma.

fected 129 GIX⁻ mice, retroviral transcripts are reduced by 80% in comparison to 129 GIX⁺ mice (Levy et al. 1982). Therefore, in order to extend this study, we repeated these experiments using the wild mouse M. spretus (Morocco). Examination of these mice for retrovirus-related transcripts shows that in all tissues examined, no retrovirus-related transcripts could be identified, even the 3 kilobase (kb) env message universally expressed in other inbred and wild mice (Khan et al., 1987; Levy et al, 1985) (Fig. 1). No retrovirus-related RNA was detected after very long exposures, or after poly(A)+ selection. Expression could not be induced in spleen cells following treatment with 5-iododeoxyuridine, an inducer of retrovirus gene expression, and the mitogens concanavalin A and lipopolysaccharide, which are known to stimulate different populations of spleen cells, and in the case of lipopolysaccharide, to induce expression of xenotropic proviral genes (Kozak and Rowe 1980). It is not yet known whether the lack of provirus expression in these mice is related to the presence of a Gv-1 like trans-acting suppressive gene, or whether these mice contain transcriptionally defective proviruses. However, Southern blot analysis of M. spretus DNA suggests that all 5 proviruses carried by this mouse are full-length and contain LTR sequences.

a b c d e

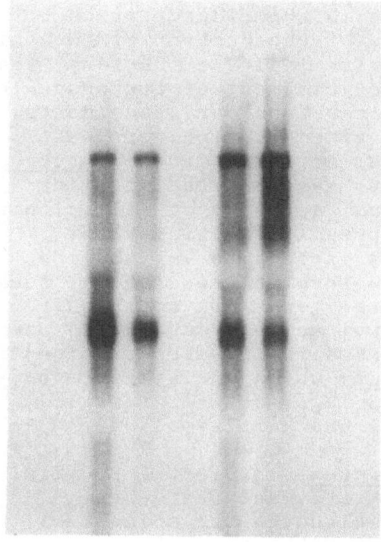

Fig. 2. Northern blot of RNA
isolated from M. spretus
mice 5 and 9 weeks after
inoculation with MoMuLV
using the pXenv probe. Lane
a, spleen, 9 weeks; b,
thymus, 9 weeks; c, liver, 9
weeks; d, spleen, 5 weeks;
e, thymus, 5 weeks.

M. spretus mice were inoculated at one to three days of age with MoMuLV
and examined for viral transcripts, MCF virus, and signs of neoplastic
disease at various times after inoculation. As shown in Fig. 2,
abundant levels of RNA reactive with an MCF viral env probe were
detected as 8.4 and 3.0 kb species in mice at 5 and 9 weeks after Mo-
MuLV inoculation. The pXenv hybridization probe does not react with the
ecotropic MoMuLV. The MCF-related transcripts were confined to the
spleen and thymus and could not be detected in other tissues such as
liver from the same animals (Fig. 2). Infectious MCF virus was also
isolated from thymus and spleen of 5 and 9 week old M. spretus mice and
lymphomas were observed in some animals by 9 weeks (Table 1).

CHARACTERIZATION OF MCF VIRUS ISOLATES

In order to confirm that the MCF viruses were true recombinants, MCF
virus was isolated from MoMuLV infected 129 GIX⁻ and M. spretus mice
and grown in mink lung cells. DNA was isolated from the virus infected
cells, digested with various restriction enzymes known to produce internal fragments from known MuLVs, and compared with fragments generated from the germline viruses of both mice. Results confirmed that the
isolated MCFs were novel recombinants since they produced unique
internal fragments. For example, digestion of mink cells infected with
either the M. spretus or 129 GIX⁻ MCF MuLVs produced a 3.1 kb BglII
fragment, whereas all 5 spretus germline copies produced a 5.9 kb
fragment, and DNA from 129 GIX⁻ mice contained 4.2 and 2.9 kb env related fragments. These studies also showed that the MCF viruses differed from MoMuLV within their env regions but not in their LTRs.

CONCLUSIONS

We can conclude from these experiments that production of recombinant MCF viruses can readily occur in mice in which the transcription of germline viruses is suppressed. Replication of the ecotropic MoMuLV is unaffected in these mice, and our results also indicate that any viral intermediates generated in the multistage development of leukemogenic MCFs are similarly unaffected. It is not clear from our experiments, or those of others, how Gv-1 acts to suppress transcription, or what common defect may affect the transcriptional activity of the spretus proviruses. Furthermore, it is impossible to say that the germline viruses of M. spretus show no transcriptional activity at all, although we were unable to find evidence of such expression in tissues of uninoculated mice as well as cultured cells exposed to various inducers. Despite the possibility of very low level expression, it seems likely that transcriptionally active proviral genes are not required for the production of MCF virus, since MCF virus is produced and the latency period in this process is not extended in the mice examined here. In comparison, other genes (Fv-1, Rmcf) which are similar to Gv-1 in that they suppress specific MuLVs by 1-3 logs, show a dramatic effect on MCF-mediated leukemogenesis (Rowe and Hartley, 1983).

Our data thus show that 129 GIX⁻ and M. spretus contain the proviral sequences necessary for production of MCF MuLVs, and that those sequences are available for recombination. Although the molecular mechanisms involved in the generation of MCF MuLVs are unknown, several models have been proposed (Linial and Blair 1985). Our data are clearly incompatible with one of these models which suggests that recombination occurs at the RNA level between viral RNAs which are co-packaged into heterozygous virions.

Finally, these studies indicate that M. spretus may prove to be a useful animal in studies of viral leukemogenesis. This mouse has no endogenous ecotropic or xenotropic MuLVs and only 5 copies of germline MCF related sequences (Kozak and O'Neill 1987). In contrast, many inbred strains contain ecotropic MuLVs, and all contain multiple copies of xenotropic and MCF MuLVs (O'Neill et al. 1986). Our data clearly show that M. spretus is susceptible to virus-induced leukemogenesis and therefore, the reduced number and restricted type of germline retroviral genes in this mouse, as well as their lack of expression may make it easier to describe the events leading to production of MCF MuLVs, and to identify specific germline sequences involved in recombination.

ACKNOWLEDGEMENTS

129 GIX⁺ and 129 GIX⁻ congenic mouse stocks were obtained from the Congenic Mouse Production Facility of Memorial Sloan-Kettering Cancer Center through the generosity of Dr. E.A. Boyse and were maintained at Microbiological Associates in Bethesda, MD. M. spretus mice were kindly provided by Dr. M. Potter from his colony at Hazelton Laboratories, Rockville, MD.

REFERENCES

Cloyd MW, Chattopadhyay SK (1986) A new class of retrovirus present in many murine leukemia systems. Virology 151:31-40
Cloyd MW, Evans LH (1987) Endogenous retroviral env expression in primary murine leukemia. Lack of xenotropic antigens in the presence

of distinct mink cell focus-forming _env_ subtypes correlating with
ecotropic virus inoculated and mouse strain. J Natl Cancer Inst
78:181-189

Hartley JW, Yetter RA, Morse HC III (1983) A mouse gene on chromosome 5
that restricts infectivity of mink cell focus forming recombinant
murine leukemia viruses. J Exp Med 158:16-24

Hoggan MD, O'Neill RR, Kozak CA (1986) Nonecotropic murine leukemia
viruses in BALB/c and NFS/N mice: Characterization of the BALB/c
Bxv-1 provirus and the single NFS endogenous xenotrope. J Virol
60:980-986

Holland CA, Hartley JW, Rowe WP, Hopkins N (1985) At least four viral
genes contribute to the leukemogenicity of murine retrovirus MCF 247
in AKR mice. J Virol 53:158-165

Kai K, Ikeda H, Yuasa Y, Suzuki S, Odaka T (1976) Mouse strain
resistant to N-, B- and NB-tropic murine leukemia viruses. J Virol
20:436-440

Kozak CA O'Neill RR (1987) Diverse wild mouse origins of xenotropic,
mink cell focus-forming and two types of ecotropic proviral genes. J
Virol 61:3082-3088

Kozak CA, Rowe WP (1980) Genetic mapping of xenotropic murine leukemia
virus-inducing loci in five mouse strains. J Exp Med 152:219-228

Levy DE, Lerner RA, Wilson MC (1982) A genetic locus regulates the
expression of tissue-specific mRNAs from multiple transcription
units. Proc Natl Acad Sci USA 79:5823-5827

Levy DE, Lerner RA, Wilson MC (1985) The _Gv-1_ locus coordinately
regulates the expression of multiple endogenous murine retroviruses.
Cell 41:289-299

Linial M, Blair D (1985) Genetics of retroviruses. In: Weiss R, Teich
N, Varmus H, Coffin J (eds) RNA tumor viruses: Molecular biology of
tumor viruses, 2nd edn. Cold Spring Harbor Laboratory, Cold Spring
Harbor, New York p 649

Moloney JB (1960) Biological studies on a lymphoid and leukemic virus
extracted from sarcoma 37. I. Original and introductory
investigation. J Natl Cancer Inst 24:933-951

Obata Y, Ikeda H, Stockert E, Boyse EA (1975) Relation of GIX antigen
of thymocytes to envelope glycoprotein of murine leukemia virus. J
Exp Med 141:188-197

Quint W, Boelens W, van Wezenbeek P, Cuypers T, Maadag ER, Selten G,
Berns A (1984) Generation of AKR mink cell focus-forming viruses: A
conserved single-copy xenotrope-like provirus provides recombinant
long terminal repeat sequences. J Virol 50:432-438

Rowe WP, Hartley JW (1983) Genes affecting mink cell focus-inducing
(MCF) murine leukemia virus infection and spontaneous lymphoma in AKR
F1 hybrids. J Exp Med 158:353-364

Stockert E, Sato H, Itakura K, Boyse EA, Old LJ, Hutton JJ (1972)
Location of the second gene required for expression of the leukemia-
associated mouse antigen GIX. Science 178:862-863

Suzuki S (1975) _Fv-4_: A new gene affecting the splenomegaly induction
by Friend leukemia virus. Jpn J Exp Med 45:473-478

Tung JS, Vitetta ES, Fleissner E, Boyse EA (1975) Biochemical evidence
linking the GIX thymocyte surface antigen to the gp69/71 envelope
glycoprotein of murine leukemia virus. J Exp Med 141:198-205

Reverse Genetics Approaches for Cloning *RIL-1*, a Major Locus Involved in Susceptibility to Leukemia

N.M.B. Amari, S. Scandalis, D. Zhang, C.L. Pampeno, S. Arant, and D. Meruelo

INTRODUCTION

The mechanism by which fractionated-x-irradiation (FXI) induces leukemia has been much debated. Kaplan and Brown (1952) first showed that fractionated doses of x-irradiation can cause leukemia in mice. Gross (1958), and Lieberman and Kaplan (1959), subsequently reported the transfer of neoplasia by radiation-induced leukemia virus, RadLV, obtained from FXI-induced leukemias. However, despite the identification of type-C RNA particles in FXI-induced leukemias and the demonstration that such particles can, when injected into young mice, cause lymphomas, several investigators have taken exception with the concept of a viral etiology for FXI-induced leukemia (Ihle et al., 1976, 1976a, 1978; Haran-Ghera 1977; Pazmino et al., 1978; Mayer and Dorsch-Hasler 1982). The etiological mechanism(s) of this disease however remains unclear.

Our laboratory's approach to try to understand the mechanism by which FXI induces leukemia avoids making any assumptions regarding the viral etiology of FXI-induced leukemia. Rather it focuses on defining, localizing, and understanding the mode of action of genes involved in susceptibility to the FXI-induced disease.

Our studies to date have indicated that multiple genes control the process of leukemogenesis. Loci on chromosome 1, 4 and 15 (Ril-3, Ril-2 and Ril-1, respectively) are involved in susceptibility to FXI-induced leukemia (Meruelo et al., 1981, 1987). Ril-1 has the overriding influence in susceptibility to the disease.

Spira et al. (1980) have shown that the distal portion of chromosome 15 is critical in the development of T-leukemias. Many of the leukemias arising in diseased mice were pseudodiploid with two normal chromosomes 15. However, an extra duplicated segment of bands D, E, and F (the segment which encodes Ril-1) of chromosome 15 was actually present, but translocated to another chromosome.

Spira et al. (1980) and Weiner et al. (1980) demonstrated that the genetic content of chromosome 15, and not its translocated state, determines the relative importance of the two reciprocal duplications for leukemia development. This hypothesis implies allelic variation between different mouse strains with regard to the critically important locus. This is precisely what has been demonstrated in the case of Ril-1 (Meruelo et al. 1981, 1983, 1987; Meruelo and Rossomando, 1986).

In this manuscript we will focus our attention on our approach to cloning and characterizing Ril-1. Our approach to clone Ril-1 is based on the methods and rationale of "reverse genetics" which allows the isolation of a gene without reference to a specific protein or without any reagents or functional assays useful in its detection.

Department of Pathology and Kaplan Cancer Center, New York University Medical Center, 550 First Avenue, New York, New York 10016.

Current Topics in Microbiology and Immunology, Vol. 137
© Springer-Verlag Berlin · Heidelberg 1988

For phase I of the studies, just as we have done for Ril-1, the strategy is to first establish the map position of the gene and then identify a specific gene within this region in which mutations or allelic variations are strictly correlated with the disease. Restriction fragment length polymorphisms (RFLPs) (Botstein et al., 1980), in combination with genetic methods, helps establish the initial map assignment. A variety of recently developed methodologies come into play in phase II. These include pulse gradient gel electrophoresis, chromosome walking and hopping techniques, cDNA library construction and subtractive hybridization, as well as genomic subtractive hybridization methodologies such as PERT.

MATERIALS AND METHODS

Mice:

All mice were bred at the New York University Medical Center.

Leuokemogenic FXI:

Mice (4 to 5 weeks old) were irradiated unanesthetized with a ^{137}Cs source (model A Gammator; Radiation Machines Corp., Parsippany, N.J.) at 175 rads weekly for 4 weeks.

Cell Culture:

In vitro-adapted tumors of C57B1/6 and B6.C-H-30^C X-irradiated tumors were maintained in Dulbecco modified Eagle medium supplemented with 10% fetal bovine serum, 1% penicillin-streptomycin solution, and 0.1% Fungizone.

Molecular Probes:

The DNA probes used for Southern hybridization were as follows:

(a) pKL6.1-2R contains a 750bp insert specific for Ly-6. It was cloned into the EcoRI site of pUC19 and kindly provided by Dr. A. Bothwell of the Howard Hughes Medical Institute Research Laboratories, Yale University School of Medicine, New Haven, Connecticut; (b) a PstI/XbaI fragment from a Simian sarcoma virus clone that corresponds to v-sis; (c) the pSFFV probe was a 600 bp PstI fragment in pBR322 kindly provided by Dr. Dino Dina and contains sequences specific for the spleen focus-forming virus (SFFV) defective env gene (gp52).

DNA Sample Preparation:

The DNAs used in our studies were isolated by the procedure of Blin and Stafford (1976). All DNA concentrations were determined spectrophotometrically by the diphenylamine method as previously described (Rossomando et al. 1986).

Southern Blots:

Restriction enzyme-digested DNA (10 µg) was separated by electrophoresis on 0.8% agarose gels and transferred to nylon membranes (Biotrace, Gelman Sciences, Inc.) as described by Southern (Southern 1975). Hybridization and washing of filters were done as described previously (Amari 1987).

Fluorescence-Activated Cell Sorter Analysis:

Thymocytes from newly sacrificed mice were washed twice in Phosphate Buffered Saline (PBS)-1%, Bovine Serum Albumin (BSA)-0.1% sodium azide, then resuspended in the same solution at 3×10^6 cells/ml. Anti-Ly-6 monoclonal (kindly provided by Ethan Shevach, NIH, Bethesda) was added at optimum concentration and the cells left at room temperature for 30 minutes. Cells were pelleted by centrifugation and resuspended in anti-Rat fluorescein labelled IgG at optimum concentration. The cells were left at room temperature for 30 minutes in the dark. The cells were subsequently washed three times and resuspended in PBS-1% BSA-0.1% sodium azide for analysis.

Results

Linkage of Ril-1 to H-30, Pol-5 and Ly-6 and identification of two pairs of congenic strains differing at Ril-1.

Even though no probe currently exists that would allow identification of Ril-1 we have been able, by in vivo susceptibility studies, to link this locus to the minor histocompatibility H-30 and lymphocyte antigen-6 (Ly-6) loci (Meruelo et al., 1981; 1983; 1987). Confirming the validity of these linkages and the proposition that Ril-1 plays a dominant role in susceptibility to FXI-induced leukemia, congenic mice differing at H-30 (C56BL/6By and B6.C-H-30^c) as well as congenic mice differing in their Ly-6 genotype (C3H/HeJ and C3H.B-Ly6^b) vary markedly in their susceptibility to FXI-induced leukemia (Fig. 1).

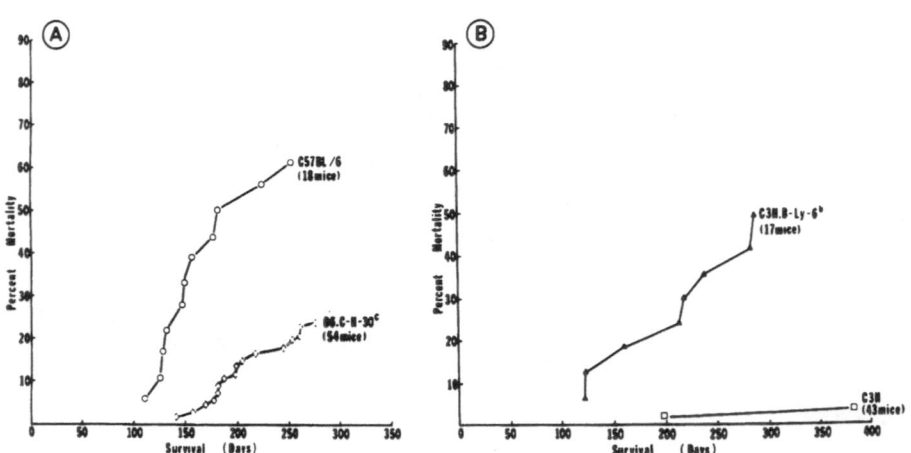

Fig. 1 A and B. Evidence that Ril-1, Ly-6 and H-30 are tightly linked. A. Ril-1 mediated susceptibility to FXI by B6.C-H-30^c is markedly less than that by C57Bl/6By mice. B. Similarly, susceptibility to FXI encoded by Ril-1 is markedly less in C3H/HeJ than in congenic C3H.B-Ly-6^b mice. Hence, Ril-1 must be linked to both H-30 and Ly-6.

The Ly-6--Ril-1--H-30 complex was unambiguously assigned to chromosome 15 (Meruelo et al., 1987), by using a 358 bp subclone (Rossomando and Meruelo 1986) derived from an endogenous retroviral polymerase (Pol-5) to probe a panel of somatic cell hybrids that carried various combinations of C57BL/6J (Pol-5[b] positive) mouse chromosomes on a constant Chinese hamster or rat background (Fournier and Moran 1983; Killary and Fournier 1984). This result was confirmed and approximate distances established between these loci, by analysis of four sets of RI strains. The order of these loci, most concordant with all the data is currently thought to be Ly-6--Ril-1--Sis--Pol-5--H-30-- Ins-3--Krt-1--Int-1--Gdc-1. This complex is located in the distal end of chromosome 15.

Functional studies: Effects of FXI on the Ly-6--Ril-1--Pol-5 region.

One obvious question that can be asked, given the availability of molecular and serological reagents for several loci in the vicinity of the Ril-1, is whether FXI has any effect on the expression or DNA structure of genes in this segment of chromosome 15. From the data shown in Fig. 2-5 it would appear that the answer is affirmative, with the entire region spanning Sis, Pol-5 and Ly-6 affected. These studies suggest that expression, methylation and DNA arrangements of these genes are significantly altered by FXI. While it is clear that much more needs to be done to understand the significance of these findings and their potential relationship to the mechanism of Ril-1 action, these results are per se intriguinging.

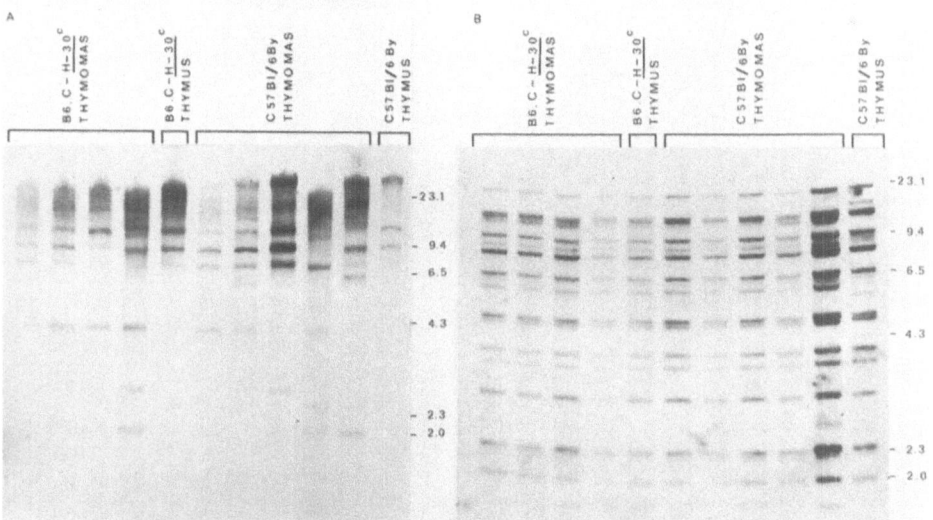

Fig. 2 A and B.   FXI-induced thymomas in C57B1/6 and in B6.C-H-30[c] mice are less methylated than normal thymus tissue. A. Ten micrograms of HpaII- digested normal thymus or thymoma DNAs per lane was used. B. Ten micrograms of MspI-digested normal thymus and thymoma DNAs per lane was used. A ^{32}P-labeled, nick translated pKLy-6.1 probe was used for both digests. Migration of lambda HindIII markers on the gels is indicated. Similar results were obtained using SmaI and XmaI digests of normal thymus and thymoma DNAs (data not shown).

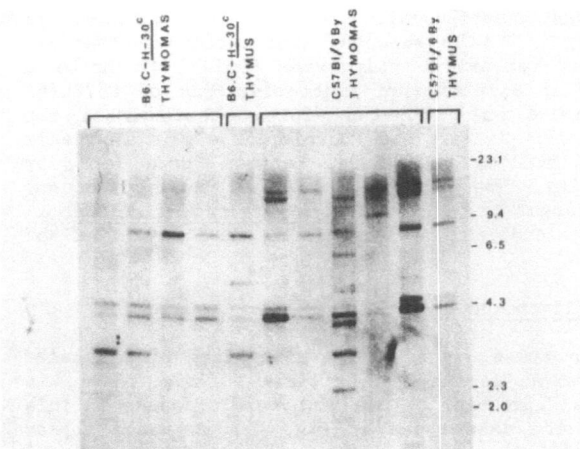

Fig. 3. The Sis region is more methylated in C57Bl/6 and B6.C-H-30^c FXI-induced thymomas. Ten micrograms of HpaII-digested normal thymus or thymoma DNAs per lane was used. A ^{32}P-labeled, nick translated Sis probe was used. Migration of lambda HindIII markers on the gels is indicated. The same observation was made using SmaI and XmaI digested normal thymus and thymoma DNAs (data not shown).

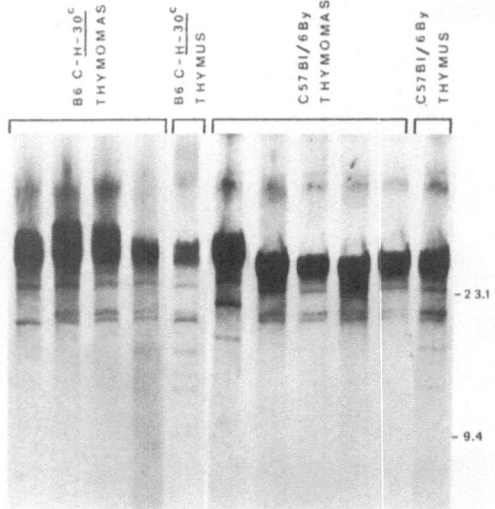

Fig. 4. The majority of C57Bl/6By FXI-induced tumors have a rearrangement detected by an SFFV probe. Five micrograms of SstII-digested normal thymus or thymoma DNAs per lane was used. Migration of lambda HindIII markers on the gels is indicated.

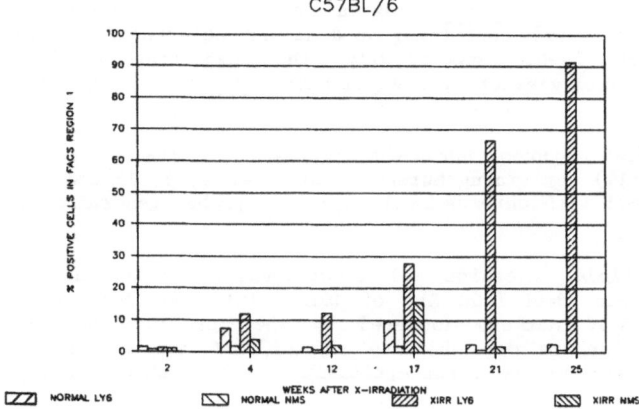

Fig. 5. Phenotypic changes in Ly-6 expression accompanies disease progression.
Time course studies of X-irradiatd mice beginning at 2 weeks post-X-irradiation
and ending at 25 weeks post-X-irradiation demonstrated a steady increase of
Ly-6 expression. A dramatic increase was noted 21 weeks post-X-irradiation
which is the time period in which tumors become apparent. This observation
may correlate with the fact that the Ly-6 region appears to be less methylated
than the normal thymus.

DISCUSSION

Clearly significant progress has been made in many aspects of the research
needed to successfully complete identification and isolation of Ril-1.

We are pursuing several strategies in order to complete the goal of cloning
Ril-1. This involves the use of several methodologies which include the PERT
technique (Kunkel et al., 1985). This method involves phenol-accelerated
competitive DNA reassociation using C57B1/6 By, and B6.C-H-30^C DNAs). This
would result in isolating H-30 region-specific clones. These clones will
hopefully generate probes closer to Ril-1.

A cDNA subtractive library has also been created from an X-irradiated tumor
cell line. This library will be screened with subtractive cDNA probes (i.e.
tumor cell lines minus normal thymus RNA from B6.C-H-30^C). This
procedure will result in the identification of clones which fall into two
categories: Those which are "tumor" specific but are not located in the
(Ly-6--Ril-1--Sis) region, and more importantly, those located within the
(Ly-6--Ril-1--Sis region). The latter, if not resulting in Ril-1 will allow
the development of probes mapping closer to Ril-1 than those presently
available (i.e. Ly-6 and Sis) and eventually lead to the cloning of this gene.

Insertional mutagenesis of the Ly-6---Ril-1 region is also being employed. More cell lines will be generated containing a dominant selectable marker integrated in or around Ly-6, specifically the amphotrophic Neo^r retrovirus. This approach would generate probes flanking Ly-6 thereby getting closer to Ril-1.

In addition, an ABM 14 cosmid library has been prepared from the hamster - mouse hybrid cell line (ABM14) containing murine chromosomes 2, 6, 15 and 17. This library will be screened with chromosome 15 specific probes generated by the above methodologies.

Lastly, we are employing field inversion gel electrophoresis which allows restriction mapping over more than 1000 Kbp of DNA. This technique will bridge the genetically linked markers isolated by the methods discussed above. Comparison of the linkage maps between the C57BL/6 and B6.C-H-30^c congenic strains, which differ in their susceptibility to X-irradiation, may help identify the Ril-1 locus.

REFERENCES

Amari NMB, Meruelo D (1987) Murine thymomas induced by fractionated-x-irradiation have specific T cell receptor rearrangements and characteristics associated with day 15-16 thymocytes. Mol Cell Biol 7:4159-4168

Blin N, Stafford DW (1976) Isolation of high molecular weight DNA. Nucleic Acids Res 3:2303-2308

Botstein, D, White RL, Skolnick M, Davies, RW (1980) Construction of a genetic linkage map in man using restriction fragment length polymorphism. Am J Hum Gent 32:314-331

Fournier REK, Moran RG (1983) Complementation mapping in microcell hybrids: localization of Fpgs and Ak-1 on Mus musculus chromosome 2. Somatic Cell Genetics 9:69-84

Gross L (1958) Attempt to recover filterable agent from x-ray-induced leukemia. Acta Haematol (Basel) 19:353-361

Haran-Ghera N (1977) Target cells involved in radiation and radiation leukemia virus leukemogenesis. In JF Duplan, ed, "International Symposium on Radiation-induced leukemogenesis and related viruses" (INSERM Symposium No 4). Elsevier North Holland Biomedical Press, Amsterdam, Holland, p 79-89

Ihle JN (1978) Experimental models and conceptual approaches to studies of lymphomas and leukemia-etiology, biology and control. Sem Hematol 15:95-115

Ihle JN, McEwan R, Bengali K (1976) Radiation leukemia in C57BL/6 mice. I. Lack of ecotropic virus in pathogenesis. J Exp Med 144:1391-1405

Ihle JN, Joseph DR, Pazmino NH (1976a) Radiation leukemia in C57BL/6 mice. II. Lack of serological evidence for the role of endogenous ecotropic virus in pathogenesis. J Exp Med 144:1406-1423

Kaplan HS, Brown MB (1952) A quantitative dose-response study of lymphoid tumor development in irradiated C57 black mice. J Natl Cancer Inst 13:185-208

Killary AM, Fournier REK (1984) A genetic analysis of extinction: trans-dominant loci regulate expression of liver-specific traits in hepatoma hybrid cells. Cell 38:523-534

Kunkel, LM, Monaco, AP, Middlesworth, W, Ochs, HD, Latt, SA (1985) Specific cloning of DNA fragments absent from the DNA of a male patient with an X chromosome deletion. Proc Natl Acad Sci USA 82:4778-4782

Lieberman M, Kaplan HS (1959) Leukemogenic activity of filtrates from radiation-induced lymphoid tumors of mice. Science 130:387-388

Mayer A, Dorsch-Hasler K (1982) Endogenous MuLV infection does not contribute to onset of radiation or carcinogen-induced murine thymoma. Nature 295:253-255

Meruelo D, Offer M, Flieger N (1981) Genetics of susceptibility to radiation-induced leukemia. Mapping of genes involved to chromosome 1, 2, and 4 . Implications for a viral etiology in the disease. J Exp Med 154:1201-1211

Meruelo D, Offer M, Rossomando A (1983) Induction of leukemia by both fractionated-x-irradiation and radiation leukemia virus involves loci in the chromosome 2 segment coding for H-30 -- Agouti. Proc Natl Acad Sci USA 80:462-466

Meruelo D, Rossomando A (1986) A molecular and genetic approach to understanding the mechnaisms by which fractionated x-irradiation induces leukemia in mice. Leuk Research 10:819-832

Meruelo D, Rossomando A, Scandalis S, D'Eustachio P, Fournier REK, Roop DR, Saxe D, Blatt C, Nesbitt MN (1987) Assignment of the Ly-6--Ril-1--Sis--H-30--Pol5/Xmmv72--Ins-3--Ker-1--Int-1--Gdc-1 region to murine chromosome 15. Immunogenetics 25:361-372

Pazmino NH, McEwan R, Ihle JN (1978) Radiation leukemia in C57BL/6 mice. III. Correlation of altered expression of terminal deoxynucleotidyl transferase to induction of leukemia. J Exp Med 148:1338

Rossomando A, Meruelo D (1986) Viral sequences are associated with many histocompatibility genes. Immunogenetics 23:233-245

Southern EM (1975) Detection of specific sequences among DNA fragments separated by gel electrophoresis. J Mol Biol 98:503-517

Spira J, Babonits M, Weiner F, Ohno S, Wirschubski Z, Haran-Ghera N, Klein G (1980) Nonrandom chromosomal changes in the Thy-1 positive and the Thy-1 negative lymphomas induced by 7,12 demethyl benzantracene in SJL mice. Cancer Res 40:2609-2616

Wiener F, Babonits M, Haran-Ghera N, Klein G (1980) Non-random duplication of chromosome 15 in murine T cell leukemias: Further studies on translocation heterozygotes. Int J Cancer 26:661-668

Genetic Map Location of *Afr-1*: Results From Four Genetic Crosses

E. P. Blankenhorn[1], R. Duncan[2], C. Teuscher[3], and M. Potter[2]

INTRODUCTION

Afr-1 is a genetic locus in mice that controls the adult level of serum alpha-fetoprotein. Under normal circumstances, AFP synthesis is repressed shortly after birth, from levels approaching 10 million nanograms/milliliter to adult levels of only several hundred ng/ml (Olsson et al., 1977). In the special case of BALB/cJ mice however, this down-regulation of AFP synthesis is ten- to twenty-fold less efficient, resulting in circulating AFP levels of several thousand ng/ml in 15-week old mice (Olsson et al., 1977). The recessive allele of Afr-1 responsible for this persistance of AFP (Afr-1^b) is found only in BALB/c mice of the Jackson substrain, and not in any other mouse tested to date (Blankenhorn et al., 1985).

The work presented here will center on experiments designed to map Afr-1 to a mouse chromosome. Three separate genetic crosses have been employed to discover and confirm that Afr-1 is located on mouse Chromosome 15, near the myc-1 locus. In addition, related results will be presented which bear on some of the properties of Afr-1 and high AFP expression in these mice.

RESULTS AND DISCUSSION

In previous work, Afr-1$^{b/b}$ progeny were distinguished by radioimmunoassay from Afr-1$^{a/-}$ mice in F2 crosses between BALB/cJ and either C57Bl/6J or DBA/2 (Blankenhorn et al., 1985). Because Afr-1^b is recessive, only b/b homozygotes were analyzed further. We chose to look for linkage to Gdc-1, a marker on chromosome 15 (Kozak and Birkenmaier, 1983), because BALB/cJ mice differ from other BALB/c sublines in the expression of this enzyme (glycerol-3-phosphate dehydrogenase) (Kozak 1985), and it is a reasonable assumption that the expression of Gdc-1 might be controlled by at least one cis-linked regulatory element (also on 15). Alleles for the structural Gdc-1 gene are easily screened using a PstI restriction fragment length polymorphism. In both sets of F2 crosses, Afr-1^b segregated with the parental Gdc-1^c allele in about 70% of the progeny. This result allowed further study for more closely linked markers.

Afr-1 is more closely linked to a group of chromosome 15 markers (Meruelo et al 1987; LeClair et al. 1987), containing the structural genes for Ly-6,c-sis, and pol-5. Dr. Meruelo kindly agreed to test our Afr-1$^{b/b}$ BALB/cJ x C57Bl/6 F2 segregants; the results showed that Afr-1 is approximately 15 map units from Ly-6 and slightly further from c-sis (about 20 cM). These results were confirmed using a third genetic cross (an F2 cross between BALB/cJ and CLA; see R. Duncan, this volume), which was scored for Afr-1, Gdc-1, Ly-6, Sis and the Mupm-1 locus. In these mice, as with the BALB/cJ x DBA/2 cross, Afr-1 and Gdc-1 appeared to be about 25 cM apart (cf. 32 cM in the BALB/cJ x B6 F2 experiment), and the map distances between Afr-1 and the more proximal markers were also correspondingly shorter. Such discrepancies, when using F2 mice for testing,

---

[1]Department of Microbiology and Immunology, Hahnemann University, Philadelphia, PA 19102; [2]Laboratory of Genetics, National Cancer Institute, Bethesda, MD 20205; [3]Department of Reproductive Biology, University of Pennsylvania School of Medicine, Philadelphia, PA 19104

---

may or may not have scientific significance.

The advantage of using the BALB/cJ x CLA F2 mice is that more restriction fragment length polymorphisms (RFLPs) can be scored, one of which involved the Myc-1 locus. CLA and BALB/cJ can be distinguished for Myc-1 by digestion of their DNA with Taq1 (Huppi, K., Duncan, R., and Potter, M., submitted 1987). Of 21 mice scored as having Afr-1$^{b/b}$, only one mouse had a non-parental allele for Myc-1, and this mouse was Myc-1 heterozygote. The array of other typing results for this sole recombinant favors the same map order determined from the other two crosses, summarized here:

Centro----/ /--- Mupm-1 --- Afr-1 -- Myc-1 -- Ly-6 ---- Sis ---------- Gdc-1
  mere   7   2.4   2   5   14 cM

Mice from the BALB/c x CLA cross were also scored for Mupm-1, a modifier of mouse urinary protein expression (R. Duncan, et al, this volume). From previous work we had suspected that Afr-1 and this trait were associated, and they were found to segregate together very frequently in these progeny. Of 27 male mice scored for both markers, only four showed separation of the parental phenotypes; two mice were Afr-1$^{b/b}$ and had the CLA allele (presumably in the heteroygous form) at Mupm-1 (all other linked markers were of the BALB/cJ type: Myc-1, Ly-6, c-sis, and Gdc-1), and two mice had a BALB/cJ-like expression of Mupm-1, but were heterozygous for Afr-1, Myc-1, and Ly-6. The placement of Mupm-1 with respect to other chromosome 15 markers has been confirmed in a series of experiments described elsewhere (R. Duncan, R. Matthai, K. Huppi, T. Roderick, and M. Potter, submitted, 1987).

The separation of the Afr-1 and Mupm-1 loci in these mice indicates strongly that they are independently controlled traits and not the result of a single pleiotropic gene perhaps exhibiting variable penetrance; this assumption is currently being tested in backcross mice in our laboratories.

Two differences in AFP expression due to Afr-1 with respect to sex are apparent in our studies. Adult male AFP levels are significantly higher than those found in females (Table 1), a finding that has been reported previously (Pollard et al., 1982). It is interesting that this 2 - 3 fold higher male AFP expression occurs irrespective of the genetic background of the non-BALB/cJ parent. However, this genetic background was important in one case: in female progeny of the BALB/cJ x CLA F2 cross, there was a significant deficit of Afr-1$^{b/b}$ animals. This could be due to poor penetrance of the Afr-1$^{b/b}$ allele in the presence of CLA background genes, or to lethality of Afr-1$^{b/b}$ or linked markers in these mice, or to failure to detect the Afr-1$^{b/b}$ females in the radioimmunoassay. The likelihood of lethality could be tested be an examination of the ratios of myc-1 alleles (closely linked to Afr-1) in female BALB/cJ x CLA F2 progeny; the Mupm-1 allele characteristic of BALB/cJ is difficult to score in females (R. Duncan, personal communication).

One further point about Afr-1 deserves mention here. In an unrelated study, 63 backcross mice were scored for inheritance of Afr-1$^{b/b}$ {and thus circulating levels of AFP in excess of 2000 ng/ml (and sometimes 7000 ng/ml)} and for the inheritance of susceptibility to one of two autoimmune syndromes: experimental autoimmune orchitis (EAO) or experimental allergic encephalomyelitis (EAE). These susceptibility traits have been shown to distinguish several sublines of BALB/c mice (Teuscher et al 1985). In this study, there was absolutely no genetic association between the gene responsible for high levels of circulating AFP and the gene affording "protection" from autoimmune attack (C. Teuscher, E. P. Blankenhorn, and W. F. Hickey, in press 1987). Therefore, it is hard to find support for the supposed role of AFP as an immunosuppressive agent in mice (Murgita and Tomasi, 1975), especially in unmanipulated animals in which AFP is synthesized entirely naturally.

Table 1. Sex-associated differences among BALB/cJ crosses

	MALES			FEMALES	
Cross	Ratio	AFP/ml		Ratio	AFP/ml
(B6 x J)F2	3.0 : 1	5700 ng		4.4 : 1	2000 ng[a]
(J x D2)F2	3.7 : 1	3900 ng		2.6 : 1	2630 ng[a]
(J x By) x J	1.3 : 1	5980 ng		1.6 : 1	3170 ng[a]
(J x CLA)F2	3.3 : 1	4100 ng		12.0 : 1[c]	2180 ng[b]

[a], $p < 0.005$ compared to male AFP level
[b], $p < 0.05$ compared to male AFP level
[c], $p < 0.02$ compared to male ratio of $Afr-1^{a/-}$ to $Afr-1^{b/b}$
By = BALB/cBy subline mice, J = BALB/cJ, D2 = DBA/2J, B6 = C57B1/6, and CLA = Centerville Light (M. musculus domesticus).

TABLE 2. Syntenic groups of mouse and human markers

Mouse genes	Human genes
Chromosome 15	Chromosome 8
Gpt-1	GPT (q13-qter)
Myc-1	MYC (q24)
Afr-1	
pvt-1	
	Chromosome 22
C-sis	SIS (q12.3-q13.1)
Ly-6	
Dia-1	DIA1 (q13.31-qter)
ars-a	ARSA (q13.31-qter)
	Chromosome 12
Gdc-1	GPD1
Int-1	INT1 (pter-q14)
Ela-1	ELA1 (p prox)
keratin	
Caracul	
Velvet	
Hox-3	HOX3 (q11)

All designations and sources for genetic mapping found in O'Brien, 1987, and McKusick, 1986.

In conclusion, we have demonstrated the following points:

<1> Afr-1 is on chromosome 15, closely linked to myc-1, in a group of mouse markers which have a corresponding syntenic group on human chromosome 8. (Table 2). The only human case of hereditary persistance of AFP was described by Dr. S. Tilghman and her colleagues, and the gene responsible for this condition appears to be linked to the structural gene for human AFP (in Vogt et al., 1987), which is not in this syntenic group.

<2> Afr-1 control of AFP in serum is affected by gender: in all crosses reported, males have significantly higher levels than females. In addition, in one combination only, significantly fewer females than expected were found to be homozygous for the Afr-1^b allele in the BALB/cJ x CLA F2 cross.

<3> Models of Afr-1 have been proposed which state that this locus encodes a tissue-specific (Belayew and Tilghman, 1982), trans-activating product, and our mapping data lend support to this hypothesis. Any models for how Afr-1 works must take into account that the mutant Afr-1^b allele is affected by sex, probably liver-specific (Vogt, et al., 1987), and largely ineffective when compared with the normal decline of AFP synthesis (Afr-1^b homozygotes still repress AFP synthesis 1,000-fold, as compared to 10,000-fold in Afr-1$^{a/-}$ mice).

REFERENCES

Belayew A, Tilghman SM (1982) Genetic analysis of alphafetoprotein synthesis in mice. Mol Cell Biol 2: 1427 - 1435

Blankenhorn EP, Wax, JS, Matthai, R, Potter, M (1985) Genetic analysis of alphafetoprotein levels in BALB/c sublines. Curr Top Micro Immunol 122:53-57

Kozak LP, Berkenmeier EH (1983) Mouse sn-glycerol-3-phosphate dehydrogenase: Molecular cloning and genetic mapping of a cDNA sequence. Proc Natl Acad Sci (USA) 80: 3020-3024

Kozak LP (1985) Genetic variation of catecholamine responsive metabolic pathways - a hypothesis for a common regulatory mechanism in BALB/c sublines. Curr Top Micro Immunol 122: 66-70

LeClair KP, Rabin M, Nesbitt MN, Pratcheva D, Ruddle FH, Palfree RGE, Bothwell A (1987) Murine Ly-6 multigene family is located on chromosome 15. Proc Natl Acad Sci (USA) 84: 1638-1642

McKusick VA (1986) The Human Gene Map. Clin Gen 29:545-588

Meruelo D, Rossomando A, Scandalis S, D'Eustachio P, Fournier REK, Roop DR, Saxe D, Blatt C, Nesbitt MN (1987) Assignment of the Ly-6--Ril-1--Sis--H30 --Po15/Xmnv-72--Ins3--Krt-1--Int-1--Gdc-1 region to mouse chromosome 15. Immunogenetics 25: 361-372

Murgita RA, Tomasi TB (1975) Suppression of immune response by alpha-fetoprotein. J Exp Med 141:440-452

O'Brien SJ Genetic Maps 1987. Cold Spring Harbor Laboratory.

Olsson M, Lindahl G, Ruoslahti E (1977) Genetic control of alphafetoprotein synthesis in the mouse. J Exp Med 145: 819-827

Pollard DR, Woodward B, Gupta K (1982) Strain and sex differences in serum alpha-fetoprotein levels in Mus musculus. Can J Genet Cytol 24: 343-346

Teuscher C, Potter M, Tung KSK (1985) Differential susceptibility to experimental autoimmune orchitis in BALB/c substrains. Curr Top Micro Immunol 122: 181-188

Vogt TF, Solter D, Tilghman SM (1987) Raf, a trans-acting locus, regulates the alpha-fetoprotein gene in a cell-autonomous manner. Science 236: 301-303.

The Effect of the *nude* Gene on Plasmacytoma Development in BALB/cAn Mice

L. Byrd, M. Potter, B. Mock, and K. Huppi

INTRODUCTION

The role of the T-lymphocyte in the development of plasma cell tumors may be investigated by attempting to induce these tumors in mice that lack a mature T-cell population. The nude mutation in mice is a recessive gene and homozygous mice (nu/nu) lack both a thymus (Pantelouris, 1968) and a hair coat (Flanagan, 1966). The absence of functional thymus glands in nu/nu mice results in a severe deficiency of mature T-lymphocytes throughout life (Scheid, et al. 1975; Chen et al. 1984). Consequently, these mice have defective immune responses which involve T-lymphocytes and have commonly been used to demonstrate the role of T-lymphocytes in a variety of immune responses (Eckels, et al., 1979; Jacobson, et al., 1974; Kindred, 1978). A congenic strain with the nu gene on the BALB/cAn background, the BALB/cAn·nu/nu, was utilized to determine whether nude mice would develop plasmacytomas (PCTs) and if so, at what incidence. In addition, we determined whether the BALB/cAn·nu/nu was genetically identical (with the possible exception of genes flanking the nude mutation on chromosome 11) to the BALB/cAnPt subline which is commonly used in PCT induction experiments.

METHODS

Mice: The BALB/cAn·nu/nu congenic strain used in this report was developed by Dr. Carl Hansen (NIH). The nude gene was placed on the BALB/cAnN background from the NIH:Swiss·nu/nu stock by a backcross-intercross system to backcross 10 (N10). A breeding stock of these BALB/cAn·nu/nu N10's was sent to the Frederick Cancer Research Facility (FCRF) in 1981 and are maintained by mating female BALB/cAn·nu/+ to male BALB/cAn·nu/nu under Specific Pathogen-free (SPF) conditions (Clarence Reeder, personal communication). All BALB/cAn·nu/nu and BALB/cAn·nu/+ in this report were obtained from FCRF. The BALB/cAnPt mice were originally obtained from Dr. H.B. Andervont (NIH) in 1964 by Michael Potter and have been maintained as inbred stock in a closed but conventionally maintained colony. The NIH:Swiss mice were obtained from the Small Animal Division, NIH.

Plasmacytoma Inductions: PCTs were induced with three 0.5ml i.p. injections of pristane in BALB/cAnPt mice, BALB/cAn·nu/nu mice and BALB/cAn·nu/+ mice on days 0, 60, and 120 according to previously reported protocols (Anderson and Potter (1969)). All mice were maintained in isolated mouse colonies under NIH

Laboratory of Genetics, National Cancer Institute, National Instiues of Health, Bethesda, Maryland.

Current Topics in Microbiology and Immunology, Vol. 137
© Springer-Verlag Berlin · Heidelberg 1988

contract #N01-CB-25584 at Hazleton Laboratories America, Rockville, Maryland. All BALB/cAn·nu/nu and one-half of the
BALB/cAn·nu/+ mice were maintained under SPF conditions. The
other half of the BALB/cAn·nu/+ and the BALB/cAnPt mice were
maintained under conventional housing conditions. Ascites fluid
was examined by cytofuge preparations every two weeks beginning
at day 130 for the presence of PCTs. In addition, sections of
intestinal mesentery, liver, spleen, Peyer's patches, pancreas,
and mediastinal lymph nodes were taken at the termination of the
experiments (days 214 and 325) and examined for the presence of
plasma cells.

Genetic Profiles: High molecular weight DNAs prepared from
BALB/cAn·nu/nu, BALB/cAn·nu/+, BALB/cAnPt, and NIH:Swiss livers
were digested for 5 - 7 hours with restriction endonucleases and
electrophoretically separated on 0.8% horizontal agarose gels at
voltage gradients of approximately 1 V/cm in 40mM Tris-acetate,
20mM sodium acetate, 1mM EDTA, pH 7.4. After staining with
ethidium bromide and photography under UV light, the gels were
blotted onto nitrocellulose. Blots were hybridized for 16 hours
with the probes listed in Table I. Each of the probes were
labelled with ^{32}P-dCTP by nick-translation. After hybridization,
filters were washed 4 times at 65°C in 0.3x SSC for 30 min. each.

RESULTS

Plasmacytoma Induction Studies: No evidence of plasmacytoma
development was seen by cytospin preparation in 19 BALB/cAn·nu/nu
observed until day 214 nor in 48 BALB/cAn·nu/nu observed until
day 325. In contrast, 48% (11/23) of the BALB/cAnPt control mice
observed until day 325 developed PCT's. Somewhat surprisingly,
none of the conventionally housed or SPF housed BALB/cAn·nu/+
followed for 214 days developed PCTs. In addition, only one of
the 27 (4%) SPF nu/+ and 5 of the 26 (19%) conventionally housed
nu/+ mice developed PCTs by day 325.

Genetic Testing: The present study used probes which detect loci
on chromosomes 1, 2, 4-7, 11-13, 15-19, and Y (Table 1). Most of
the probes showed no restriction fragment length polymorphisms
(RFLPs) between BALB/cAn·nu/nu and BALB/cAnPt, however a Ula-
associated sequence did show an RFLP between the BALB/cAn·nu/nu
congenic strain and the BALB/cAnPt inbred strain. A sequence
associated with Ula hybridized to a 4.0kb band in BALB/cAn·nu/nu
DNA; this band was absent in BALB/cAnPt (Figure 1).

DISCUSSION

The initial purpose of this study was to determine whether
the lack of mature T-lymphocytes affected the development of IgA
secreting plasma cell tumors in BALB/cAn mice by testing the
susceptibility of an athymic BALB/cAn mouse, the BALB/cAn·nu/nu
mouse. Although the standard regimen of PCT induction studies
(monitoring PCT development over 365 days) was not followed due
to the compromised immune system of the nu/nu, the mice were
observed until day 214 and day 325 by which time resistance would
be recognizable as a significant reduction in PCT formation. The
lack of PCT development in control BALB/cAn·nu/+ mice made us

question both the role of the SPF conditions under which these mice are maintained (studies in progress) and the genetic profile of the BALB/cAn·nu/nu.

Most inbred strains and the strains on which the nu gene is carried are resistant to plasmacytoma induction. There are also past reports of genetically contaminated BALB/cAn·nu/nu strains (Gubbels, et al., 1985). Susceptibility to plasmacytoma induction has been demonstrated to be under complex genetic control involving multiple genes (several studies have implicated at least three unlinked loci) that influence susceptibility or resistance (Morse et al.,1980; Potter et al., 1975; 1984; 1985; Potter and Wax 1981; 1985). The genes controlling plasmacytoma susceptibility have not been mapped, although genes on chromosomes 4 (Potter and Wax, 1985), 15 and 17 have been implicated (Potter, CTMI, this volume). Therefore, the genetic profile of the congenic BALB/cAn·nu/nu is necessary in evaluating the role of the athymic state in plasmacytoma formation.

BALB/cAn·nu/nu male breeders are routinely tested by the FCRF for possible genetic drift from the BALB/cAn type. The isoenzymes routinely tested (Table 2) showed no detectable differences between BALB/cAn and BALB/cAn·nu/nu in their last report (November 1986, Clarence Reeder, personal communication). Further testing of the major and minor histocompatibility loci was accomplished by utilizing a Strain Restricted Typing Sera (SRTS) (Arn et al., 1982) for serologic monitoring of the genetic integrity of a BALB/c strain. The antiserum was produced by immunizing BALB/cAn mice with a combination of 3 or 4 hybrids made by crossing non-BALB/c parental strains with each other. This highly sensitive antiserum detects the presence of multiple histocompatibility antigens including MHC, minor histocompatibility differences, and other cell surface differentiation antigens (Arn et al., 1982). The antiserum is assayed by a complement-mediated cytotoxicity assay using peripheral blood lymphocytes. No significant difference between the congenic strain BALB/cAn·nu/nu and the inbred strain BALB/cAnPt was found with this antiserum. This data combined with the genetic profile from the present study has determined that 41 loci on a total of 18 autosomes and the Y chromosome in addition to many undetermined minor histocompatibility loci are indistinguishable between BALB/cAnPt and BALB/cAn·nu/nu. These observations suggest that no major chromosomal segments of NIH:Swiss background (other than genes closely linked to nu/nu) have been carried over in the construction of the congenic BALB/cAn·nu/nu. This is consistent with the prediction that 99% of the genetic background in congenic mice should be host genes by backcross generation 10.

However, differences have been noted between the BALB/cAn and BALB/cAn·nu/nu. Skin grafts between male BALB/cAn·nu/nu breeders and BALB/cAn hosts were rejected 70 days after the initial operation (Clarence Reeder, personal communication). This was the first difference found between BALB/cAn and BALB/cAn·nu/nu mice in 6 years of monitoring the congenic strain. We have also found an RFLP difference between BALB/cAn·nu/nu and BALB/cAnPt using a Ula-associated sequence whose chromosomal location has not been determined.

CONCLUSIONS

The BALB/cAn·nu/nu congenics obtained from FCRF are resistant to pristane induced plasmacytomagenesis. In addition, both the SPF housed and conventionally housed BALB/cAn·nu/+ show reduced susceptibility (4% and 19%) when compared to the susceptible strain BALB/cAnPt (48%) housed in the same room.

Thus far, BALB/cAnPt and BALB/cAn·nu/nu have similar polymorphic alleles at most loci tested. Detailed analysis of chromosome 11 is in progress. The possibility that a gene near nu on chromosome 11 determines resistance to plasmacytomagenesis has not been ruled out. We are currently testing conventionalized BALB/cAn·?/+ mice obtained by breeding BALB/cAn·nu/+ x BALB/cAn·nu/+ for plasmacytoma susceptability.

The role of T-cells in plasmacytomagenesis cannot be assessed from these experiments and will require appropriate reconstitution of the BALB/cAn·nu/nu mouse with functional T-cells.

Acknowledgements

We would like to thank J. Mullins, L. Kozak, B. Callahan, P. Pitha, B. Hogan, A. Joyner, E. Howard, W. Held, L. Flaherty, W. Roeker and D. Loh for the use of the cDNA probes in this study.

Figure 1: Southern blot hybridization of Bam HI digested DNA from BALB/cAnPt and BALB/cAn·nu/nu with a Ula-associated sequence. Lane 1) BALB/cAnPt DNA; Lane 2) BALB/cAn·nu/nu DNA. BALB/cAn·nu/nu DNA hybridizes with an extra band around 4kb (shown by the <).

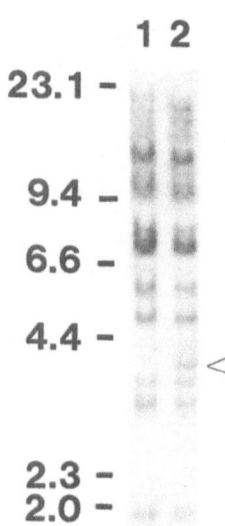

TABLE 1. Probes used to determine genetic profiles of BALB/cAnPt, BALB/cAn·nu/nu, and NIH:Swiss mice. The DNA probes and restriction enzymes used as well as the fragment name and chromosomal assignment are indicated. Numbers in parenthesis after the probe name refer to the original reference.

Probe	Restriction Enzyme	Fragment Name	B/c[*]	nu[**]	Sw[***]	Chr. #
Anf[(24)]	Pvu II	Anf	+	+	−	4
Gdc-1[(13)]	Bgl II	9.3kb	+	+	−	15
MMTV[(3)]	Eco RI	Mtv-6	+	+	+	16
MMTV[(31)]	Eco RI	Mtv-8	+	+	+	6
MMTV[(3)]	Eco RI	Mtv-9	+	+	+	12
MMTV[(19)]	Eco RI	Mtv-16	−	−	+	4
pIl-3[(37)]	Eco RI	Il-3	+	+	ND[%]	11
pMc-myc54[(35)]	Eco RI	myc	+	+	+	15
pMIF1204[(17)]	Eco RI	Ifa	+	+	+	4
pPE220[(21)]	Eco RI	SPARC	+	+	ND	11
pRRF51[(22)]	Taq I	Hox 2.1	+	+	ND	11
pUla-236[#] [(14)]	Eco RI	3.8kb	+	+	ND	11
pUla-236[@]	Bam HI	4.0kb	−	+	ND	ND
pX$_{env}$[(36)]	Pvu II	Xmmv-42	−	−	−	19
pX$_{env}$	Pvu II	Xmmv-48	−	−	+	ND
pX$_{env}$[(36)]	Pvu II	Xmmv-50	−	−	−	12
pX$_{env}$[(36)]	Pvu II	Xmmv-52	+	+	−	5
pX$_{env}$	Pvu II	Xmmv-53	−	−	+	ND
pX$_{env}$	Pvu II	Xmmv-54	+	+	+	ND
pX$_{env}$[(13)]	Pvu II	Xmmv-72	−	−	+/−[o]	15
pX$_{env}$	Pvu II	Xmmv-60	+	+	+	ND
pX$_{env}$[(36)]	Pvu II	Xmmv-61	+	+	+/−	1
pX$_{env}$[(36)]	Pvu II	Xmmv-62	−	−	−	4
pX$_{env}$	Pvu II	Xmmv-65	+	+	−	ND
pX$_{env}$	Pvu II	Xmmv-69	+	+	−	ND
pX$_{env}$	Pvu II	Xmmv-70	+	+	+	ND
pX$_{env}$[(9)]	Hind III	Xmmv-Y	+	+	+	Y
p499[(20)]	Stu I	Mup	+	+	+	4
S-15[(7)]	Xba I	Qa-2[a]	−	−	+	17
Tnf[(10)]	Pst I	Tnf	+	+	ND	17
V$_H$J606[(12)]	Eco RI	7.0kb	+	+	−	12
Vk21[(15)]	Eco RI	Igk	+	+	+	6
v-src[(32)]	Eco RI	src	+	+	+	2,4
V$_T$τ5[(34)]	Eco RI	Tcrg	+	+	+	13
Vττ11[(5)]	Eco RI	Tcra	+	+	+	14

* BALB/cAnPt; ** BALB/cAn·nu/nu and BALB/cAn·nu/+; *** NIH:Swiss; % ND = Not determined; # a 560bp insert; @ a 480bp insert; o One NIH:Swiss showed the restriction fragment while another did not.

Table 2: BALB/cAn·nu/nu male breeders are routinely tested by the
Frederick Cancer Research Facility for possible genetic drift
from the BALB/cAn type. The testing involves electrophoretic
techniques which detect different mobilities of enzymes indicating differences in alleles. Listed below are the isoenzymes
routinely tested and their chromosomal location. The last report
(November 1986) showed no detectable differences between BALB/cAn
and BALB/cAn·nu/nu.

Isozyme	Chromosome location
Idh-1	1
Pep-3	1
Car-2	3
Gpd-1	4
Pgm-1	5
Gpi-1	7
Hbb	7
Es-1	8
Mod-1	9
Es-3	11
Es-10	14

REFERENCES

1) Anderson, P.N. and M. Potter.(1969) Induction of plasma cell
   tumours in BALB/c Mice with 2,6,10,14-Tetramethylpentadecane
   (pristane). Nature, 222;994 - 995.
2) Arn, J.S., S.E. Riordan, D. Pearson, and D.H. Sachs.(1982)
   Strain Restricted Typing Sera (SRTS) for Use in Monitoring
   the Genetic Integrity of Congenic Strains. Journal of
   Immunological Methods, 55;141 - 153.
3) Callahan, R., D. Gallahan, and C. Kozak.(1984) Two genetically
   transmitted BALB/c mouse mammary tumor virus genomes located
   on chromosomes 12 and 16. Journal of Virology, 49(3);1005-
   1008.
4) Chen, W., R. Scollay, D. Shortman, M. Skinner, and J. Marbrook.
   (1984) T-cell development in the absence of a thymus: the
   number, the phenotype, and the functional capacity of T-
   lymphocytes in nude mice. The American Journal of Anatomy,
   170;339 - 347.
5) Chien, Y.H., D.M. Becker, T. Lindsten, M. Okamura, D.J. Cohen,
   and M.M. Davis(1984) Third type of murine T cell receptor
   gene. Nature, 312:31 - 35.
6) Eckels, D.D., M.E. Gershwin, J. Drago and L. Faulkin.(1979)
   Comparative Patterns of Serum Immunoglobulin levels in
   Specific-Pathogen-Free Congenitally Athymic (nude), Heredi-
   tarily Asplenic (Dh/+), congenitally Athymic-Asplenic
   (lasat) and Splenectomized Athymic Mice. Immunology, 37:777
   - 783.
7) Flaherty, L., K. DiBiase, M.A. Lynes, J.G. Seidman, O. Weinber-
   ger, and E.M. Rinchik.(1985) Characterization of a Q
   subregion gene in the murine major histocompatibility
   complex. Procedures of the National Academy of Science,
   U.S.A., 82;1503 - 1507.
8) Flanagan, S.P.(1966) 'Nude", a new hairless gene with pleiotropic effects in the mouse. Genetic Research, 8;295 - 309.

9) Gallahan, D., J. Robbins, L. Byrd, and R. Callahan.(1985) The genetic stability of endogenous type B and C retroviruses in BALB/c sublines. in <u>Current Topics in Microbiology and Immunology</u>, Vol. 122. Ed. M. Potter. Springer-Verlag, Berlin.

10) Gardner, S.M., B. Mock, J. Hilgers, K. E. Huppi, W.D. Roeder.- (1987) Mouse lymphotoxin and tumor necrosis factor: structure analysis of the cloned genes, physical linkage, and chromosomal position. <u>Journal of Immunology</u>, 139(2);476- 483.

11) Gubbels, E., R. Poort-Keesom, and J. Hilgers.(1985) Genetically contaminated BALB/cNude mice. in <u>Current Topics in Microbiology and Immunology</u>, Vol. 122.Ed. M. Potter. Springer-Verlag, Berlin.

12) Hartman, A.B. and S. Rudikoff.(1984) V_H genes encoding the immune response to β-(1,6)-galactan: somatic mutation in IgM molecules. <u>The EMBO Journal</u>. 3(12);3023 - 3030.

13) Hogarth, P.M., I.F.C. McKenzie, V.R. Sutton, K.M. Curnow, B.K. Lee, and E.M. Eicher.(1987) Mapping of the mouse <u>Ly-6</u>, <u>Xp-14</u>, and <u>Gdc-1</u> loci to chromosome 15. <u>Immunogenetics</u>, 25;21 - 27.

14) Howard, E.F., S.K. Michael, J.E. Dahlberg, and E. Lund.(1987) Functional, developmentally expressed genes for mouse U1a and U1b snRNAs contain both conserved and non-conserved transcription signals, in press.

15) Huppi, K. E. Jouvin-Marche, C. Scott, M. Potter, and M. Weigert.(1985) Genetic polymorphism at the <u>k</u> chain locus in mice: comparisons of restriction enzyme hybridization fragments of variable and constant region genes. <u>Immunogenetics</u>, 21;445 - 457.

16) Jacobson, E.B., L.H. Caporale, and G.J. Thorbecke.(1974) Effect of Thymus Cell Injections on Germinal Center Formation in Lymphoid Tissues of Nude (Thymusless) Mice. <u>Cellular Immunology</u>, 13;416 -430.

17) Kelley, K.A., C.A Kozak, F. Dandoy, F. Sor, D. Skup, J.D. Windass, J. DeMaeyer-Guignard, P.M. Pitha, and E. DeMaeyer.(1983) Mapping of murine interferon-α genes to chromosome 4. <u>Gene</u>, 26;181 - 188.

18) Kindred, B.(1978) The Nude Mouse in Studying T Cell Differentiation. in <u>The Nude Mouse in Experimental and Clinical Research</u>. Ed: Jorgen Fogh and Beppino C. Giovanella. Academic Press. 111 -134.

19) Kozak, C.A., R. Callahan, G. Peters, V. Morris, R. Michalides, J. Dudley, M. Green, M. Davisson, O. Prakash, A. Vaidya, J. Hilgers, A. Verstraeten, N. Hynes, H. Diggelman, D. Peterson, J.C. Cohen, C. Dickson, N. Sarker, and R. Nusse.(1987) A revised nomenclature for endogenous mouse mammary tumor viruses. <u>Journal of Virology</u>,(in press).

20) Kuhn, N.J., M. Woodworth-Gutai, K.W. Gross, and W.A. Held. (1984) Subfamilies of the mouse major urinary protein (MUP) multi-gene family: sequence analysis of cDNA clones and differential regulation in the liver. <u>Nucleic Acids Research</u>, 12(5);6073 - 6091.

21) Mason, I.J., D. Murphy, M. Munke, U. Francke, R.W. Elliott, and B.L.M. Hogan.(1986) Developmental and transformation-sensitive expression of the Sparc gene on mouse chromosome 11. <u>The EMBO Journal</u>, 5(8);1831 - 1837.

22) Mock, B., J. Hilgers, K. Huppi and L. D'Hoostelaere.(1987) A <u>Taq</u> I restriction fragment length polymorphism at the

Hox-2.1 locus cosegregates with the <u>Dlb-1</u> locus on mouse chromosome 11. <u>Nucleic Acids Research</u>, 15(5);2397.

23) Morse III, H.C., J.W. Hartley, and M. Potter.(1980) Genetic considerations in plasmacytomas of BALB/c, NZB, and (BALB/c x NZB)F_1. <u>Progress in Myeloma</u>, Ed. M. Potter. Elsevier/North Holland, Inc. 263 - 279.

24) Mullins, J.J., Q. Zeng, and K.W. Gross.(1987) Mapping of the mouse ANF gene. <u>Mouse News Letter</u>, 77;152 - 153.

25) Pantelouris, E.M.(1968) Absence of thymus in a mouse mutant. <u>Nature</u>, 217;370 - 371.

26) Potter, M., J.G. Pumphrey, and D.W. Bailey.(1975) Genetics of susceptibility to plasmacytoma induction. I. BALB/cAnN (C), C57Bl/6N (B6), C57Bl/Ka (BK), (C x B6)F_1, (C x BK)F_1, and C x B recombinant-inbred strains. <u>Journal of the National Cancer Institute</u>, 54(6);1413 - 1417.

27) Potter, M. and J.S. Wax.(1981) Genetics of susceptibility to pristane-induced plasmacytomas in BALB/cAn: reduced susceptibility in BALB/cJ with a brief description of pristane-induced arthritis. <u>The Journal of Immunology</u>, 127(4):1591 - 1595.

28) Potter, M., J.W. Hartley, J.S. Wax, and D. Gallahan.(1984) Effect of MuLV-related genes on plasmacytomagenesis in BALB/c mice. <u>Journal of Experimental Medicine</u>, 160;435-440.

29) Potter, M., J.S. Wax, and E. Blankenhorn.(1985) BALB/c subline differences in susceptibility to plasmacytoma induction. in <u>Current Topics in Microbiology and Immunology</u>, Vol. 122. Ed. M. Potter. Springer-Verlag, Berlin.

30) Potter, M. and J.S. Wax.(1985) Role of genes in the susceptibility to plasmacytomas. <u>Genetic Control of Host Resistance to Infection and Malignancy</u>, Alan R. Liss, Inc. 793 - 804.

31) Robbins, J.M., D. Gallahan, E. Hogg, C. Kozak, and R. Callahan. (1986) An endogenous mouse mammary tumor virus genome common in inbred mouse strains is located on chromosome 6. <u>Journal of Virology</u>, 57(2);709 - 713.

32) Sakaguchi, A.Y., P.A. Lalley, B.U. Zabel, R.W. Ellis, E.M. Scolnick, and S.L. Naylor.(1984) Chromosome assignments of four mouse cellular homologs of sarcoma and leukemia virus oncogenes. <u>Procedures of the National Academy of Science, U.S.A.</u>, 81;525 - 529.

33) Scheid, M.P., G. Goldstein, and E.A. Boyse.(1975) Differentiation of T cells in nude mice. <u>Science</u>, 190;1211 -1213.

34) Snodgrass, H.R., Z. Dembic, M. Steinmetz, and H. von Boehmer. (1985) Expression of T-cell antigen receptor genes during fetal development in the thymus. <u>Nature</u>,315;232 - 233.

35) Stanton, L.W., R. Watt, K. B. Marcu.(1983) Translocation, breakage, and truncated transcripts of <u>c-myc</u> oncogene in murine plasmacytomas. <u>Nature</u>, 303;401 - 406.

36) Wejman, J.C., B.A. Taylor, N.A. Jenkins, and N.G. Copeland. (1984) Endogenous xenotropic murine leukemia virus-related sequences map to chromosomal regions encoding mouse lymphocyte antigens. <u>Journal of Virology</u>, 50(1);237 - 247.

37) Yokota, T., F. Lee, D. Rennick, C. Hall, N. Arai, T. Mosmann, G. Nabel, H. Cantor, and K. Arai.(1984) Isolation and characterization of a mouse cDNA clone that expresses mast-cell growth-factor activity in monkey cells. <u>Procedures of the National Academy Science, U.S.A.</u>, 81;1070 - 1074.

Organization of the Distal End of Mouse Chromosome 4

K. Huppi, B. A. Mock, P. Schricker, L. A. D'Hoostelaere, and M. Potter

INTRODUCTION

BALB/cAn and NZB/B1NJ mice are unique among mouse inbred strains in their increased susceptibility to the induction of plasma cell tumors (Potter and Wax, 1981). The inability to produce plasmacytomas in DBA/2N or (BALB/cAn x DBA/2N)F$_1$ mice for example, indicates that one or more resistance (R) genes can be associated with the development of plasmacytomas (Potter and Wax, 1985). Similarly, plasmacytoma induction studies among a broad panel of BALB/cAn.DBA/2N (C.D2) congenic strains, originally selected for allelomorphic markers that differ between BALB/cAn and DBA/2N indicate some regions fortuitously harbor R genes of DBA/2 origin. C.D2 congenic mice carrying single resistance genes from DBA/2N are partially resistant to plasmacytoma induction, e.g., C.D2 Fv-1^n mice (Potter et al., 1984). The C.D2Fv-1^n congenic has also been found to carry a locus (Rep-2) derived from DBA/2N which confers more efficient chromatin repair than the BALB/cAn strain (Potter et al., 1988). This has been determined by studies of efficiency of DNA repair following x-irradiation induced damage. Thus, the region on the distal end of mouse chromosome 4 in the vicinity of Fv-1 harbors not only genes associated with DNA repair but also genes involved in increased resistance to plasmacytomagenesis.

The distal portion of mouse chromosome 4, in the vicinity of the Fv-1 locus, carries one of the largest regions of synteny between man and mouse (Nadeau and Taylor, 1984). Several loci including phosphoglucomutase (Pgm-2) alkaline phosphatase (akp-2), atrianatriuretic factor (Anf), adenylate kinase 2 (ak-2), phosphogluconate dehydrogenase (Pgd) and glycerol-3-phosphate dehydrogenase (Gpd-1), which map to the telomere of mouse chromosome 4 also reside in a conserved linkage group on the short arm of human chromosome 1 (p32-36) (for review, see Lalley and McKusick, 1985).

As the initial step towards the eventual isolation of DNA repair genes and/or genes involved in plasmacytoma resistance, we have ordered the distal end of mouse chromosome 4 with respect to the following molecular probes: major urinary protein (Mup-1), Interferon α (Ifa), units 11 and 13 of mouse mammary tumor virus (Mtv-13), an anonymous DNA sequence (D4Rpl) lymphocyte tyrosine kinase (Lck), and atrianatriuretic factor (Anf). Previous reports have positioned Mup-1 (Bennett et al., 1982), Ifa (Kelley et al., 1983), D4Rpl (Berger et al., 1984) and Anf (Mullins, 1987) on mouse chromosome 4 primarily by the strain distribution pattern (SDP) generated between C57BL/6J by DBA/2J (BXD) or BALB/cByJ by C57BL/6ByJ (CXB) recombinant inbred (RI) strains of mice.

In the present study, we have adopted the BXD (Bailey, 1971) and CXB (Taylor, 1980) RI strains for comparison of these loci with the loci Mtv-13 and Lck and Anf, which most likely map within the conserved linkage group of human chromosome 1p and mouse chromosome 4 (Morris et al., 1979, Marth et al., 1986, Mullins, 1987). Some loci were also compared for the SDP generated among RI strains of BALB/cHeA and STS/A parental mice as well as a series of backcross mice generated between C57BL/10ScSn and SWR/J.

Laboratory of Genetics, National Cancer Institute, National Institutes of Health, Bethesda, Maryland 20892

Current Topics in Microbiology and Immunology, Vol. 137
© Springer-Verlag Berlin · Heidelberg 1988

Determining the gene order for distal chromosome 4 allowed us to examine the extent of DBA/2 contained within the C.D2-Fv-1^n congenic at different generations of backcross by RFLP analysis. As a result, we can delimit the region which potentially harbors DNA repair genes and/or plasmacytoma resistance genes to a region of approximately 17 cM surrounding the Fv-1 locus.

MATERIALS AND METHODS

Mice

The following inbred strains of mice are maintained at the Hazleton facility, Rockville, MD (contract #N01-CB-71085): AKR/N BALB/cAnPt, C57BL/10N DBA/2N, NZB/B1NJ and SJL/JLWPt. The inbred strains C57BL/6J, C57L/J, C58/J, BALB/cByJ, DBA/2J and SWR/J were obtained from the Jackson Laboratories. The inbred strains, STS/A and BALB/cHeA were kindly provided by J. Hilgers (Amsterdam).

Genetic Crosses

The C57BL/6J by DBA/2J (BXD) and C57BL/6ByJ by BALB/cByJ (CXB) RI series consist of 26 and 7 inbred strains, respectively. The BALB/cHeA by STS/A (CXS) RI strains provide 14 additional strains which have been brother-sister mated for 30 generations (Hilgers and Arends, 1987). The 38 males or females of the (SWR/J x C57BL/10ScSn)F$_1$ x SWR/J backcross were kindly provided by J. Blackwell and were tested for frequency of recombination among progeny. The generation of BALB/cAn. DBA/2N-Fv-1^n/Fv-1^n (C.D2-Fv-1^n) congenic mice was by successive backcross of (Fv-1^n/Fv-1^b) mice to BALB/cAn and selection for the Fv-1^n phenotypes of DBA/2N origin. At the 6th and 10th generation of backcross, mice were tested for susceptibility to the induction of plasmacytomas.

Recombination Frequency

Estimates of gene order and genetic distance were determined by the statistical method of Silver and Buckler (1986). The recombination frequencies were generated from RI strains (cumulative totals) and backcross mice.

Preparation of DNA and Southern Hybridization Probes

The preparation of high molecular weight DNA from liver tissue has been described (Huppi et al., 1985). The restriction digestion conditions, gel electrophoresis and subsequent procedures for Southern transfer are as previously described. The molecular DNA probes used in this study are listed in Table 1 along with their sources and references. All final wash stringencies were 0.2 x SSC (1 x SSC = 0.15 M sodium chloride, 0.015 M sodium citrate) at 65°C for 30 minutes.

RESULTS

The positions of Mup-1 and Ifa loci have been well established on chromosome 4 (Davisson and Roderick, 1981; Nadeau et al. 1987) and were used as reference points for comparison with more distal markers. The positions of these loci have been generated by examination of recombination frequencies among BXD, CXB and CXS RI strains, as well as among other RI strains of mice. For the purpose of direct comparison, RFLPs were generated, when possible, between parental inbred mice of RI strains with the DNA probes for MMTV, D4Rp1 Lck and Anf.

Table 1. Chromosome 4 - Molecular Probes

Genomic locus	Probe	Insert	Reference or Source
Major urinary protein (Mup)	p499	0.8Kb Pst I	Kuhn et al. (1984)
Interferon (Ifa)	pMF1204	0.8Kb Pst I	Kelley et al. (1983)
D4Rp1	pODC1440	1.0Kb Pst I	Elliott (pers. comm.) Berger, 1984
Mouse mammary tumor locus (Mtv)	pMMTV	1.5Kb Pst I	Callahan, R. et al. (1984)
Lymphocyte tyrosine kinase (Lck)	pNT18	1.8Kb EcoRI	Marth et al. (1985)
Atrial natriuretic factor (Anf)	PcAR60	0.4Kb AccI/PstI	Davies (pers. comm.) and Mullins et al. (1987)

Mtv-13

The endogeneous mouse mammary tumor virus, MMTV, has been integrated on several mouse chromosomes into genomic sites very characteristic of a particular inbred strain. Since MMTV carries a conserved internal EcoRI restriction site, a DNA probe for MMTV will hybridize to EcoRI restriction fragment (RF) bands which comprise 5' and 3' portions of the provirus plus flanking genomic DNA (Fig. 1). Mtv proviral units have been chromosomally mapped in the DBA/2N mouse using primarily the SD pattern generated among BXD RI strains (Morris et al., 1979). The 5.8 kb and 9.0 kb EcoRI RF bands of DBA/2N (Fig. 1) refer to units 11 and 13 which segregate with a distribution pattern for the Mtv-13 provirus harboring a best fit of 19/26 concordancies with Ifa. The most likely position of Mtv-13 would be 10.5 cM (p=.85) distal to Ifa on mouse chromosome 4 (Table 2).

D4Rp1

Ornithine decarboxylase (Odc) is an enzyme found in the polyamine biosynthetic pathway and is induced by androgens in the mouse kidney. A cDNA clone, pODC1440, with a high degree of homology to Odc has been generated from a kidney cDNA library (Berger et al., 1984) and resides on mouse chromosome 4 (Elliott, 1987). This anonymous DNA probe, D4Rp1, displays no RFLPs (18 restriction endonucleases tested) between the parental strains C57BL/6J and DBA/2J. However, an EcoRI RFLP was detected among a few inbred strains including the parental strains of the CXS Recombinant Inbreds' BALB/cHeA and STS/A (Table 3). The D4Rp1[a] pattern corresponds to polymorphic EcoRI RF bands of 3.5 kb and 5.0 kb whereas the D4Rp1[b] pattern refers to a single 4.3 kb RF band (Fig. 2). For example, BALB/cHeA displays a D4Rp1[a] pattern in contrast to the D4Rp1[b] RF pattern found with STS/A. Comparison of the CXS SD pattern for D4Rp1 with Ifa shows 10 of 12 concordancies (Table 1). In addition, the D4Rp1 EcoRI RF pattern of the parental inbred strains of the CXB RI strains are also polymorphic. The CXB SDP for D4Rp1 display 6/7 concordancies with Ifa. Compilation of the CXB and CXS recombination frequencies and minimizing double crossover between Ifa and D4Rp1 shows 16 of 19 concordancies which positions D4Rp1 5.2 cM distal to Ifa (P=.838).

Fig. 1. Southern hybridization of MMTV to EcoRI restricted DNA of inbred mouse strains. Size standards of λ HindIII are denoted on the left side of upper and lower panels.

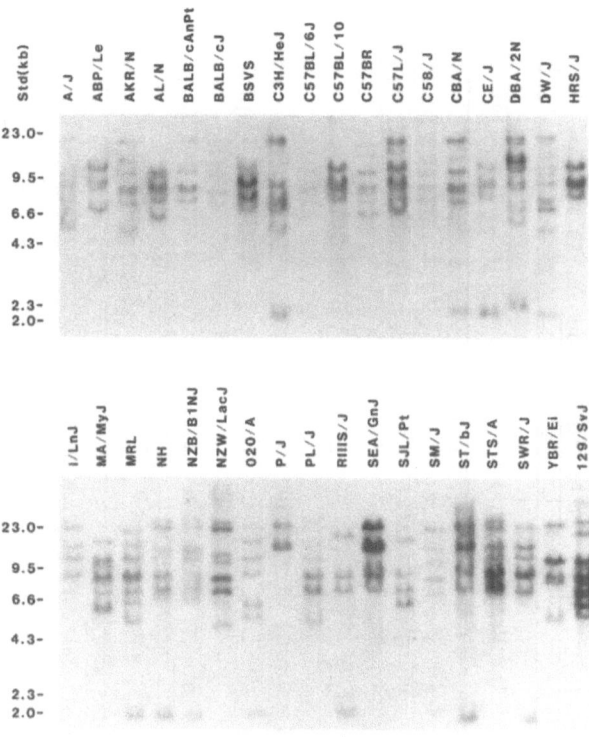

Lck

The lymphocyte specific tyrosine kinase gene (Lck) has been determined to be expressed principally in T and perhaps early B cells (Marth et al., 1986). Originally isolated as a rearranged gene in the tumor LSTRA, Lck is a cDNA probe from a C57BL/Ka thymus library and hybridizes to single copy RF bands under stringent wash conditions. Hybridization of the Lck probe to a panel of mouse inbred strains reveals RFLPs with the restriction endonuclease StuI (data not shown) or EcoRV (Fig. 2 and Table 3). Two EcoRV RF patterns are found among inbred mouse strains. The EcoRV RF band for Lck[a] is 14 kb and is found among strains including C57BL/6J. In contrast, the Lck[b] allele is found as a 23 kb EcoRV RF band in inbred strains such as BALB/c or DBA/2J (Fig. 2 and Table 3). EcoRV restricted DNA from the BXD and CXB RI strains were hybridized to Lck and compared with other chromosome 4 markers. The closest markers to Lck are Fv-1 (17/23 concordancies) and Ela-1, a pseudogene of elastase (20/25 concordancies). Comparison of the recombination frequency and assuming minimal double crossover suggests Lck most likely lies 7.2 cM (p=0.872) distal to Ela-1 and 10.9 cM (p=0.558) proximal to Fv-1. In addition, the SDP generated among CXB mice indicates that Lck probably resides distal to D4Rp1.

Table 2. Strain Distribution of Mup-1, Ifa, Mtv-11,13, Ahd-1, Ela-1, Lck and Anf in BXD Strains

	1	2	5	6	8	9	11	12	13	14	15	16	18	19	20	21	22	23	24	25	27	28	29	30	31	32
Mup-1	D	B	B	B	B	B	B	B	B	B	D	B	B	B	B	D	D	B	D	D	B	B	B	B	B	B
Ifa	D	B	B	B	B	D	B	D	D	B	D	B	B	B	B	D	D	D	D	D	D	D	D	D	B	B
Mtv-13	D	B	D	B	B	D	B	D	B	D	D	D	D	B	B	D	D	D	B	D	D	D	D	D	B	D
Ahd-1	D	B	B	B	B	B	B	D	D	D	D	D	D	B	B	D	B	D	B	B	B	D	B	D	B	D
Ela-1	D	B	B	B	B	D	B	D	D	D	D	D	D	B	B	D	B	D	B	B	B	D	D	D	B	D
Lck	D	B	B	B	D	D	D	D	D	D	B	D	.	D	B	D	B	D	B	B	B	D	B	D	B	D
Anf	D	B	D	B	D	B	B	D	D	D	B	D	D	B	B	D	B	B	B	B	D	D	B	D	.	.

D refers to DBA/2J alleles whereas B refers to alleles derived from C57BL/6J.

Figure 2. RFLPs determined by
Southern hybridization with D4Rp1,
Lck and Anf DNA probes. RF
patterns "a" or "b" are labeled
at the top of each lane.
Molecular weight size standards
of λ HindIII are on the left
panel.

Restriction Fragment Length Polymorphisms

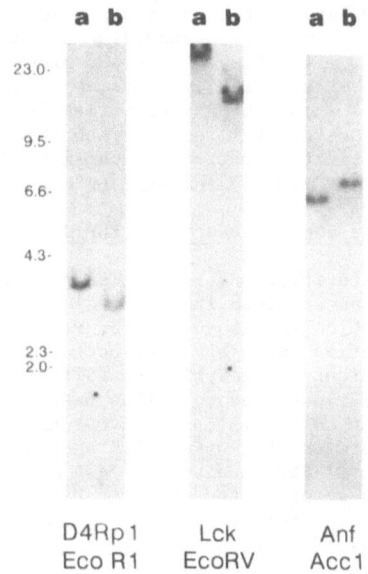

Table 3. Inbred Strain Distribution of Chromosome 4 Loci

-DNA Markers-

Inbred strains	Mup-EcoRI	Ifa-PvuII	D4Rp1-EcoRI	Lck-EcoRV	Anf-AccI
AKR/N	a	a	b	a	b
BALB/c(An,ByJ HeA)	a	a	a	a	a
C57BL/6J	b	b	b	b	a
C57BL/10ScSn	b	b	b	b	a
C57L/J	b	b	b	b	b
C58/J	–	b	b	b	b
DBA/2N	a	c	b	a	b
NZB/B1NJ	–	b	b	a	b
SJL/JLwPt	–	a	a	a	c
STS/A	b	b	b	a	–
SWR/J	b	a	b	a	d

Anf

Atrianatriuretic factor is a peptide which plays a significant role in electrolyte balance. A cDNA probe encoding Anf has been isolated and an RFLP was established among certain inbred strains of mice with the restriction endonuclease PvuII (Mullins et al., 1987). Mullins et al. (1987) have shown that Anf cosegregates with Fv-1 among the BXD RI series by utilizing the PvuII RFLP. We have detected another useful RFLP for Anf with the restriction endonuclease AccI, which generates four distinct RF patterns among inbred strains; Anf^a (6.5 kb), Anf^b (7.0 kb), Anf^c (6.3 kb and 7.0 kb) and Anf^d (7.0 kb and 8.5 kb) (Fig. 2 and Table 3).

Recombination Frequency in (SWR/J x C57BL/10ScSn)F$_1$ x SWR/J Backcross Progeny

An opportunity for more precise positioning of D4Rpl, Lck and Anf with respect to Ifa was obtained from a panel of 38 backcross mice (SWR/J x C57BL/10ScSn)F$_1$ x SWR/J, which were surveyed for recombination between these loci. The inbred strain distribution shows that for both Ifa and Anf, the restriction endonuclease PvuII is a convenient polymorphism to follow for crosses between SWR/J and C57BL/10ScSn. An EcoRI RFLP was used to follow SWR/J and C57BL/10ScSn alleles for D4Rpl whereas EcoRV was an inheritable polymorphism to use for Lck (Table 2). The recombinations found between Ifa, D4Rpl, Lck and Anf is consistent with the gene order predicted from the RI SDP results (Table 4). However, the gene order and recombination distance as predicted from the (SWR/J x C57BL/10ScSn)F$_1$ x SWR/J F2 backcross is as follows: centromere--Ifa--17.85 cM ± 7.23 cM--D4Rpl--10.71 cM ± 5.84 cM--Lck--7.14 cM ± 4.86 cM--Anf.

The DBA/2N Composition of the C.D2 Fv-1^n Congenic

The congenic C.D2-Fv-1^n at the N6, N10, N12, N17-N19 generations of backcross was surveyed for the extent of DBA/2N chromosome 4 genetic material. The following DNA probes were used in RFLP analysis with C.D2 Fv-1^n: Ifa (PvuII), MMTV (EcoRI), D4Rpl (EcoRI) and Anf (AccI). By the N6 generation of backcross, the C.D2-Fv-1^n congenic did not contain the DBA/2N RFs for Ifa or D4Rpl (Fig. 3). Furthermore, between the N6 and N10 generations of backcross, the DBA/2N region harboring Mtv-13 is lost from the C.D2-Fv-1^n congenic. Nevertheless, the Anf locus continues to co-segregate with Fv-1 through the N19 generation of backcross.

DISCUSSION

Recent studies have established the order of several loci including Ifa, interferon beta (Ifb), aminoleuvilinate dehydratase (Lv) and alpha-1 acid glycoprotein-1 and -2 (Orm-1, Orm-2) with respect to brown (b), B cell maturation factor responsiveness (Bmfr-1) and Mup-1. The most likely order as reported is: Mup-1, (Lv--b--Orml), (Orm-2--Ifa), (Ifb--Bmfr-1) (Nadeau et al. 1987). We have extended this detailed mapping to include new markers from mouse chromosome 4 more distal to Mup-1 and Ifa. These gene loci, D4Rpl, Mtv-13, Lck and Anf, have been compared to other loci from mouse chromosome 4 including Mup-1, Ifa, and Fv-1. Comparison of recombination frequencies between these loci among RI strains (CXB, BXD and/or CXS) permits us to predict a gene order as follows: centromere--Ifa--5.2 cM--D4Rpl--Mtv-13--Lck--10.9 cM--Anf. However, the probabilities clearly indicate that some of the genetic distances are not precise. This is principally shown by the recombination frequencies generated among an (SWR/J x C57BL/10ScSn)F$_1$ x SWR/J backcross experiment in which the following gene order and recombination frequences are found: Ifa--17.85 cM ± 7.23 cM--D4Rpl--10.71 cM ± 5.84 cM--Lck--7.14 cM ± 4.86 cM--Anf. The gene

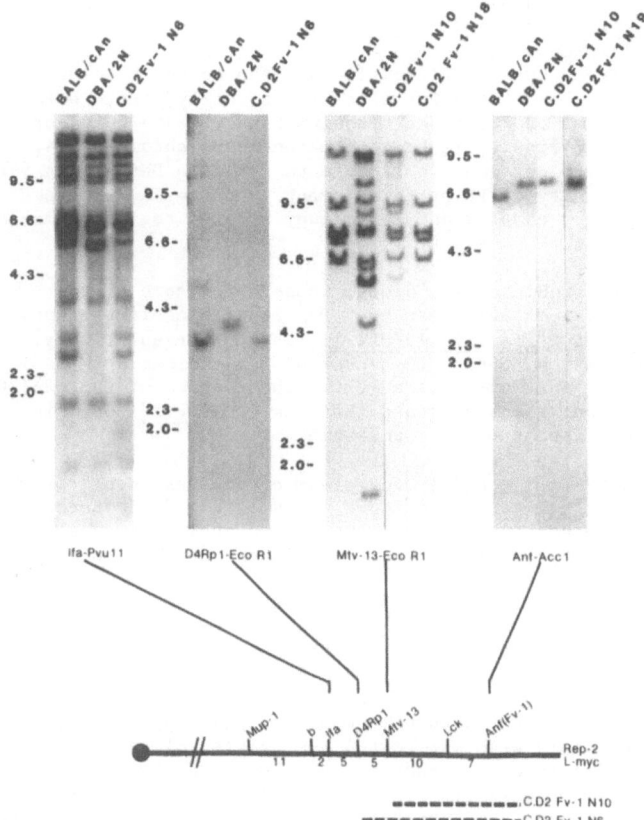

DISTAL MOUSE CHROMOSOME 4

Figure 3. Upper panel – DBA/2N content of C.D2-$Fv-1^n$ at various backcross generations. RFLPs determined at the Southern hybridization level with the probes and restriction endonucleases listed below each panel. C.D2-$Fv-1^n$ examples are shown only with the backcross generation(s) of most significance.
Lower panel – Organization of distal mouse chromosome 4 loci. The centromere is on the left and certain loci located at the distal end with recombination distances listed below the line are denoted. b refers to the brown locus and the position of Rep-2 remain to be determined. The likely extent of DBA/2N in the C.D2-$Fv-1^n$ N6 and N10 generations are shown by dotted lines below.

order predicted from the backcross experiment is identical to that found in SDPs generated among RI strains and the distances lie within >95% confidence limits. The distance between Ifa and D4Rpl varies between 5.2 and 17.5 cM. This difference in the genetic distance between loci could be due largely to low numbers of genetic progeny or to disparity between the particular parental inbred strains used in this analysis. Similar heterogeneity among conventional inbred strains and M. spretus crosses as to the positioning of Ifa and Ifb has already been reported (Nadeau et al., 1987). Furthermore, in DBA/2N may significantly alter the positioning of nearby loci in this particular inbred strain. In addition to MMTV integration sites, other viral integration sites have been found in this region of chromosome 4, namely the endogenous xenotropic Murine leukemia Virus related sequences (Blatt et al., 1983, Wejman et al., 1984) which map within 1 cM of Gpd-1. The integration of Moloney LTR sequences into a region 5' of Lck in the thymoma LSTRA led initially to the identification and subsequent cloning of the gene Lck. Since Lck is a member of the tyrosine kinase family, there have been predictions that complex families of other tyrosine kinase genes c-fgr or c-src may also map to a region physically linked to Lck on mouse chromosome 4. We are presently unable to confirm any genetic linkage to Lck with DNA probes for c-fgr or c-src due to the complexity of RF patterns among tyrosine kinase genes. This family is expected to be very complex and may occupy a large region of mouse chromosome 4.

Nevertheless, the gene order as predicted for distal mouse chromosome 4 is independently confirmed by the sequential absence of DBA/2N alleles in the back-cross generations of C.D2 $Fv-1^n$ for Ifa, D4Rpl, Mtv-13, and Anf, respectively. We have established that between the N6 and N10 backcross generations 5 cM of DBA/2 chromosome 4 between D4Rpl and Mtv-13 were lost. The absence of the DBA/2N Mtv-13 component at N17-N19, generations suggests that the C.D2-$Fv-1^n$ congenic carries approximately 17 cM or less of DBA/2 chromosome 4.

Contemporary studies of the C.D2-Fv-1 congenic for plasmacytoma resistance or DNA repair genes has demonstrated both R genes and Rep-2 genes at the N12 generation of backcross. Our data would suggest that these genes lie distal and mutually exclusive of Mtv-13 and yet remain closely associated with the Lck and Anf loci.

The region of distal mouse chromosome 4 bears synteny with the short arm of human chromosome 1. Thus loci which have been mapped to this region of human chromosome 1 (p32-p36) should correspond closely to the order found on distal mouse chromosome 4. That this is in fact the case has been elegantly shown by Searle et al. (1987). More recently, several new DNA markers including L-myc (Nau et al., 1985) have mapped to this region of human 1p32-p34. By synteny association these DNA markers should also map to the same region of distal mouse chromosome 4. This raises interesting consequences about the potential associa-tion of characteristic c-myc chromosomal translocations in mouse plasmacytomas (rcpt 12;15, rcpt6;15) and the presence of the homologous genes like L-myc in the vicinity of plasmacytoma R genes. Furthermore, the association of putative DNA repair defects with mouse plasmacytomas (Potter et al., 1988) also leads to the possible connection between DNA repair genes and plasmacytoma R genes on mouse chromosome 4. Reports of suppression of malignancy in somatic cell hybrids (Fenyo et al., 1980) also raises the possiblity that Fv-1 in its role in viral replication may also be involved in certain stages of malignancy similar to that found with leukemia (Ril-3) (Meruelo et al., 1981) or plasma cell tumors.

ACKNOWLEDGMENTS

We would like to acknowledge the excellent technical assistance of D. Siwarski and expert skills of V. Rogers in preparing this manuscript. The efforts of D. Bailey, B. Taylor (Jackson Labs), J. Hilgers (The Netherlands Cancer Inst.) and J. Blackwell (The London School of Hygiene and Tropical Medicine) in the original construction of CXB, BXD, CXS and (C57BL/10ScSn x SWR/J)F$_1$ x SWR/J mice is gratefully acknowledged. This experiment would not have been possible without the generous gifts of DNA probes from the following: W. Held (Mup), R. Elliott (D4Rpl) and J. Mullins (Anf), all of Roswell Park; P. Pitha (Ifa, J. Hopkins); J. Marth (Lck, Hutchinson Cancer Inst.), P. Davies (Anf, Vancouver) and R. Callahan (MMTV, National Cancer Institute).

Table 4.   Strain Distribution Patterns of Chromosome 4 Loci

A.   Strain Distribution of Mup-1, Ifa and D4Rp1 Among
     Among CXS RI Strains

	1	2	3	4	5	6	7	8	9	10	11	12	13	14
Mup-1	C	S	C	C	S	C	C	S	C	S	S	C	C	S
Ifa	C	S	C	C	S	C	C	S	C	S	S	C	C	.
D4Rp1	C	S	C	C	C	C	C	S	C	S	S	S	C	S

C refers to BALB/cHeA alleles whereas S refers to alleles
derived from STS/A.

B.   Strain Distribution of Mup-1, Ifa, D4Rp1
     and Lck Among CXB RI Strains

	D	E	G	H	I	J	K
Mup-1	B	C	C	C	B	C	B
b	B	B	C	C	C	C	B
Ifa	C	B	C	C	C	C	B
D4Rp1	B	B	C	C	C	C	B
Lck	C	B	C	C	B	B	B

B refers to the C57BL/6ByJ allele and C refers to alleles
derived from BALB/cByJ.

Table 4. Continued

C. (SWR/J x C57BL/10ScSn) x SWR/J Backcross

	Ifa	D4Rp1	Lck	Anf	N
SWR/J	S	S	S	S	
C57BL/10ScSn	B	B	B	B	
(B10 x SWR)F$_1$	S/B	S/B	S/B	S/B	
Backcross Progeny F1 x SWR	S/S	S/S	S/S	S/S	6
	S/B	S/B	S/B	S/B	12
	S/B	S/S	S/S	S/S	0
	S/B	S/B	S/S	S/S	1
	S/B	S/B	S/B	S/S	1
	S/S	S/S	S/S	S/B	1
	S/S	S/S	S/B	S/B	2
	S/S	S/B	S/B	S/B	5

Analysis of Recombinants

Pairs of Loci	r	N	Distance (cM) ± Standard Error
Ifa,D4Rp1	5	28	17.85 ± 7.23
Ifa,Lck	8	28	28.57 ± 8.54
Ifa,Anf	10	28	35.71 ± 9.05
D4Rp1,Lck	3	28	10.71 ± 5.84
D4Rp1,Anf	5	28	17.85 ± 7.23
Lck,Anf	2	28	7.14 ± 4.86

N=total number
r=recombinants
S=SWR/J   B=C57BL/10ScSn

REFERENCES

Bailey, D.W. (1971) Recombinant-inbred strains, an aid to finding identity, link-age, and function of histocompatibility and other genes. Transplantation 11, 325-327.

Bennett, K.L., Lalley, P.A., Barth, R.K., and N.D. Hastie (1982) Mapping the structural genes coding for the major urinary proteins in the mouse: Combined use of recombinant inbred strains and somatic cell hybrids. Proc. Natl. Acad. Sci. USA 79: 1220-1224.

Berger, F.G., Szymanski, P., Read, E., and G. Watson (1984) Androgen-regulated Ornithine Decarboxylase mRNAs of mouse kidney. J. Biol. Chem. 259: 7941-7946.

Callahan, R., Gallahan, D. and C. Kozak (1984) Two genetically transmitted BALB/c mouse mammary tumor Virus genomes located on chromosomes 12 and 16. J. Virol 49:1005-1008.

Davisson, M.T. and T.H. Roderick (1981) Recombination percentages. In Genetic Variants and Strains of the Laboratory Mouse, pp. 283-313, M. Green (ed.) Gustav Fischer, Verlag, New York.

Elliott, R. (1981) Restriction enzyme fragment polymorphisms. Mouse News Letter 64: 88.

Fenyo, E.M., Klein, G., Povey, S., Jeremiah, S.J., Spira, J., Wiener, F., and H. Harris (1980) Suppression and reappearance of N-tropic L virus production in somatic cell hybrids after introduction and loss of chromosomes carrying Fv-1^n. Eur. J. Cancer 16, 357-368.

Hilgers, J. and Arends, J. A series of Recombinant Inbred Strains Between the BALB/cHeA and STS/A Mouse Strains. In Current Topics in Microbiology and Immu-nology 121, 31-37.

Huppi, K., Jouvin-Marche, E., Scott, C., Potter, M., and M. Weigert (1985) Genetic polymorphism at the kappa chain locus in mice: comparisons of restriction enzyme hybridization fragments of variable and constant region genes. Immunogenet. 21: 445-457.

Kelley, K.A., Kozak, C.A., Dandoy, F., Sor, F., Skup, D., Windass, J.D., DeMaeyer-Guignard, J., Pitha, P.M., and E. DeMaeyer (1983) Mapping of murine interferon-α genes to chromosome 4. Gene 26, 181-188.

Kuhn, N.J., Woodworth-Gutai, M., Gross, K.W. and W.A. Held (1984) Subfamilies of the mouse major urinary protein (MUP) multi-gene family: sequence analysis of cDNA clones and differential regulation in the liver. Nucl. Acids. Res. 12, 6073-6090.

Lalley, P.A., and V.A. McKusick (1985) Report of the Committee on Comparative Mapping: Eighth International Workshop on Human Gene Mapping, Cytogenet. Cell Genet. 40, 536-566.

Marth, J.D., Peet, R., Krebs, E.G., and R.M. Perlmutter (1985) A lymphocyte specific protein-tyrosine kinase gene is rearranged and overexpressed in the murine T cell lymphoma LSTRA. Cell 43: 393-404.

Marth, J.D., Disteche, C., Pravtcheva, D., Ruddle, F., Krebs, E.G., and R.M. Perl-mutter (1986) Localization of a lymphocyte-specific protein tyrosine kinase gene

(Lck) at a site of frequent chromosomal abnormalities in human lymphomas. Proc. Natl. Acad. Sci. USA 83, 7400-7404.

Meruelo, D., Offer, M. and N Flieger (1981) Genetics of susceptibility to radiation induced leukemia. J. Exp. Med. 154, 1201-1211.

Morris, V.L., Kozak, C., Cohen, J.C., Shank, P.R., Jolicoeur, P., Ruddle, F. and H.E. Varmus (1979) Endogenous mouse mammary tumor virus DNA is distributed among multiple mouse chromosomes. Virology 92, 46-55.

Mullins, J.J., Zeng, Q. and K.W. Gross (1987) Mapping of the mouse ANF gene. Mouse Newsletter 77, 152-153.

Nadeau, J.H. and B.A. Taylor (1984) Lengths of chromosomal segments conserved since divergence of man and mouse. Proc. Natl. Acad. Sci. USA 81, 814-818.

Nadeau, J.H., Berger, F.G., Kelley, K.A., Pitha, P.M., Sidman, C.L. and N. Worrall (1987) Rearrangement of genes located on homologous chromosomal segments in mouse and man: The location of alpha and beta interferon, alpha-1 and glycoprotein-1 and -2 and aminoleulinate dehydratase on mouse chromosome 4. Genetics 104:1239-1255.

Nau, M., Brooks, B., Battey, J., Sansville, E., Gasdar, A., Kirsh, I., McBride, O., Bertness, V., Hollis, G. and J. Minna (1985) L-myc, a new myc-related gene amplified and expressed in human small cell lung cancer. Nature 318:69-73.

Potter, M. and J.S. Wax (1981) Genetics of susceptibility to pristane induced plasmacytomas in BALB/cAn: Reduced susceptibility in BALB/cJ with a brief description of pristane induced arthritis. J. Immunol. 127, 1591-1595.

Potter, M., Hartley, J.W., Wax, J.S. and D. Gallahan (1984) Effect of MuLV-related genes on plasmacytomagenesis in BALB/c mice. J. Exp. Med. 160, 435-440.

Potter, M., and J.S. Wax (1985) Role of genes in the susceptibility to plasmacytomas. In Genetic Control of Host Resistance to Infection and Malignancy, pp. 793-804, Alan R. Liss, Inc.

Potter, M., Sanford, K.K., Parshad, R., Tarone, R.E., Price, F.M., Mock, B., and K. Huppi (1988) Genes on chromosomes 1 and 4 in the mouse are associated with repair of radiation-induced chromatin damage. Genomics (in press).

Searle, A.G., Peters, J., Lyon, M.F., Evans, E.P., Edwards, J.H. and V.J. Buckle (1987) Chromosome maps of man and mouse, III. Genomics 1, 3-18.

Silver, J. and C.E. Buckler (1986) Statistical considerations for linkage analysis using recombinant inbred strains and backcrosses. Proc. Natl. Acad. Sci. USA 83, 1423-1427.

Taylor, B.A. (1980) Recombinant inbred strains: use in gene mapping. In Origins of Inbred Strains, Morse, H.C. (ed.), pp. 423-428, Academic Press, New York.

Terao, M., Prautcheva D., Ruddle, F.H. and B. Mintz (1988) Mapping of the gene encoding mouse placental alkaline phosphatase to chromosome 4. Somatic Cell and Molecular Genetics, in press.

Wejman, J.C., Taylor, B.A., Jenkins, N.A. and N.G. Copeland (1984) Endogenous, xenotropic murine leukemia virus-related sequences map to chromosomal regions encoding mouse lymphocyte antigens. J. Virol. 50, 237-247.

Susceptibility and Resistance to Plasmacytomagenesis: Possible Role of Genes That Modify Efficiency of Chromatin Repair

M. Potter, K. K. Sanford, R. Parshad, K. Huppi, and B. Mock

The responsiveness of inbred mice to microbial pathogens and tumor-inducing agents can vary with individual strains. Thus, the genotype of a given strain can determine whether the mouse will be susceptible or resistant to the development of a disease process. In many cases the phenotype is controlled by more than one gene. Identification of specific genes usually requires that two reference strains, a susceptible and resistant one, be used in the genetic analysis and the genes defined are referable to the two strains compared. The responses to pathogenic agents can be broken down into two general steps: the first (afferent pathway) governs how a specific strain of mice interacts with the pathogenic agent(chemical or microbial) and the second set of responses relates to the damage incurred and how the damaged cells cope with the agent or its effects (efferent pathway).

We have been attempting for several years to analyse the genetic basis of susceptibility to the induction of plasmacytomas in the BALB/cAn mouse by the intraperitoneal injection of paraffin oils or related pure alkanes such as pristane (2,6,10,14-tetramethyl-pentadecane). BALB/cAn, in contrast to most other strains, is highly susceptible to developing these tumors. When adult BALB/c mice are given three intraperitoneal injections of 0.5ml each at bi-monthly intervals, 61% of the mice develop plasmacytomas with a mean latent period of approximately 210-220 days (Potter and Wax,1983). In most other inbred strains few plasmacytomas are induced (Potter 1984).

We have also tested 8 different sublines of BALB/c and found that all except BALB/cJ are highly susceptible (Blankenhorn et al 1985) Only 10% of BALB/cJPt mice develop plasmacytomas after receiving pristane (Potter and Wax 1981). BALB/cAn and J sublines of mice share a large number of common allelomorphic genes (Roderick et al.1985)which makes it very unlikely that the genetic differences between these two strains are due to genetic contamination. Instead, BALB/cAn and BALB/cJ accumulated genetic differences over the 50 years that they have been separated (Potter 1985). The comparison of responses between the two BALB/c sublines provides a useful model system for analyzing genetic differences that govern susceptibility and resistance to pathogenic agents. We are in the process of developing congenic strains of BALB/cAn.J based on the few known genotypic differences: Qa2 (chr 17); Afr-1 (chr 15) Mup-ml (chr 15) and Mup-1 (chr 4) [Blankenhorn et al. 1988; Duncan et al. 1988].

A second model system for finding susceptibility/resistance (S/R) genes in our laboratory involves the analysis of plasmacytoma-resistant strains. We have focused on DBA/2N as the Fl hybrids (BALB/cAn x DBA/2N)F1 are also solidly resistant indicating that resistance is dominant. The incidence of plasmacytomas induced in 101 first generation backcross progeny from BALB/cAn x CDF1 was 11%

National Cancer Institute, N.I.H., Bethesda, MD 20892 and Howard University, Washington D.C. 20059

(Potter et al. 1984). This low incidence suggests that resistance to plasmacytomagenesis is a multigenic trait. It is difficult to determine how many gene differences there are between these two strains because each gene may have a different quantitative effect. If the genes controlling resistance in DBA/2 have very strong effects, then 2, or possibly 3, such genes could account for the differences. However, if each DBA/2 resistance gene has only a weak effect, many more genes may be required to establish resistance.

Because BALB/cAn mice appear to carry several recessive genes that govern susceptibility to plasmacytomagenesis it is difficult to locate susceptibility (S) genes through linkage analysis. Thus we resorted to making BALB/cAn.DBA/2 congenic strains to find DBA/2 resistance (R) genes, reasoning that the allelomorphs of R genes may be S genes. BALB/c and DBA/2 have a large number of allelic differences involving genes on almost every chromosome. We began constructing congenic strains by backcrossing single or linked genes onto the BALB/cAn background. A variable and sometimes large amount of chromatin can be introduced and maintained during introgressive backcrossing (i.e. the swept radius around the marker). Routinely markers were introduced for 6 consecutive backcrosses (N6) and then the mice were crossed to generate an N6F1 from which homozygotes were selected. If the congenic proved interesting the backcrossing was continued to N20.

Using this approach we have screened over 10 markers and found a continuum of responses (Potter and Wax 1985; Potter et al. 1984). Among the more susceptible strains were: C.D2-Idh-1,Pep-3 (N10); C.D2-Rmcf(N10) and C.D2-CC.(N10) Partially resistant strains were : C.D2-Qa2(N6), C.D2-Fv-1(N10) and C.D2-Ly6(N14) (Potter et al 1985] . The BALB/c-Ly6(N14) mouse was originally developed by Horton and Sachs(1979) at the London Hosptial Medical College and was named BALB-DAG. The DAG marker was placed on BALB/cLAC(Festenstein and Berumen 1984),however it is not clear what subline of BALB/c was used as the background strain for this congenic. However the stock we obtained from J.A. Sachs is $Qa2^-$ and $Afr-1^a$ strongly suggesting it was not BALB/cJ. We have recently begun constructing congenics with combinations of specific markers from existing congenic stocks. A congenic carrying $Qa2^+$(N6) and $Fv-1^n$(N10) was developed and is more resistant to plasmacytoma induction than either of the two single congenics. This suggests that each of these resistance genes has a weak effect, and further that BALB/cAn and DBA/2 differ by multiple genes affecting the S/R phenotype.

Finding specific markers that are linked to S/R genes may provide clues about the function of the S or R gene. However, a more practical use of these congenics is to look for relevant phenotypic differences. An important characteristic of plasmacytomas induced by pristane is the fact that virtually 100% of them have chromosomal rearrangements involving the region around the c-myc locus and one of the Ig loci (Potter 1984 for refs). We have also found that plasmacytomagenesis can be strikingly inhibited by administering the non-steroidal anti-inflammatory agent indomethacin in the drinking water (Potter et al. 1985). This result suggests that indomethacin mimics the resistant state. Indomethacin-treated mice develop oil granulomatous tissue much like untreated mice but apparantly some factor produced by the chronic inflammatory tissue is suppressed. One hypothesis is that the production of reactive oxygen intermediates and other organic radicals is inhibited in indomethacin treated mice. Essentially BALB/cAn mice may not be able to deal with DNA damage as effectively as other strains; this would increase the chances for mice of this strain to develop genetic damage leading to chromosomal rearrangements.

We (R.P and K.K.S.) have developed a cytogenetic assay system that detects differences in the ability of human and mouse cells to repair X-ray induced double-stranded DNA breaks incurred during the G2 phase of the mitotic cycle (Parshad et al. 1982;1984 Potter et al. 1988 Recently adapted skin fibroblasts are utilized as the target cells although in some experiments we have studied LPS B-lymphoblasts (Sanford et al. 1986). The cells are x-irradiated with 1Gy(100rad) and then sampled at 50 minutes and 115 minutes for the number of chromatid breaks and gaps.

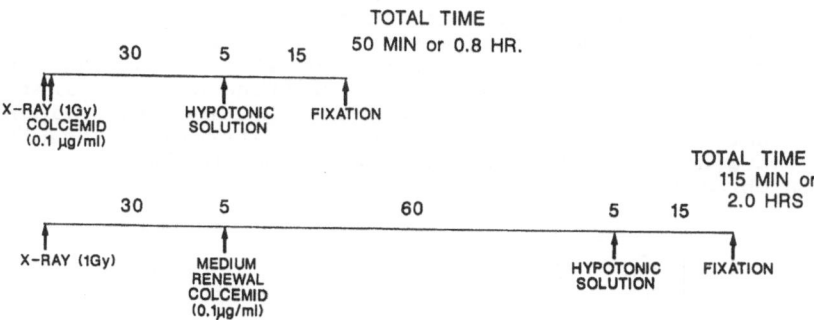

Figure 1. Protocol for the X-irradiation of Cells.

In a survey of 8 different inbred strains two phenotypes were found. The common phenotype that characterized most strains was the induction of 98 to ~110 chromatid breaks per 100 metaphases at the 50 minute post-irradiation time point followed by a reduction to 28 to 35 breaks at the 115 minute timepoint. In contrast, the cells from BALB/cAn mice had similar high numbers of chromatid breaks at the 50 minute time but by 115 minutes the number of chromatid breaks had not changed appreciably. The common phenotype was called the efficient repair phenotype while the BALB/cAn phenotype was the inefficient repair phenotype. DBA/2N and (BALB/cAn x DBA/2)F1 hybrids had efficient repair phenotypes. Accordingly, we tested the C.D2 congenic strains that had demostrated partial resistance to pristane-induced plasmacytomagenesis and found two congenics, C.D2-Idh-1,Pep-3 (N12 and N20) and C.D2-Fv-1(N10 and N19), had the efficient repair phenotype of DBA/2. A C.D2-Pep-3 mouse that had been derived from the C.D2-Idh-1,Pep-3(N19) strain by outcrossing to BALBcAn also had the DBA/2 phenotype. In contrast C.D2-Qa2+(N6), and C.D2-Ly6(N14) had the BALB/c or inefficient repair phenotype. We have tentatively named these genes Rep-1 (linked to Pep-3 on chr 1 and Rep-2 (linked to

<u>Fv-1</u> on chr 4). A summary of the results is shown in Table 1.

Table 1. Phenotypes of BALB/cAn, DBA/2N, and C.D2 congenic strains to plasmacytoma-induction and repair of chromatin damage

STRAIN	PLASMACYTOMAGENESIS	CHROMATIN REPAIR
BALB/cAnPt(C)	S	Inefficient
DBA/2N (D2)	R	Efficient
(C X D2)F1	R	Efficient
C.D2-<u>Ly6</u> (chr-15)	PR	Inefficient
C.D2-<u>Qa2+</u> (chr-17)	PR	Inefficient
C.D2-<u>Pep-3</u> (chr-1)	S	Efficient
C.D2-<u>Fv-1</u> (chr-4)	PR	Efficient

S=suceptible; R=resistant; PR=partial resistance

As may be seen, C.D2-<u>Fv-1</u> mice are partially resistant to plasmacytoma induction by pristane and have the efficient repair phenotype of DBA/2, thus suggesting that these two phenotypes are linked. Further detailed linkage studies will be necessary to establish this point. Conversely, two other strains that have partial resistance to plasmacytoma induction by pristane have the inefficient repair phenotype (i.e. C.D2-<u>Ly-6</u> and C.D2-<u>Qa2</u>). Thus the evidence suggests that one of the genes involved in determining resistance to plasmacytomagenesis may be associated with the ability to repair breaks in chromatin.

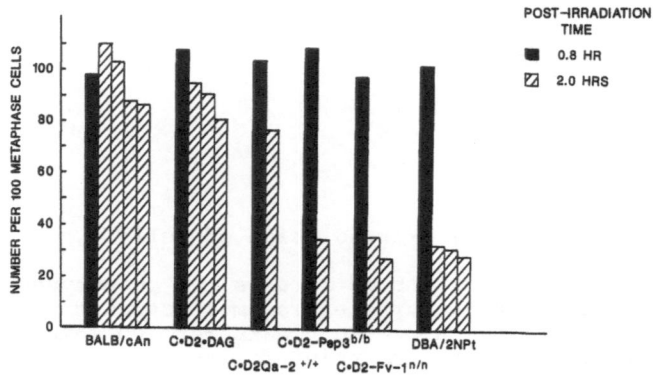

Figure 2. Chromatid Breaks in Skin Fibroblasts After G2 Phase X-irradiation (1Gy)

BALB/cAnPt and BALB/cJPt fibroblasts also differ in their responses to 1Gy X-ray. BALB/cJPt shows an efficient repair phenotype. We do not yet have evidence of linkage to any of the known markers that distinguish the BALB/c sublines.

Summary and Conclusions

The findings indicate that the C.D2-<u>Fv-1</u>(N19) mouse carries both a gene on the distal end of chr-4 that determines partial resistance to plasmacytoma development and a gene for efficient chromatin repair.

This suggests the possibility that both phenotypes are controlled by the same gene. If so, one of the genes that determines the S phenotype of BALB/cAn mice may operate by increasing the chances for the development of DNA damage that might predispose to the formation of chromosomal translocations. This must be regarded as speculative for a number of reasons. First the distal end of chr-4 contains approximately 10cM or more of DBA/2 chromatin in C.D2-Fv-1 mice. BALB/cAn and DBA/2N then could differ in several different allelomorphic genes in this region of the chromosome. Second we have not tested the C.D2-Fv-1 N19 mouse for partial resistance to plasmacytoma induction. The C.D2-Fv-1 N10 mouse did express partial resistance but during continued backcrossing the C.D2 Fv-1(N19) mouse no longer had the DBA/2 allele of Mmtv-13. Thus, it is possible that the plasmacytoma R gene could be more closely linked to the Mmtv-13 locus and hence is no longer present in the N19 mouse.

The working hypothesis is that the inefficient repair phenotype is associated with an inability to correct double stranded DNA breaks. The assay system we have employed specifically examines chromatid breaks that are a result of double-stranded DNA breaks incurred during G2 phase of the cell cycle. While the assay system only determines the capability for repair during G2, similar lesions that develop in other stages of the cell cycle may also be inefficiently repaired. Chromatid breaks that are unrepaired in G2 may lead to lethality during subsequent mitoses if significant losses of DNA are sustained. If, however, double-stranded breaks occur in different chromosomes that happen to be neighbors during G1 to S phase then other factors may promote illegitimate recombinations such as are seen in reciprocal translocations. The primary effect of the inefficient Rep allele may be to delay normal repair processes and permit the formation of illegitimate recombination.

The data summarized here suggests that there may be multiple genes in the mouse that affect the efficiency of DNA repair and susceptibility to pristane induced plasmacytoma formation. We have a C.D2 congenic mouse that coincidently has the phenotype of partial resistance to plasmacytoma induction and efficient repair of X-ray induced chromatid breaks. Further analysis will be required to determine if these are controlled by the same or different genes.

References

Blankenhorn, E.P., Duncan, R., Huppi, K., and Potter, M. (1988) Chromosomal location of the regulator of mouse alphafetoprotein Afr-1. Genetics, in press.

Blankenhorn, E.p., Wax, J.s., Matthai, R., and Potter, M. (1985) Genetic analysis of alphafetoprotein levels in BALB/c sublines. Current Topics in Microbiology and Immunology 122: 53-57.

Duncan, R., Matthai, R., Huppi, K., Roderick, T., and Potter, M. Genes that modify the expression of major urinary proteins. (Submitted)

Horton, M.A., and Sachs, J.A. (1979) Identity of murine lymphocyte alloantigens DAG, ALA-1, Ly-8 ,and Ly-6? Immunogenetics 9: 273-280.

Huppi, K., Duncan, R., and Potter, M. (1988) Myc-1 is centromeric

294

to the linkage group Ly-6-Sis--Gdc-1 on mouse chromosome 15.
Immunogenetics in press.

Mock, B.A., Givol, D., D'Hoostelaere, L.A.D., Huppi, K., Seldin, M.F., Gurfinkel, N., Unger, T., Potter, M., and Mushinski, J.F. (1988) Mapping of the bcl-2 oncogene on mouse chromosome 1. Cytogenet. Cell. Genet. 47:in press.

Parshad, R., Gantt, R., Sanford, K.K., Jones, G.M., and Tarone, R.E. (1982) Repair of chromosome damage induced by x-irradiation during G2 phase in a line of normal human fibroblasts and its malignant derivative. J. Natl. Cancer Inst. 69: 409-414.

Parshad, R., Gantt, R., Sanford, K.K., and Jones, G.M., (1984) Chromosomal radiosensitivity of human tumor cells during the G2 cell cycle period. Cancer Res. 44: 5577-5582.

Potter, M. (1984) Genetics of susceptibility to plasmacytoma development in BALB/c mice. Cancer Surveys 3: 247-264.

Potter, M. (1985) History of the BALB/c Family. Current Topics in Microbiology and Immunology 122: 1-5.

Potter, M., Hartley, J.W., Wax, J.S., and Gallahan, D. (1984) Effect of MuLV-related genes on plasmacytomagenesis in BALB/c mice. J. Exp. Med. 160: 435-440.

Potter, M., O'Brien, A.D., Skamene, E., Gros, P., Forget, A., Kongshavn, P.A.L. and Wax, J.S. (1983) A BALB/c congenic strain of mice that carries a genetic locus (Ity^r) controlling resistance to intracellular parasites. Infection and Immunity 40: 1234-1235.

Potter, M. and Wax, J.S. (1981) Genetics of susceptibility to pristane-induced plasmacytomas in BALB/cAn: Reduced susceptibility in BALB/cJ with a brief description of pristane-induced arthritis. J. Immunol. 127:1591-1595.

Potter, M. and Wax J.S. (1983) Peritoneal plasmacytomagenesis in mice: comparison of different pristane dose regimens. J. Natl. Can. Inst. 71: 391-395.

Potter,M., and Wax J.S. (1985) Role of genes in the susceptibility to plasmacytomas. In Genetic Control of Host Resistance to Infection and Malignancy pp. 793-804 E. Skamene (Ed) Alan R. Liss New York

Potter, M., Wax, J.S., Anderson, A.O., and Nordan, R.P. (1985) Inhibition of plasmacytoma development in BALB/c Mice by indomethacin. J. Exp. Med. 161: 996-1012.

Roderick T.H., Langley S.H. and Leiter E.H. (1985) Some unusual genetic characterisitics of BALB/c and evidence for genetic variation among BALB/c substrains. Current Topics in Microbiol. and Immunol. 122: 9-18.

Sanford, K.K., Parshad, R., Potter, M., Jones, G.M., Nordan, R.P., Brust, S.E., and Price, F.M. (1986) Chromosomal radiosensitivity during G2 phase and susceptibility to plasmacytoma induction in mice. Current Topics in Microbiology and Immunology, 132: 202-208.

A Molecular Characterization of BALB/c Congenic C.D2-*Idh-1*^{b}, *Lsh*^{r}, *Rep-1*^{b}, *Pep-3*^{b} Mice

B. Mock and M. Potter

INTRODUCTION

The region of murine chromosome 1 surrounding the biochemical markers, Idh-1 and Pep-3 (band C) contains segments of homology with genes on human chromosomes 1, 2 and 18 (Lalley and McKusick 1985; Mock et al., in press). This 27 cM region of chromatin contains sites of endogenous proviral loci (Emv-16,17; Buchberg et al., 1986), an oncogene (bcl-2; Mock et al., 1987; in press) which, in man, is consistently rearranged in follicular lymphomas (Bakshi et al., 1985; Cleary and Sklar 1985; Tsujimoto et al., 1985), a cytolytic T-cell associated sequence (Ctla-4; Brunet et al., 1987) and genes involved in the serum complement system (Cfh and C4bp; Seldin in press; D'Eustachio et al. 1986), murine embryogenesis (En-1; Joyner et al. 1985), muscle development (Myl-1; Robert et al. 1984), the repair of chromatin breaks (Rep-1, Potter et al. in press) and the resistance/ susceptibility to Leishmania (Lsh, Bradley et al. 1979), Salmonella (Ity, Plant and Glynn 1976; Taylor and O'Brien 1982) and Mycobacterium (Bcg, Gros et al. 1981).

BALB/c and DBA/2 mice have been found to differ in in vivo susceptibility to visceral leishmaniasis, salmonellosis and leprosy (Potter et al. 1983). In addition, their fibroblasts have also been found to differ in vitro with respect to their ability to repair radiation-induced breaks in chromatin (Potter et al. in press). The focus of this study was to characterize, by restriction fragment length polymorphism (RFLP) analysis, the swept radius of the region of DBA/2 chromatin introgressively backcrossed onto the BALB/c background during the production of a series of chromosome 1 congenics which have been used to study these in vivo and in vitro responses.

MATERIALS AND METHODS

Construction of the C.D2 Congenic Strains. A series of chromosome 1 congenics were developed by the introgressive backcrossing of DBA/2N genes onto a BALB/cAnPt background (Potter et al. 1983). The C.D2-Idh-1^b, Pep-3^b congenic was derived through the selection of DBA/2N alleles for Idh-1 and Pep-3 at each backcross generation. After the seventh, twelfth and twentieth introgressive backcross generations (N7, 12 and 20), the mice were made homozygous for Idh-1^b and Pep-3^b. At each of these generations, the mice were tested for susceptibility to S. typhimurium (Alison O'Brien), L. donovani (P. Kongshavn, J. Blackwell, B. Mock) and Mycobacterium bovis (P. Gros, E. Skamene) and found to carry the r (resistant) allele of DBA/2 origin. The C.D2-Idh-1^b, Ity^r congenic was derived from the N6 backcross generation during the production of the C.D2-Idh-1^b, Pep-3^b strain and carries the BALB/c a allele for Pep-3. Similarly, the C.D2-Pep-3^b strain was also derived from the C.D2-Idh-1^b, Pep-3^b strain at backcross generation N21. Both the C.D2-Idh-1^b, Pep-3^b and C.D2-Pep-3^b congenic strains were found to carry the DBA/2 b allele for Rep-1, a gene involved in the efficient repair of chromatin breaks (Potter et al. in press, CTMI, this volume). Two other chromosome 1 congenics were derived independently. They were selected for Idh-1^b only

Laboratory of Genetics, Building 37, Room 2B-21, NCI, NIH, Bethesda, MD 20892

(C.D2-Idh-1[b]) and Pep-3[b], Akp-1[b] (C.D2-Pep-3[b], Akp-1[b]). These congenics were produced and maintained under NCI contract N01-CB-71085 at Hazleton Laboratories (Rockville, MD).

Gel electrophoresis, DNA Transfer and Hybridization. High molecular weight DNAs prepared from mouse livers or kidneys were digested for 5-7 h with restriction endonucleases and electrophoretically separated on 0.7% horizontal agarose gels at voltage gradients of approximately 1 V/cm in 40 mM Tris-acetate, 20 mM sodium acetate, 1 mM EDTA, pH 7.4. After staining with ethidium bromide and photography under UV light, gels were blotted onto nitrocellulose for 20 h and then hybridized for 16 h with probe inserts which were labeled with ^{32}P-dCTP by nick translation to specific activities of 1-2 x 10^8 cpm/ μg. After hybridization, filters were rinsed in 3XSSC, washed in 1XSSC at 65°C for 10 min and subsequently washed for 30 min in 0.2XSSC at 65°C. Filters hybridized to the Fn probe were washed with a final stringency of 0.2XSSC at 55°C for 30 min.

Hybridization Probes. The mouse Myl-1 cDNA probe (pGLC101) was a 450 bp EcoRI-Hind III fragment (Robert et al. 1984). The mouse Ctla-4 cDNA probe (F41F4) was subcloned into the Pst I site of puc 9 (Brunet et al. 1987) and the 2.0 kb Hind III-EcoRI fragment was used in this study. The mouse Cryg cDNA probe (pMγ2) was a 614 bp Pst I insert (Breitman et al. 1984). The mouse bcl-2 cDNA probe (Ncm4) was a 1.4 kb EcoRI-Hind III insert (Gurfinkel et al. 1987). The mouse Ren-1,2 cDNA probe (pDD-1D2) was a 1.4 kb Pst I insert (Field et al. 1984). The mouse Ly-17 cDNA probe [γ2b/γ1 FcRα (J774)] was a 1.3 kb Pst I insert (Ravetch et al. 1986).

RESULTS AND DISCUSSION

The RFLPs which were established for BALB/cAnPt and DBA/2N genomic DNAs upon hybridization with various chromosome 1 probes is illustrated in Table 1. The extent of DBA/2N chromatin present in the various chromosome 1 congenics, as determined by RFLP analysis, is presented in Table 2 and Fig. 1.

Table 1. RFLPs observed between BALB/cAnPt and DBA/2N DNAs, restricted with the indicated enzyme, upon hybridization with inserts of various cDNAs localized to mouse chromosome 1

| Probe for | Enzyme | Restriction fragment (kb) | |
		BALB/cAnPt	DBA/2N
Myl-1	BamHI	2.3	--
Ctla-4	XbaI	18.0	10.0
Cryg	EcoRI	5.2	5.0
bcl-2	XbaI	5.0	5.8
Ren-1,2	EcoRI	--	4.3
Ly-17	BamHI	9.8	9.4

Table 2. The allelic composition of C.D2 congenics for a variety of chromosome 1 loci. Isozyme analyses for Idh-1 and Pep-3 were performed by Hazleton Laboratories and Animal Genetic Systems. In vivo susceptibility to intracellular pathogens was determined by Potter et al. (1983). In vitro ability to repair chromatin damage was assessed by Potter et al. (in press). The presence (D), absence (C) of DBA/2 chromatin in the C.D2 congenics, for the remainder of the chromosome 1 loci indicated, was determined by RFLP analysis.

Strain	Ctla-4	Myl-1	Cryg	Idh-1	Bcg Ity Lsh	bcl-2	Rep-1	Ren-1,2	Pep-3	Ly-17
BALB/cAnPt	C	C	C	C	C	C	C	C	C	C
DBA/2N	D	D	D	D	D	D	D	D	D	D
C.D2-Idh-1	D	D	D	D	C	C	-	C	C	C
C.D2-Idh-1,Ity	C	D	D	D	D	D	-	C	C	C
C.D2-Idh-1,Pep-3	C	D	D	D	D	D	D	D	D	C
C.D2-Pep-3	C	C	C	C	D	-	D	D	D	C
C.D2-Pep-3,Akp-1	C	C	-	C	-	D	-	D	D	D

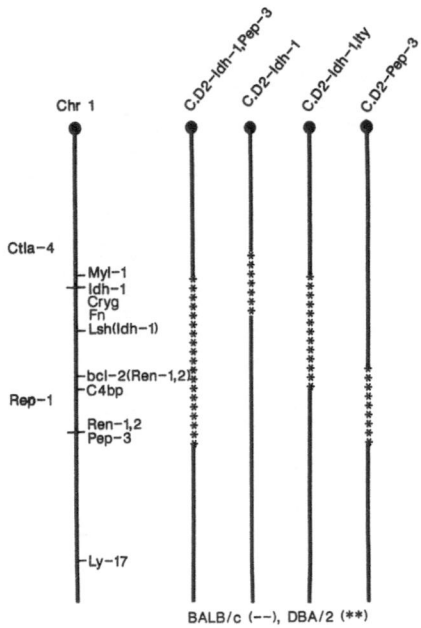

Fig. 1. The swept radius of
DBA/2N chromatin intro-
gressively backcrossed onto
the BALB/cAnPt background
during the production of a
series of C.D2 chromosome 1
congenics. Relative distances
between loci are based on
Davisson and Roderick (1986)
Mock et al. (1987), Seldin
et al. (1987) and unpublished
data (Mock and Seldin).

Both the in vivo susceptibility to infection with a set of diverse intracellular pathogens and the in vitro inefficiency in repair of radiation-induced
chromatin damage exhibited by BALB/cAn macrophages and fibroblasts, respectively,
provide interesting phenotypes to characterize molecularly. We have been interested in identifying RFLPs which could be useful in reverse genetic approaches
to isolating these two genes (Lsh and Rep-1) which reside on mouse chromosome 1
and have not been characterized at the molecular or protein product level.

The initial molecular characterization of the C.D2 congenics in this study
provides a basis for establishing a molecular map of murine chromosome 1, band C.
We have generated a few hundred backcross progeny from a cross between C.D2-Idh-
1$^{a/b}$, Lsh$^{r/s}$, Rep-1$^{a/b}$, Pep-3$^{a/b}$ N22 and BALB/cAnPt (Idh-1$^{a/a}$, Lsh$^{s/s}$, Rep-1$^{a/a}$,
Pep-3$^{a/a}$) mice to examine the extent of allelic consegregation of molecular
markers with Lsh and Rep-1 phenotypes. These studies will provide a detailed
multipoint linkage analysis of recombination rates between a number of chromosome
1 loci in this 27 cM region.

Acknowledgements

We thank David Givol, Pierre Golstein, Kenneth Gross, Joram Piatigorsky,
Jeffrey Ravetch and Benoit Robert for hybridization probes, Naomi Ruff and John
Shaughnessy for technical assistance, Judith Wax, Linda Byrd, Roberta Matthai,
Simon Leath and Richard Bamford for the production and maintenance of mice, Jean-Louis
Guenet and Jenefer Blackwell for helpful discussions and Victoria Rogers for typing
the manuscript.

REFERENCES

Bakhshi A, Jensen JP, Goldman P, Wright JJ, McBride OW, Epstein AL, Korsmeyer SJ (1985). Cloning the chromosomal breakpoint of t(14;18) human lymphomas: clustering around J_H on chromosome 14 and hear a transcriptional unit 18. Cell 41: 899-906.

Bradley DJ, Taylor BA, Blackwell JM, Evans EP, Freeman J (1979) Regulation of Leishmania populations within the host, III. Mapping of the locus controlling susceptibility to visceral leishmaniasis in the mouse. Clin. Exp. Immunol. 37: 7-14.

Breitman ML, Lok S, Wistow G, Piatigorsky J, Treton JA, Gold RJM, Tsui L-C (1984) γ -Crystallin family of the mouse lens: Structural and evolutionary relationships PNAS 81: 7762-7766.

Brunet J-F, Benijot F, Luciani M-F, Roux-Dosseto M, Suzan M, Mattei M-G, Golstein P (1987) A new member of immunoglobulin superfamily CTLA-4. Nature 328: 267-270.

Buchberg AM, Taylor BA, Jenkins NA, Copeland NG (1986) Chromosomal localization of Emv-16 and Emv-17, two closely linked ecotropic proviruses of RF/J mice. J. Virol. 60: 1175-1178.

Cleary ML, Sklar J (1985) Nucleotide sequence of a t(14;18) chromosomal breakpoint in follicular lymphoma and demonstration of a breakpoint-cluster region near a transcriptionally active locuson chromosome 18. PNAS, USA 82: 7439-7443.

Davisson MT, Roderick TH (1986) Linkage map of the mouse. Mouse News Lett. 75: 12-15.

D'Eustachio P, Kristensen T, Wetsel RA, Riblet R, Taylor B, Tack BF (1986) Chromosomal location of the genes encoding complement components C5 and factor H in the mouse. J Immunol 137: 3990-3995.

Field LJ, McGowan RA, Dickinson DP, Gross KW (1984) Tissue and gene specificity of mouse renin expression. Hypertension 6: 597-603.

Gros P, Skamene E, Forget AJ (1981) Genetic control of natural resistance to Mycobacterium bovis (BCG) in mice. J. Immunol. 127: 2417-2421.

Gurfinkel N, Unger T, Givol D, Mushinski JF (1987) Expression of the bcl-2 gene in mouse B lymphocytic cell lines is differentiation stage specific. Eur. J. Immunol. 17: 567-570.

Joyner AL, Kornberg T, Coleman KG, Cox DR, Martin GR (1985) Expression during embryogenesis of a mouse gene with sequence homology to the Drosophila engrailed gene. Cell 43: 29-37.

Lalley PA, McKusick VA (1985) Report of the committee on comparative mapping. Eighth International Workshop on Human Gene Mapping. Cytogenet. Cell Genet. 40: 536-566.

Mock BA, Givol D, D'Hoostelaere LA, Huppi K, Gurfinkel N, Unger T, Potter M, Mushinski JF (1988) Mapping of the bcl-2 oncogene on mouse chromosome 1. Cytogenet. Cell Genet. 47: in press.

Mock BA, Givol D, D'Hoostelaere LA, Huppi K, Gurfinkel N, Unger T, Potter M, Mushinski JF (1987) Mapping of the mouse bcl-2 gene. Mouse News Lett. 78: 63.

Plant JE, Glynn A (1976) Genetics of resistance to infection with Salmonella typhimurium in mice. J. Infect. Dis. 133: 72-78

Potter M, O'Brien AD, Skamene E, Gros P, Forget A, Kongshavn PAL, Wax JS (1983) A BALB/c congenic strain of mice that carries a genetic locus (Ity^r) controlling resistance to intracellular parasites. Infect. Immunity 40: 1234-1235.

Potter M, Sanford KK, Parshad R, Tarone RE, Price FM, Mock B, Huppi K (1988) Genes on chromosomes 1 and 4 in the mouse are associated with repair of radiation-induced chromatin damage. Genomics, in press.

Ravetch JV, Luster AD, Weinshank R, Kochan J, Pavlovec A, Portnoy DA, Hulmes J, Pan Y-CE, Unkeless, JC (1986) Structural heterogeneity and functional domains of murine immunoglobulin G Fc receptors. Science 234: 718-725.

Robert B, Daubas P, Akimenko M-A, Cohen A, Garner I, Guenet J-L, Buckingham M (1984) A single locus in the mouse encodes both myosin light chains 1 and 3, a second locus corresponds to a related pseudogene. Cell 39: 129-140.

Seldin MF, Morse HC, D'Hoostelaere LA, Britten JL, Steinberg AD (1987) Mapping of alpha-spectrin on distal mouse chromosome 1. Cytogenet Cell Genet 45: 52-54.

Seldin MF, Morse HC, Reeves JP, Scribner CL, LeBoeuf RC, Steinberg AD (1988) Genetic analysis of "autoimmune" gld mice: I. Identification of a restriction fragment length polymorphism closely linked to the gld mutation within a conserved linkage group. J. Exp. Med., in press.

Taylor BA, O'Brien AD (1982) Position on mouse chromosome 1 of a gene that controls resistance to Salmonella typhimurium. Infect. Immunity. 36: 1257-1260.

Tsujimoto Y, Cossman J, Jaffe E, Croce CM (1985) Involvement of the bcl-2 gene in human follicular lymphoma. Science 228: 1440-1443.

Analysis of *Lsh* Gene Expression in Congenic B10.L-*Lsh*^r Mice

J.M. Blackwell, S. Toole, M. King, P. Dawda, T.I.A. Roach, and A. Cooper

INTRODUCTION

Although it has been the subject of continued investigation by several laboratories over the past decade, the macrophage resistance gene (Lsh/Ity/Bcg), located between Idh-1 and Pep-3 on mouse chromosome 1, enters its second decade without having been characterized either at the level of a protein gene product or at the mRNA/DNA level. While the different laboratories have all at one time or another recognised the potential importance of the gene as a natural resistance mechanism operating against a broad range of phylogenetically distinct macrophage pathogens, recent observations that a cluster of linked genes including Idh-1 (Narahara et al., 1985), Myl-1 (Robert et al., 1985), fibronectin (Jhanwar et al., 1986), villin (Rousseau-Merck et al., 1988), collagen (COL3A1, COL5A2, COL6A3) (Weil et al., 1988), glucagon (Schroeder et al., 1984), elastin (Emanuel et al., 1985), acetylcholine receptor (Heidmann et al., 1986) and gamma-crystallin (Len-1) (Shiloh et al., 1986) have been conserved onto the long arm of human chromosome 2 (around 2q31–qter) has refuelled interest in identification of an Lsh gene homologue in man. In 1975 we commenced production of a congenic mouse strain bearing the Lsh resistant allele from C57L mice on a C57BL/10ScSn (=B10) genetic background. This strain we hoped would one day be useful in characterization of the gene/gene product at the molecular level. This meeting provides an opportunity for us to describe production and initial characterization of the strain, and to review its use in functional analysis of Lsh gene expression at the cellular level. Some new data on T cell-independent macrophage activation events are presented which suggest that these studies may yet provide the functional basis for identification of a gene product and/or characterization of the gene at the DNA level.

PRODUCTION OF THE B10.L-Lsh^r STRAIN

To produce the B10.L-Lsh^r strain, the resistant allele from C57L mice was transposed onto the genetic background of C57BL/10ScSn (=B10) mice by repeated backcrossing of heterozygous resistant male progeny to homozygous Lsh^s female B10 mice. Selection of the male parents for each successive backcross was made retrospectively since the mice had to be infected and killed 15 days later to determine their genotype. Although the C57L strain carried alternative alleles for the two linked loci Idh-1 and ln, these were never used in choosing parents for the next generation. Idh-1 typing was used, however, to monitor progress

Department of Tropical Hygiene, London School of Hygiene and Tropical Medicine, Keppel Street, London WC1E 7HT, U.K.

Current Topics in Microbiology and Immunology, Vol. 137
© Springer-Verlag Berlin · Heidelberg 1988

in production of the congenic strain at generations 9 and 10 of
backcrossing (Table 1). After 10 generations (=N10) of
backcrossing, heterozygous mice (determined by test-crossing to
B10 mice and typing a minimum of 10-12 progeny per cross) were
crossed with each other and the homozygous resistant progeny
(determined by further test crosses) mated together to obtain a
homozygous $\underline{Lsh}^r$ line on the B10 genetic background. Typing for
$\underline{Idh-1}$ and $\underline{ln}$ in congenic mice confirmed that, in the generation
10 mice chosen to produce the congenic strain, the C57L alleles
had been replaced by B10 alleles at least to distances within 6
centimorgans (cM) proximal and 8 cM distal to $\underline{Lsh}$ respectively.
However, the fact that (a) 37% of heterozygous $\underline{Lsh}^{r/s}$ generation
10 backcross progeny still carried a C57L allele at $\underline{Idh-1}$ (Table
1), and (b) one out of six ($\underline{Lsh}^{r/s}$ x $\underline{Lsh}^{r/s}$) N10 selfings gave
homozygous $\underline{ln}$ offspring, suggests that the break points were very
close to the two linked marker genes. On theoretical grounds
(Johnson, 1981), there is 39 to 63% probability that the segment
of chromosome transferred includes genes within 5 to 10 cM on
either side of the $\underline{Lsh}$ gene. The 14 cM segment actually
transferred is a close approximation to this. The N10 congenic
strain and further generations of backcross progeny are currently
being typed for a much larger range of linked markers by analysis
of restriction fragment length polymorphisms (RFLPs) (B. Mock and
J.M. Blackwell).

Table 1. Proportion of heterozygous $\underline{Lsh}^{r/s}$ N9 and N10 progeny
carrying B10 ($\underline{Idh-1}^a$) versus C57L ($\underline{Idh-1}^b$) alleles at $\underline{Idh-1}$
during production of the congenic B10.L-$\underline{Lsh}^r$ strain.

Generation	$Idh-1^{a/a}$	$Idh-1^{a/b}$	Total
9	10(0.30)	23(0.70)	33
10	17(0.63)	10(0.37)	27

CELLULAR ASPECTS OF $\underline{Lsh}$ GENE EXPRESSION

Work from several laboratories (reviewed Blackwell, 1985) has
shown that expression of $\underline{Lsh}/\underline{Ity}/\underline{Bcg}$ resistance against
Leishmania donovani, Salmonella typhimurium, or Mycobacterium
bovis, does not require a functional T cell population and can be
transferred with the donor haematopoietic system in reciprocal
radiation bone marrow chimaeras. Using the L. donovani infection
model and the B10.L-$\underline{Lsh}^r$ strain (or phenotypically resistant
(B10xB10.L-$\underline{Lsh}^r$)F1 mice) we have published the following
observations on Lsh gene expression in vivo and in vitro:-

1. In terms of microbistatic activity against the parasite, the
gene is expressed most clearly at the level of the infected
resident tissue macrophage (e.g. Kupffer cells of the liver) and
is poorly expressed in immature macrophage populations (e.g.
monocytes; resident peritoneal macrophages) (Crocker et al.,
1987).

2. There is a 2-3 day time lag in expression of resistance in vivo and in vitro, i.e. parasites multiply equally well in susceptible and resistant liver macrophages for the first 2-3 days after infection (Crocker et al., 1984; 1987).

3. Resistance is enhanced in vivo by prior administration of small doses of S. typhimurium lipopolysaccharide or purified L. donovani membranes (Crocker et al., 1984) suggesting that expression of resistance involves T cell-independent macrophage priming/activation pathways.

4. Differential responses to activation signals can be measured in terms of enhanced Ia expression on splenic adherent cells isolated from resistant mice within the first week of infection, and in 3-day rested peritoneal macrophages activated with recombinant interferon gamma in vitro (Kaye et al., 1988).

5. Splenic adherent cells from naive resistant and susceptible mice stimulate equivalent mixed lymphocyte responses across H-2 barriers and equivalent antigen specific secondary proliferation of T cells from day 7 infected B10 mice. Splenic adherent cells from day 7 infected resistant mice stimulate higher antigen-specific proliferative responses both on a cell per cell basis and in terms of antigen concentration compared to splenic adherent cells from similarly infected susceptible mice (Kaye et al. , 1988).

With respect to these various pleiotropic effects of T cell-independent macrophage activation, similar observations have been made by Skamene and coworkers (reviewed in this volume) using the M. bovis infection model. One question which has always intrigued us is how the three phylogenetically unrelated microorganisms, L. donovani, S. typhimurium, and M. bovis, stimulate expression of this T cell-independent macrophage activation.

CR3-MEDIATED T CELL-INDEPENDENT MACROPHAGE ACTIVATION

Recent studies by Wright and coworkers (Ding et al., 1987; Wright and Detmers, 1988) suggest that the family of adhesion promoting receptor molecules, CR3, LFA-1, and p150,95, might not only control targeting of macrophages to sites of infection, but may also regulate T cell-independent macrophage priming/activation. Each of these cell surface dimeric glycoprotein molecules has a distinct alpha chain (150-190 kD) but they share a common beta chain (95 kD). Our own demonstration that CR3 was involved in binding Leishmania to macrophages (Blackwell et al., 1985), probably via an LPS-like glycolipid molecule on the parasite surface (Handman and Goding, 1985; Cooper et al., 1988), together with the observation that the lipid A portion of bacterial LPS binds to all members of the receptor family (Wright and Jong, 1986), tempted us to speculate that this family of molecules might mediate T cell-independent macrophage activation in resistant mice in response to infection. This was coupled with the tantalizing possibility that the clustering of linked genes encoding extracellular matrix proteins (e.g. fibronectin), which bind to other members of the larger integrin family of receptors and, in the case of fibronectin, activate CR3 (Wright et al.,

304

1984), might have some functional relevance to <u>Lsh</u> gene expression. This might, for example, explain the differential expression of <u>Lsh</u> resistance in resident tissue macrophages compared to immature macrophage populations (Crocker et al., 1987). In pursuing this line of thought we have made the following preliminary observations:

1. Since the beta chain of the adhesion promoting receptor family had already been mapped elsewhere (human 21, Marlin et al., 1986), we first considered whether <u>Lsh</u> resistance might result from a polymorphism in the alpha chain of CR3. Immunoprecipitation of CR3 from B10 and (B10xB10.L-<u>Lsh</u>^{r})F1 using two different anti-CR3 monoclonal antibodies, M1/70 (Beller et al., 1982) and 5C6 (Rosen and Gordon, 1987), failed to show any protein polymorphism on 1-D SDS PAGE analysis (T.I.A. Roach and J.M. Blackwell, unpublished). This is being pursued at the protein level by 2-D SDS PAGE analysis (T.I.A. Roach) and at the DNA level by analysis of RFLPs using alpha chain specific probes (B. Mock and J.M. Blackwell).

2. The anti-CR3 mAb M1/70, which in our hands inhibits lectin-like complement-independent binding of peanut agglutanin (PNA) negative stationary phase promastigotes of <u>Leishmania</u> to the LPS binding site of CR3 (Cooper et al., 1988), has been employed in 48 hour activation experiments (Ding et al., 1987) using resident peritoneal macrophages from B10(<u>Lsh</u>^{s}) and (B10xB10.L-<u>Lsh</u>^{r})F1 mice. Figure 1 shows that, at low doses of M1/70 (3ug/ml),

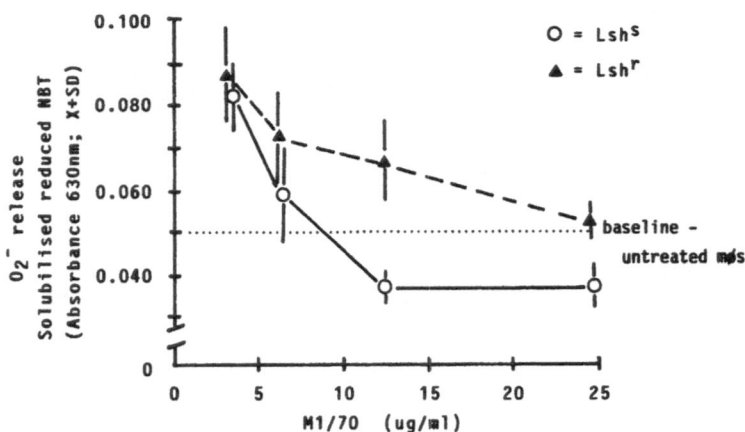

Fig. 1. PMA-elicited O_2^- release in resident peritoneal macrophages from B10(<u>Lsh</u>^{s}) (o) and (B10 x B10.L-<u>Lsh</u>^{r})F1 (▲) mice activated for 48 hours with increasing concentrations of M1/70. Equivalent numbers of cells (10^6/well) were plated into 96 well tissue culture plates in RPMI 1640 containing 10% heat inactivated low endotoxin foetal calf serum (Gibco Biocult Ltd). Non adherent cells were removed after 1 hour and M1/70 added to test wells. PMA-elicited O_2^- release was measured 48 hours later by the method of Rook et al. (1985). Results show mean $\pm$ S.D. for six wells per treatment.

macrophages from the two strains respond equally in terms of PMA-elicited superoxide anion release following activation.
Interestingly, high doses of M1/70 apparently depress activation and do so more efficiently in Lsh^S macrophages. Dose-dependence required to reach maximal activation at lower concentrations of M1/70 requires further examination. In terms of antileishmanial activity, 48 hour activation with 5ug/ml M1/70 followed by amastigote infection results in a transient (between 1 hour and 24 hours post infection) reduction in amastigote numbers in M1/70 activated (B10xB10.L-Lsh^r)F1 macrophages but not in macrophages from B10(Lsh^S) mice (Fig. 2).

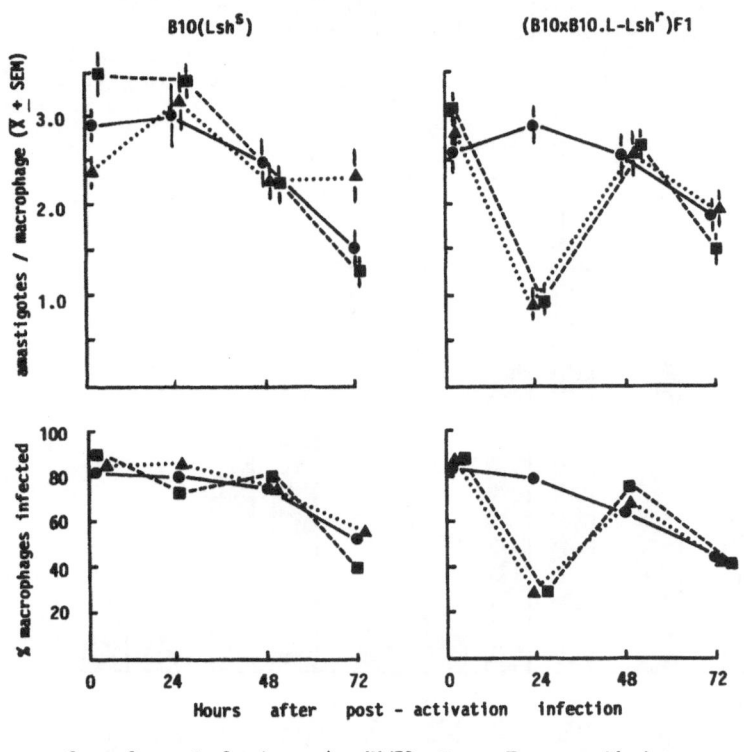

Fig. 2. Shows amastigotes per macrophage and % macrophages infected in control peritoneal macrophages (●) or in macrophges activated for 48 hours with 5ug/ml M1/70 (▲) or 10^5/well PNA negative L. donovani promastigotes (■). After the 48 hour activation period, cells were infected with 10^6 amastigotes/well for 1 hour, washed and examined (MtOH/Giemsa) at time points as indicated. Promastigote activated macrophages had zero background parasite counts at the time of amastigote infection. A minimum of 100 macrophages was scored on duplicate coverslip preparations examined per treatment per time point.

These results are interesting for two reasons. Firstly, this is the first evidence we have for Lsh gene controlled antileishmanial activity in resident peritoneal macrophages. Secondly, the antileishmanial activity is manifest at least in part as cidal activity since many digested parasites are seen in the macrophages at the 24 hour time point. Nevertheless, the rise in parasites per macrophage and percent macrophages infected thereafter almost certainly results from lysis and reinfection since the fastest doubling times observed even in susceptible mice are usually around 48 hours (Crocker et al., 1984). These experiments are currently being repeated with infection followed in the continuous presence of the activating signal (M1/70).

3. In parallel with M1/70 activation experiments, resident peritoneal macrophages from B10(Lsh^s) and (B10xB10.L-Lsh^r)F1 mice were also activated with recombinant interferon gamma and with low numbers (<1 parasite/macrophage) of logarithmic (>80% PNA +ve) or stationary (<20% PNA +ve) phase L. donovani promastigotes (Fig. 3). As mentioned, binding of PNA negative stationary phase

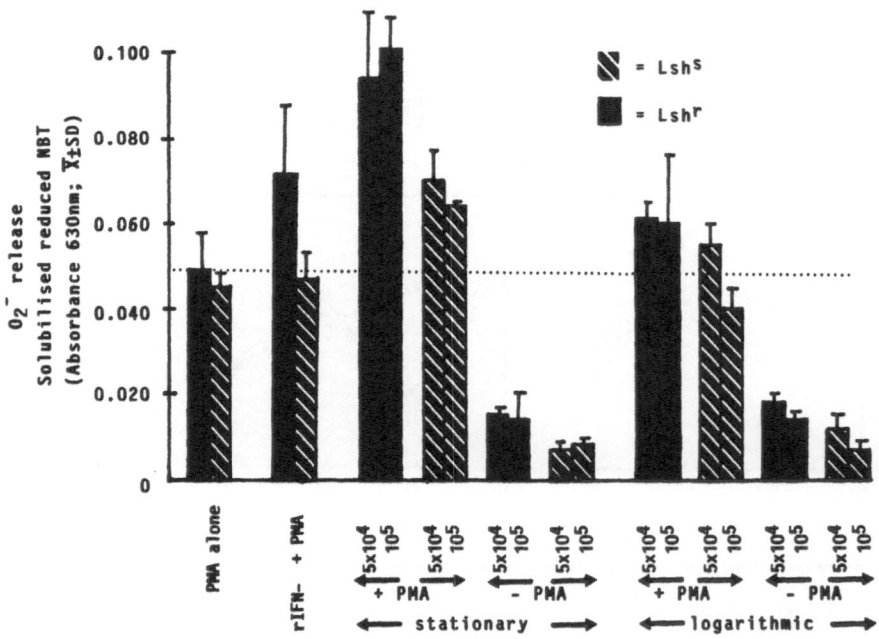

Fig. 3. PMA-elicited O_2^- release in resident peritoneal macrophages from B10(Lsh^s) (◨) and (B10 x B10.L-Lsh^r)F1 (■) mice activated for 48 hours with recombinant interferon gamma (100U/ml), or cultures of <20% or >80% PNA positive promastigotes (5x10^4 or 10^5/well), as indicated. Cell culture and assay conditions as per fig. 1.

parasites appears to be via the M1/70 inhibitable LPS binding site of CR3 whereas binding of logarithmic PNA positive parasites is via 5C6 and sodium salicyl hydroxamate inhibitable complement-mediated binding to the iC3b binding site on the CR3 molecule (Cooper et al., 1988). Logarithmic phase parasites failed to activate either macrophage population in terms of PMA-induced superoxide anion release (Fig. 3), whereas stationary phase organisms differentially activated resistant macrophages both in terms of superoxide anion release (Fig. 3) and for antileishmanial activity (Fig. 2). Resistant macrophages also responded better to recombinant interferon gamma than macrophages from susceptible mice (Fig. 3).

4. Since resistant macrophages respond differentially to a range of activation signals including interferon gamma it is likely that Lsh gene control of the macrophage priming/activation process is at a level subsequent to ligand binding to activation receptors. The fact that resident Kupffer cells express Lsh gene activity against Leishmania more efficiently than any other macrophage population examined (Crocker et al., 1987) and yet do not express CR3 on their surface (Flotte et al., 1985) also suggests that CR3 may not be the only member of the adhesion/activation promoting receptor family which might mediate differential T cell-independent priming/activation of resistant macrophages. To get a handle of some of the biochemical events subsequent to ligand (M1/70, parasite)-mediated activation we are currently examining PMA-induced and particle/parasite induced myristoylation and phosphorylation of proteins in macrophages (peritoneal, Kupffer cells) from resistant and susceptible mice. In earlier studies Aderem and coworkers (1986) have shown that LPS, PMA and zymosan induce myristoylation of specific macrophage proteins (e.g. the catalytic subunit of the cAMP-dependent protein kinase and possibly protein kinase C) involved in the priming signal. Wright and Detmers (1988) have also observed phosphorylation of CR3 itself as the receptor becomes activated.

CONCLUSIONS

Studies presented here span a decade of work pursuing molecular characterization of the Lsh/Ity/Bcg macrophage resistance gene by functionally relevant analysis of its expression in vivo and in vitro. Although at an early stage, some of our own and others observations on binding characteristics of Leishmania glycolipid molecules and bacterial LPS-like molecules to adhesion and activation-promoting macrophage receptors, which we here show results in differential activation of Lsh resistant and susceptible macrophages, encourages us to believe that we may finally be making some progress towards uncovering the Lsh resistance mechanism at the cellular/protein level. This we hope will parallel studies at the DNA level such that transcribed proteins from any putative cloned gene can be functionally verified as the Lsh gene product.

ACKNOWLEDGEMENTS

Work presented here is supported by grants from the Medical Research Council and the Wellcome Trust. J.M. Blackwell is a Wellcome Trust Senior Lecturer.

REFERENCES

Aderem AA, Keum MM, Pure E, Cohn ZA (1986) Bacterial
  lipopolysaccharides, phorbal myristate acetate, and zymosan
  induce the myristoylation of specific macrophage proteins.
  Proc Natl Acad Sci USA 83:5817-5821
Beller DI, Springer TA, Schreiber RD (1982) Anti Mac-1
  selectively inhibits the mouse and human type three complement
  receptor. J Exp Med 156:1000-1009
Blackwell JM (1985) Genetic control of discrete phases of
  complex infections: Leishmania donovani as a model. Prog Leuk
  Biol 3:31-49
Blackwell JM, Ezekowitz RAB, Roberts MB, Channon JY, Sim RB,
  Gordon S (1985) Macrophage complement and lectin-like
  receptors bind Leishmania in the absence of serum. J Exp Med
  162:324-331
Cooper A, Wozencraft AO, Roach TIA, Blackwell JM (1988)
  Different epitopes of the macrophage type three complement
  receptor (CR3) are used to bind Leishmania promastigotes
  harvested at different phases of their growth cycle. In:
  Leishmaniasis: The First Century (1885-1985) New Strategies for
  Control (ed DT Hart), NATOASI Workshop, Plenum Publishers, NY,
  in press
Crocker PR, Blackwell JM, Bradley DJ, (1984) Expression of the
  natural resistance gene Lsh in resident liver macrophages.
  Infect Immun 43:1033-1040
Crocker PR, Davies EV, Blackwell JM (1987) Variable expression
  of the murine natural resistance gene Lsh in different
  macrophage populations infected in vitro with Leishmania
  donovani. Parasite Immunol 9:705-719
Ding A, Wright SD, Nathan C (1987) Activation of mouse
  peritoneal macrophages by monoclonal antibodies to Mac-1
  (complement receptor type 3). J Exp Med 165:733-749
Emanuel BS, Cannizzaro L, Ornstein-Goldstein N, Indik ZK, Yoon K,
  May M, Oliver L, Boyd C, Rosenbloom J (1985) Chromosomal
  localization of the human elastin gene. Am J Hum Genet 37:
  873-882
Flotte TJ, Springer TA, Thorbek GJ (1983) Dendritic cell and
  macrophage staining by monoclonal antibodies in tissue sections
  and epidermal sheets. Am J Pathol 111:112-124
Handman E, Goding JW (1985) The Leishmania receptor for
  macrophages is a lipid containing glycoconjugate. Embo J
  4:329-336
Heidmann O, Buonanno A, Geoffrey B, Robert B, Guenet JL, Merlie
  JP, Changeux JP (1986) Chromosomal localization of muscle
  nicotinic acetylcholine receptor genes in the mouse. Science
  234:866-868
Jhanwar SC, Jensen JT, Kaelbling M, Chaganti RSK, Klinger HP
  (1986) In situ localization of human fibronectin (FN) genes to
  chromosome regions 2p14-p16, 2q34-q36, and 11q12.1-q13.5 in
  germ line cells, but to chromosome 2 sites only in somatic
  cells. Cytogenet Cell Genet 41:47-53
Johnson LL (1981) At how many histocompatibility loci do
  congenic mouse strains differ? J Heredity 72, 27-31
Kaye PM, Patel NK, Blackwell JM (1988) Acquisition of cell
  mediated immunity to Leishmania. II. Lsh gene regulation of
  accessory cell function. Immunology, submitted
Marlin SD, Morton CC, Anderson DC, Springer TA (1986) LFA-1
  immunodeficiency disease. Definition of the genetic defect and
  chromosomal mapping of α and β subunits of the lymphocyte

function-associated antigen 1 (LFA-1) by complementation.
J Exp Med 164:855-867

Narahara K, Kimura S, Kikkava Y, Takahashi Y, Wakita Y, Kasai R, Nagai S, Nishibayashi Y, Kimoto H (1985) Probable assignment of soluble isocitrate dehydrogenase (Idh-1) to 2q33.3. Human Genet 71:37-40

Robert B, Barton P, Minty A, Daubas P, Weydert A, Bonhomme F, Catalan J, Chazottes D, Guenet JL, Buckingham M (1985) Investigation of genetic linkage between myosin and actin genes using an interspecific backcross. Nature 314:181-183

Rook GAW, Steele J, Umar S, Dockrell HM (1985) A simple method for the solubilisation of reduced NBT, and its use as a colorimetric assay for activation of human macrophages by gamma interferon. J Immunol Methods 82:161-167

Rosen H, Gordon S (1987) Monoclonal antibody to the murine type 3 complement receptor inhibits adhesion of myelomonocytic cells in vitro and inflammatory cell recruitment in vivo. J Exp Med 166:1685-1701

Rousseau-Merck MF, Simon-Chazottes D, Arpin M, Pringault E, Louvard D, Guenet JL, Berger R (1988) Localization of the villin gene on human chromosome 2q35-q36 and on mouse chromosome 1. Hum Genet, in press

Schroeder WT, Lopez LC, Harper ME, Saunders GF (1984) Localization of the human glucagon gene (GCG) to chromosome segment 2q36-37. Cytogenet Cell Genet 38:76-79

Shiloh Y, Donlon T, Bruns G, Breitman ML, Tsui L-C (1986) Assignment of the human gamma-crystallin gene cluster (CRYG) to the long arm of chromosome 2, region q33-36. Hum Genet 73: 17-19

Weil D, Mattei MG, Passage E, NGuyen Van Cong, Pribula-Conway D, Mann K, Deutzmann R, Timpl R, Chu ML (1988) Assignment of the three genes coding for the different chains of type VI collagen (COL6A1,COL6A2,COL6A3). Abstract 304, Ninth International Workshop on Human Gene Mapping. Cytogenet. Cell Genet., in press.

Wright SD, Detmers PA (1988) Adhesion-promoting receptors on phagocytes. In: Proceedings from the Macrophage Plasma Membrane Symposium, Oxford 1987 (ed S Gordon), in press

Wright SD, Jong MTC (1986) Adhesion-promoting receptors on human macrophages recognize Escherichia coli by binding to lipopolysaccharide. J Exp Med 164:1876-1888

Wright SD, Licht MR, Craigmyle LS, Silverstein SC (1984) Communication between receptors for different ligands on a single cell. Ligation of fibronectin receptors induces a reversible alteration in the function of C3 receptors in cultured human monocytes. J Cell Biol 99:336-339

Identification of a Linkage Group Including the *Bcg* Gene by Restriction Fragment Length Polymorphism Analysis

E. Schurr[1], E. Skamene[2], M. Nesbitt[3], R. Hynes[4], and P. Gros[1]

INTRODUCTION

Inbred strains of mice greatly differ in their ability to control the proliferation of Mycobacterium bovis (BCG) in their reticulo-endothelial organs (liver and spleen, reviewed by Skamene, 1983) and can be classified into two non-overlapping groups as resistant and susceptible to the infection. This difference in susceptibility is most evident when mice are injected intravenously with a low dose (10,000 bacilli) of live BCG and the number of colony forming units (CFU) in the spleen of the infected animals is determined 3 weeks later: susceptible animals show CFU counts 100 to a 1000 fold higher than their resistant counterparts. A kinetic analysis of bacterial growth revealed that the difference in bacterial load is due to a limited ability of susceptible mice to control the growth of the bacteria in the initial phase of the infection. A systematic typing of inbred mouse strains showed that approximately half of the strains were either resistant or susceptible while none of the investigated strains showed a pattern of intermediate bacterial growth (Forget et al. 1981). Moreover, classical Mendelian analysis showed that the trait of BCG-resistance is under the control of a single, autosomal dominant gene, which was designated Bcg (Gros et al. 1981). Using a panel of BXD- and BXH- recombinant inbred strains (RIS) the Bcg gene was mapped to mouse chromosome 1 at a proximal position between Idh1 and Pep3 (Skamene et al. 1982). The mapping studies also showed a close linkage of Bcg with the Lsh and Ity genes which expression determines the innate resistance or susceptibility to infections with Leishmania donovani and Salmonella typhimurium, respectively (Skamene et al. 1982). Thus far, no recombinants have been observed between the three host resistance genes. It is therefore assumed that the genomic sequences encoding the Bcg gene have a pleiotropic effect as they control the natural resistance of mice to at least three taxonomically, genetically and antigenically different groups of intracellular parasites.

The aim of our ongoing studies is to generate and position a large group of polymorphic markers in the portion of mouse chromosome 1 carrying the Bcg gene. We have taken the general

[1] Department of Biochemistry, McGill University, 3655 Drummond, Montreal, Quebec H3G 1Y6, Canada
[2] Montreal General Hospital, Montreal, Quebec H3G 1A4, Canada
[3] Department of Biology, University of California at San Diego, La Jolla, CA, USA
[4] Center for Cancer Research, MIT, Cambridge, MA, U.S.A.

Current Topics in Microbiology and Immunology, Vol. 137
© Springer-Verlag Berlin · Heidelberg 1988

approach of firstly, identifying RFLPs in that region of mouse 1 chromosome and secondly, determining their distance to Bcg by segregation analysis in backcross animals or in recombinant inbred mice of known Bcg genotype. RFLPs were first determined for a number of gene probes in a pair of inbred strains, C57BL/6J and A/J. Subsequently, the distance of these DNA probes to Bcg were approximated by estimating their ability to segregate with the gene in N6, N12 and N20 congenic B10.A-Bcg^r mice (not shown) or on DNA blots derived from a limited number of AXB/BXA RIS DNA. Three cDNA probes for the Len1, Len2 and Fn genes seemed to map within a distance of <10 cMg, from the Bcg and were selected for further segregation analysis within a large set of AXB/BXA RIS.

MATERIALS AND METHODS

C57BL/6J and A/J mice were obtained from the Jackson Labs. AXB and BXA recombinant inbred strains, originally developed by Dr. M. Nesbitt (University of California in San Diego), were maintained in our animal breeding facility.

High molecular weight DNAs was isolated from mouse livers according to standard protocols (Maniatis et al. 1982). Genomic DNA samples were digested for 2 hrs with a total of 7 units of restriction endonucleases (BRL, Pharmacia) per microgram of genomic DNA under conditions recommended by the supplier. Great care was taken to ensure that DNA digestions were complete. The genomic DNA digests were separated on 0.8 - 1% horizontal agarose gels containing 40 mM Tris acetate, 20 mM sodium acetate, 20mM EDTA at pH 7.6. The gels were denatured, neutralized and blotted onto nylon membranes (Hybond N). The blots were hybridized for 48 hrs in 5 x SSPE, 5 x Denhart's and 50% formamide at 42 °C in the presence of individual ^{32}P - labelled DNA probes. DNA probes used for hybridization were the PstI fragments of pM γ-1Cr2 (Len1 probe), the AccI/BamHI- fragment of pUC9 γ-2.1 (Len 2 probe; both plasmids were kindly provided by Dr. L.-C. Tsui, Toronto) or a 1.5 kb rat fibronectin cDNA clone (Patel et al. 1987). Each of the probes was labelled by random primer labelling (Feinberg and Vogelstein, 1983) to specific activities of 3-5x10^8 cpm/µg DNA. Subsequent to hybridization, the blots were rinsed in 2XSSC and washed for 30 min at 65 °C in 2XSSC, 0.1% SDS and for another 30 min at 65°C in 0.1XSSC before being exposed on XAR-films (Kodak).

RESULTS

We have used RFLP analysis to identify genetic markers closely linked to Bcg. In this analysis, two loci already assigned to this portion of mouse 1 (Len1 and Len2) and a locus not previously mapped (Fn) were analysed. Our experimental procedure consisted in 1) identifying restriction enzymes generating polymorphic differences between our test mouse strains ; 2) screening genomic DNA from RI strains segregating at these loci; 3) comparing the respective strain distribution patterns of the loci to determine the extent of linkage. A DNA polymorphism for Len1 was identified on TaqI digested genomic DNA from A/J and C57BL/6J: Our cDNA probe detected hybridizing fragments of 2.3,

2.2, 1.1, 0.9 and 0.6kb in A/J DNA and fragments of 4.0, 2.2,
1.2, 0.9 and 0.6kb in C57BL/6J DNA. On the other hand, a RFLP
was identified with Msp1 for the Len2 gene in the same strain
combination: Msp1 hybridizing fragments of size 20, 10 and 2.2kb
were detected in A/J DNA while fragments of size 10, 4 and 2.2kb
were detected in C57BL/6J DNA. Finally, a polymorphism for the
third gene, Fn, was revealed by EcoRI in A/J and C57BL/6J. The
Fn-probe hybridized to two polymorphic fragments of 4.4 kb in A/J
- and 4.6 kb in C57BL/6-DNA. Furthermore, the Fn probe
hybridized to a 15 kb and a 1.8 kb fragment in both A/J and
C57BL/6J DNA. Typical results of such analyses are presented in
figure 1 for the Fn probe.

To determine the map position of the detected RFLPs and the
linkage to Bcg, the strain distribution patterns (SDP) of the
different alleles were determined for a set of 45 AXB/BXA RIS
(Figure 1, Table 1) and compared with the Bcg phenotype
(resistance or susceptibility to infection) of 30 AXB/BXA RIS
(Table 1). When the SDPs were arranged in a way to minimize
recombinational events, the gene order Bcg - Fn - Len2 - Len1 -
centromere was obtained (Table 1). In this linkage group Bcg is
most distal whereas Fn maps between the Len gene family and Bcg:
Based on the data in Table 1, we calculated the following map
distances, Bcg to Fn 5.5cMg, (concordance in 25 out of 30
strains); Fn to Len2 and Len2 to Len1, 1.2cMg (43 of 45); Bcg to
Len1, estimated 11cMg (22 of 30).

DISCUSSION

We have initiated a molecular genetic approach to the study of
the host resistance gene, Bcg and have defined a linkage group on
the proximal region of mouse chromosome 1 which includes 4
polymorphic markers: Bcg, Fn, Len1 and Len2. Further linkage of
the mouse gamma crystallin genes with Idh1 is well established
for mouse chromosome 1. Synteny for Fn, Len and Idh1 was also
observed in cattle (Skow L.C. private communication) and has been
described in man (Bootsma and Kidd 1984; Willard et al. 1985).
In the latter instance, all three genes map at the long arm of
human chromosome 2 (Bootsma and Kidd 1984; Henry et al. 1985;
Shiloh et al. 1986). Our results provide further evidence that
this region has been conserved during mammalian evolution and
suggest the possibility that a human equivalent to the mouse Bcg
gene may exist.

Results summarized in this communication form the basis of a two
fold study of the Bcg gene and its implication in natural
resistance to infections with intracellular parasites such as
mycobacteria. Firstly, we would like to use the kind of analysis
described here to generate a large number of polymorphic markers
mapping in the most immediate vicinity of the gene. These
markers would be first mapped within our panels of RI strains,
interspecies hybrids and congenic lines, to test their ability to
segregate with Bcg. Finer mapping and evaluation of the physical
distance of the RFLPs to the gene will be done by techniques such
as pulse field gel electrophoresis. Cloning of genomic sequences

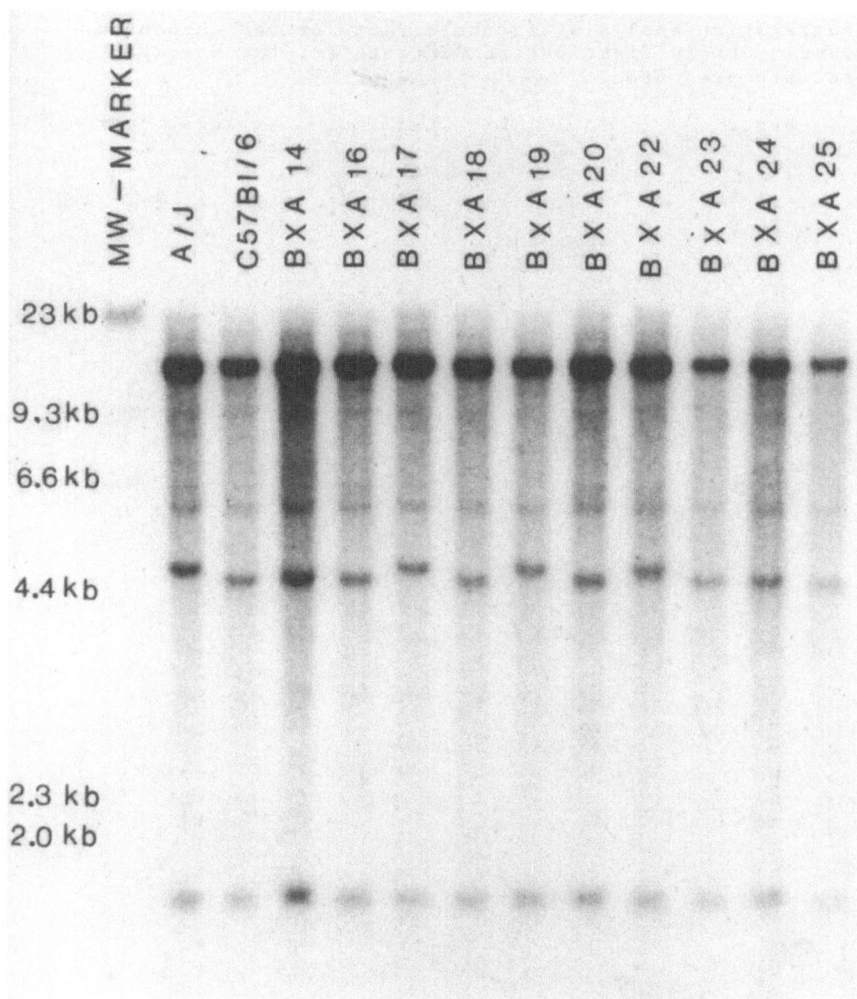

Fig. 1. Representative Southern blot illustrating restriction fragment length polymorphism analysis as described in the text for the fibronectin probe (Fn). The molecular weights markers are in kb and represent the HindIII fragments of lambda phage DNA.

Table 1. Segregation analysis of four markers on the chromosome 1 of the mouse. Strain distribution patterns for the Bcg, Fn, Len1 and Len2 are presented.

Gene	Bcg		Fn		Len2		Len1
RIS							
A/J	+		+		+		+
C57BL/6	-		-		-		-
AXB 1	-		-		-		-
AXB 2	+		+		+		+
AXB 3	-		-		-		-
AXB 4	+		+		+		+
AXB 5	+		+		+		+
AXB 6	-		-		-		-
AXB 7	+		+		+		+
AXB 8	+		+		+		+
AXB 9	+		+	x	-		-
AXB 10	+		+		+		+
AXB 11	nd		-		-		-
AXB 12	+		+		+		+
AXB 13	+	x	-		-		-
AXB 14	nd		-		-		-
AXB 15	nd		-		-	x	+
AXB 17	+		+		+		+
AXB 18	-		-		-		-
AXB 19	-		-		-		-
AXB 20	-		-		-		-
AXB 21	-	x	+		+		+
AXB 22	nd		-		-		-
AXB 23	nd		+		+		+
AXB 24	nd		+		+		+
AXB 25	+		+		+		+
BXA 1	nd		+		+		+
BXA 2	+	x	-		-		-
BXA 4	+		+		+		+
BXA 6	-		-		-		-
BXA 7	nd		+		+		+
BXA 8	+	x	-		-		-
BXA 9	+		+	x	-		-
BXA 10	-	x	+		+		+
BXA 11	nd		+		+		+
BXA 12	+		+		+		+
BXA 13	+		+		+		+
BXA 14	-		-		-	x	+
BXA 16	nd		-		-		-
BXA 17	nd		+		+		+
BXA 18	nd		-		-		-
BXA 19	+		+		+		+
BXA 20	nd		-		-		-
BXA 22	+		+		+		+
BXA 23	nd		-		-		-
BXA 24	nd		-		-		-
BXA 25	-		-		-		-

overlapping the gene could then be envisioned by utilizing
chromosome walking or chromosome jumping in appropriate genomic
DNA libraries. In order to generate large numbers of RFLPs we
plan to use chromosome specific libraries obtained from somatic
cell hybrids carrying portions of mouse 1 on a primate
background. Secondly, we will test the possibility that a human
equivalent to the mouse gene exists and is phenotypically
expressed in human populations: although they are too distant to
be used for chromosome walking experiments, the fibronectin gene
and both lens crystallin genes map close enough to Bcg to be
useful for linkage analysis in human family studies. Linkage
disequilibrium of these genes with clinically manifested
tuberculosis or leprosy would suggest two points: Firstly, the
existence of a human homolog of the mouse BCG-resistance gene and
secondly, the localization of this gene at the telomeric end of
human chromosome 2q. Studies on these two points have been
undertaken in our laboratories.

REFERENCES

Bootsma D, Kidd KK (1984) Report of the committee on the genetic
    constitution of chromosomes 2, 3, 4 and 5. Cytogenet Cell
    Genet 37:22-46
Feinberg AP, Vogelstein B (1984) A technique for radiolabelling
    DNA restriction endonuclease fragments to high specific
    activity. Anal Biochem 137:266-269
Forget A, Skamene E, Gros P, Miailhe-Ac, Turcotte R (1981)
    Differences in response among inbred mouse strains to infection
    with small doses of Mycobacterium bovis BCG. Infect Immun
    32:42-47
Gros P, Skamene E, Forget A (1981) Genetic control of natural
    resistance to Mycobacterium bovis (BCG) in mice. J Immunol
    127:2417-2421
Henry I, Jeanpierre M, Bernard M, Weil D, Greschik KH, Ramirez F,
    Chu ML, Junien C (1985) The structural gene for fibronectin
    (FN) maps to 2q32.3 - qter. Cytogenet Cell Genet 40:650
Maniatis T, Fritsch EF, Sambrook J (1982) Molecular cloning Cold
    Spring Harbor Laboratory, Cold Spring Harbor, New York
Patel RS, Odermatt E, Schwarzbauer JE, Hynes R (1987)
    Organization of the fibronectin gene provides evidence for exon
    shuffling during evolution. Embo J 6, 2265-2272
Shilloh, Y, Donlon, T, Bruns, G, Breitman ML, Tsui L-C (1986)
    Assignment of the human -crystallin gene cluster (CRYG) to the
    long arm of chromosome 2, region q33-36. Hum Genet 73:17-19
Skamene E (1986) Genetic control of resistance to mycobacterial
    infection. Curr Topics Microbiol 124:49-66
Skamene E, Gros P, Forget A, Kongshavn PAL, St-Charles C, Taylor
    BA (1982) Genetic regulation of resistance to intracellular
    pathogens. Nature 297:506-510

Continuous Expression of I-A by Murine Peritoneal Macrophages IS Linked to the *Bcg* Gene

B.S. Zwilling, M. Massie, L. Vespa, M. Kwasniewski, J. Nath, and W. LaFuse

INTRODUCTION:

The expression of Major Histocompatibility Complex (MHC) class II glycoproteins is an important step in the immunological cascade. Antigen is processed and presented to antigen specific T lymphocytes by a small number of macrophages that are expressing Ia glycoproteins (Unanue, 1985). The result of this interaction leads to the induction of Ia expression by other macrophages. These macrophages are induced to express Ia by the antigen responding T cells.

Following the injection of most antigens, Ia expressed by macrophages is a transient event (Beller and Unanue, 1980). However, the injection of Mycobacterium bovis (strain BCG) into certain strains of mice leads to the induction of constitutive Ia expression by macrophages (Johnson and Zwilling, 1985). Constitutive expression of Ia is induced by several different microorganisms in strains of mice that are resistant to BCG. Macrophages from BCG susceptible strains always transiently express Ia. We have linked the constitutive expression of Ia to the Bcg gene by showing that macrophages from BCG susceptible BALB/c mice transiently express I-A while macrophages from the BALB/c congenic C.D2Bcg^r mice constitutively express I-A (Zwilling et al, 1987). We have also characterized the expression of I-A by macrophages from Bcg^r and Bcg^s mice. The results of these investigations have been reported elsewhere (Johnson and Zwilling, 1985; Vespa et al, 1987 and Zwilling et al, 1987) and are summarized below.

MATERIALS and METHODS:

Animals: C3H/HeN, DBA.2, CBA.J, C57Bl/6, C57Bl/10 and BALB/c mice were obtained from Harlan/Sprague Dawley and housed in Bioclean filtered laminar flow air isolation cages (Hazelton Systems, Aberdeen, MD.). The C.D2Bcg^r mice were kindly provided by Dr. Michael Potter, National Cancer Institute, bred in our facility and housed in the isolation cages. Animals were provided food and water ad libitum.

Reagents: Dulbecco's modified Eagle's medium and RPMI 1640 were obtained from MA Bioproducts and supplemented as described by Zwilling et al (1987). Recombinant murine interferon (IFN)-gamma was provided by Dr. Michael Shepard, Genentech, recombinant interleukin-2 (IL-2) by Dr J.D. Irr, Dupont and recombinant interleukin 4 (IL-4) by Dr. Steven Gillis, Immunex. Seed cultures of BCG were supplied by Donald Auclair (Trudeau Institiute, TMC 1019) and Corynebacterium parvum vaccine (Coparvax) by Dr. John Whisnaut (Wellcome Biotechnology). The somatic cell hybrids producing mono-

The Ohio State University, Columbus, Ohio 43210

Current Topics in Microbiology and Immunology, Vol. 137
© Springer-Verlag Berlin · Heidelberg 1988

clonal antibodies to I-A^k and I-A^d were obtained from the American Type Culture Collection and maintained as described by Zwilling et al (1987).

Peritoneal Macrophages: Peritoneal macrophages were obtained by lavage with Hanks' balanced salt solution 28 days after injection of 1x10^6 cfu BCG or 3.5mg C. parvum intraperitoneally. Macrophages elicited by the injection of 4% thioglycollate were harvested by lavage 4 days later. In order to induce I-A expression by the thioglycollate elicited macrophages the cells were allowed to adhere for 24 hours prior to the addition of IFN-gamma to the culture medium. The cultures were incubated for an additional 2 days before I-A expression was determine by indirect immunofluorescence as described by Johnson and Zwilling (1985). Binding of radio labeled IFN-gamma was determined as described by Celada et al (1984). I-A biosynthesis was determined following metabolic labeling with ^{35}S-methionine and immunoprecipitation (Zwilling et al, 1987). The presence of class II mRNA was determined by slot blot analysis of cytoplasmic RNA (Davis et al, 1986). Briefly, phenol/chloroform extractions of cytosolic preparations were precipitated with ethanol. The precipitated cytoplasmic RNA was dissolved in water. Following blotting onto nitrocellulose the denatured RNA was hybridized with a 4.7kb EcoRI-BamHI fragment from a BALB/c cosmid clone 24.2 of I-A alpha subcloned in pBR322 (Steinmetz et al, 1982).

RESULTS

Induction of Continuous I-A Expression in Different Strains of Mice Following Injection of BCG.

In order to determine the relationship of continuous I-A expression by macrophages to the BCG resistant phenotype, the duration of I-A expression by macrophages from several different strains of mice was examined. The results, in Table 1, show that macrophages from BCG resistant mice, previously immunized with BCG or with C. parvum, continued to express I-A after three days of in vitro culture while macrophages from strains of mice that are susceptible to BCG transiently expressed I-A.

Table 1. CONTINUOUS I-A EXPRESSION CORRELATES WITH BCG RESISTANCE[1]

Microorganism	Time	PHENOTYPE OF BCG GENE[2]					
		Resistant			Susceptible		
		C3H/HeN	DBA.2	CBA.J	C57B1/6	C57B1/10	BALB/c
BCG	0	68+7[2]	86+5	64+4	40+3	83+8	85+6
	3	65+12	80+3	59+8	12+8	23+5	18+7
C. parvum	0	96+1	91+8	82+6	74+2	79+9	9+4
	3	89+10	77+5	56+14	5+2	22+4	6+1

[1] Mice were injected with 10^6 cfu BCG or C. parvum. The expression of I-A by peritoneal macrophages was determined by indirect fluorescence 28 days after injection, immediately after peritoneal lavage, and and after 3 days of in vitro incubation.

[2] Percent of macrophages expressing I-A

For example, 68% of the macrophages from C3H/HeN mice expressed I-A initially and 65% continued to express I-A after 3 days. In contrast, while 85% of the macrophages from BCG susceptible, BALB/c mice expressed I-A initially, only 18% continued to express the class II glycoprotein after 3 days of culture. Similar observations were made following injection of mice with C. parvum.

The strains of mice we tested are different in several important respects including the MHC. In order to more precisely define the role of the genes linked to the Bcg gene we used macrophages obtained from congenic C.D2Bcg[r] mice and Bcg[S] BALB/c mice following injection of BCG, C. parvum or Listeria monocytogenes. The results of this experiment are presented in Table 2.

Table 2. EXPRESSION OF I-A IN CONGENIC MICE RESISTANT OR SUSCEPTIBLE TO BCG[1]

| | | PERCENT I-A POSITIVE MACROPHAGES | |
| | Day of | Strain | |
Mice Immunized With	Culture	CD.2Ity[r]	BALB/c
BCG	0	87+5	64+7
	3	71∓9	10∓5
C. parvum	0	94+7	95+4
	3	82+10	6+1
L. monocytogenes	0	52+4	48+12
	3	14+9	15+8

[1] Mice were immunized with BCG, C. parvum or L. monocytogenes 28 days previously and the percent of macrophages expressing I-A determined immediately and after 3 days of culture.

Macrophages from BALB/c mice transiently expressed I-A following injection of these microorganisms. In contrast, macrophages from the C.D2Bcg[r] mice continuously expressed I-A following injection of BCG and C. parvum and transiently expressed I-A following injection with Listeria.

Induction of Continuous Expression Does Not Correlate With The T Cell Response.

A possible explanation for our results was that the T cell response to BCG was different in mice that were resistant or susceptible to BCG. Thus, given an equal stimulus, macrophages from both resistant and susceptible mice would continuously express I-A. When we treated macrophages from Bcg[r] and Bcg[S] mice with IFN-gamma we found that we could induce continuous I-A expression (Table 3). Treatment of the macrophages with 200 units/ml of IFN-gamma resulted in the induction of continuous I-A expression while treatment with less than 200 units/ml resulted in only transient expression.

We also showed that macrophages from both Bcg[r] and Bcg[S] mice expressed 3,000 to 5,000 high affinity receptors for IFN-gamma (Figure 1). These observations reinforced our original hypothesis that differences in the T cell response to BCG antigens accounted for the differences in I-A expression that we observed.

Table 3.   EFFECT OF RECOMBINANT INTERFERON-GAMMA ON THE EXPRESSION
OF I-A BY MACROPHAGES FROM Bcg[r] AND Bcg[s] MICE[1]

Units IFN-gamma	Bcg[r] [2]		Bcg[s] [3]	
	0	5	0	5
100	87+10	69+12	83+10	64+8
10	67∓13	19∓8	56∓20	15∓7
7	39∓20	7+3	30∓14	9+4
1	15∓10	4∓3	18∓12	6+4
0.1	10∓6	5+2	9+3	6+2
0.01	7∓2	5∓3	7∓2	4∓3
0	7∓2	4+2	7∓2	5+1

[1] Thioglycollate elicited macrophages were allowed to adhere for 24
hours prior to the addition of IFN-gamma in 0.5 ml. The macrophages were treated with IFN-gamma for 4 days, washed and the
percentages of macrophages expressing I-A was determined
immediately and after 6 days of culture.
[2] C3H/HeN
[3] BALB/c

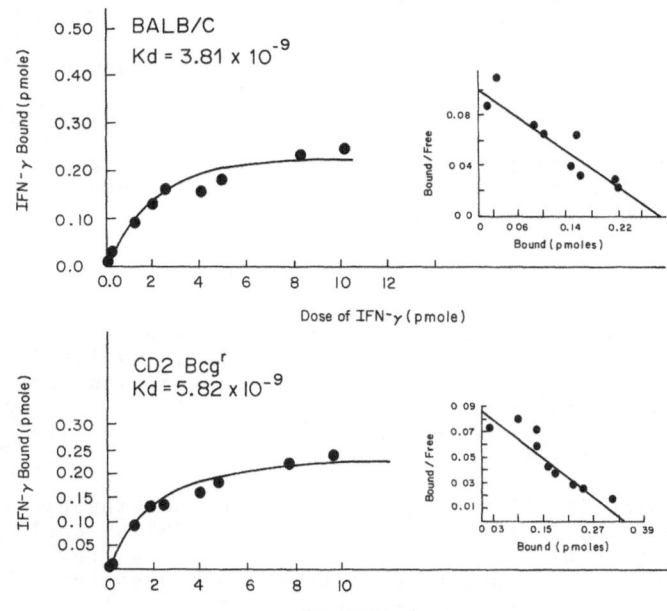

Fig. 1.   Differences in I-A Expression in Macrophages from Bcg[r] and
Bcg[s] Mice Are Not Due to Differences in Interferon-gamma
Receptors.   Interferon was labeled with ^{125}I using
iodobeads.   Receptor binding was analyzed using Ligand
(Munson and Radhard, 1980).

However, we also showed that the continued expression of I-A by macrophages from Bcg[s] mice required the continuous presence of IFN-gamma (Table 4) and was reduced by treatment of the cells with hydrocortisone (Vespa et al, 1987; Zwilling et al, 1987). In contrast, the continued expression of I-A by macrophages from Bcg[r] mice did not require the continued presence of IFN-gamma (Table 4) and was not inhibited by hydrocortisone.

Table 4. ANTIBODY TO INTERFERON-GAMMA INHIBITS CONTINUOUS I-A
          EXPRESSION BY MACROPHAGES FROM Bcg[s] MICE

	% I-A Positive Macrophages	
Treatment	Bcg[r]	Bcg[s]
1. rIFN-gamma[1]	89+5	87+6
2. rIFN-gamma + antigamma concurrently[2]	13+4	8+5
3. 3 days post rIFN-gamma[3]	82+7	71+10
4. 3 days post rIFN-gamma + antigamma[4]	85+2	16+4

[1] Thioglycollate elicited macrophages were allowed to adhere for 24 hours and then were treated with 100 U of rIFN-gamma for 2 days. The percentage of macrophages expressing I-A was determined immediately after treatment.

[2] rIFN-gamma and monoclonal antibody to murine rIFN-gamma were mixed prior to the addition to macrophage monolayers.

[3] Macrophages were treated as in 1. The cultures were then washed and incubated for an additional 3 days in medium prior to determining I-A expression.

[4] Macrophages were treated as in 1. The cultures were washed and monoclonal antigamma added for 30 minutes. The cultures were washed again and incubated in medium for 3 days prior to determining I-A expression.

This suggested that the differences in I-A expression that we observed was regulated by the macrophage. This possibility was reinforced by results of experiments presented in Table 5. While T cells from BCG immunized mice induced continuous I-A expression in vitro, when stimulated with heat killed BCG, there was no correlation between the Bcg phenotype of the T cells and their ability to induce continuous I-A expression.

T cells from some Bcg[r] mice (C.D2Bcg[r]) failed to induce continuous I-A expression in vitro while T cells from Bcg[s] mice (C57Bl/6) could induce continuous expression of I-A. The failure of T cells from C.D2Bcg[r] mice and BALB/c mice to induce continuous I-A expression was due to the lower level of IFN-gamma produced by these cells (Tyring and Lefkowitz, 1980; Kwasniewski and Zwilling, submitted for publication).

Table 5. CONTINUOUS EXPRESSION OF I-A BY MACROPHAGES DOES NOT
          CORRELATE TO THE T-CELL RESPONSE TO BCG[1]

Lymphocyte Source[2]	% I-A POSITIVE MACROPHAGES FROM					
	BALB/c			C.D2 Bcg[r]		
	0	3	HC[5]	0	3	HC[5]
C3H/HeN[3]	54±9	45±2	21±3	61±6	47±1	51±4
DBA/2[4]	51±9	48±3	16±5	52±11	54±11	49±6
C.D2Bcg[r]	nd	nd	nd	17±3	3±1	nd
BALB/c	37±4	18±7	nd	nd	nd	nd
C57Bl/6[5]	59±3	50±5	25±2	59±4	59±1	55±9

[1] 1×10^5 T-cells were incubated with 5×10^5 macrophages from BALB/c or
  C.D2 Bcg[r] mice along with 5×10^3 syngeneic macrophages. The
  syngeneic macrophages were needed to present antigen to the
  stimulating lymphocytes. Cultures without syngeneic macrophages
  resulted in no induction of continuous I-A expression.
[2] Syngeneic mixture of T-cells and macrophages yielded 77% I-A
  positive cells at day 0 and 65% at day 3.
[3] Syngeneic mixture yielded 61% at day 0 and 53% at day 3.
[4] Syngeneic mixture yielded 57% at day 0 and 48% at day 3.
[5] Three days after the induction of I-A the macrophages were treated
  with 10^{-6} M hydrocortisone for 4 hours and the percent of cells
  expressing I-A was determined.

Interleukin 2 and Interleukin 4 Act Synergistically with IFN-gamma to Induce Continuous I-A Expression.

The injection of C.D2Bcg[r] mice with BCG, as well as treatment of
peritoneal macrophages with sufficient quantities of IFN-gamma,
results in the induction of continuous I-A expression. However T
cells from these mice failed to induce continuous I-A expression in
vitro. This observation raised the possibility that other lymphokines may act with IFN-gamma to induce continuous I-A expression in
vivo. When we treated macrophages from Bcg[r] mice with a low dose of
IFN-gamma together with recombinant IL-2 or with recombinant IL-4 we
induced continous I-A expression (Table 6).

Table 6. RECOMBINANT IL-2 AND RECOMBINANT IL-4 ACT SYNERGISTICALLY
          WITH rIFN-gamma TO INDUCE CONTINUOUS I-A EXPRESSION

Treatment[1]	% I-A Positive Macrophages	
	0	3
IFN-gamma (2 U/ml)	60±8	22±9
IFN-gamma (200 U/ml)	64±8	55±5
IL-2 (200 U/ml)	8±2	6±6
IL-4 (200 U/ml)	20±5	3±3
IFN-gamma (2 U/ml) + IL-2	55±3	54±1
IFN-gamma (2 U/ml) + IL-4	57±6	60±16
none	6±1	4±3

[1] Macrophages from Bcg[r] mice were allowed to adhere for 24 hrs prior
  to the addition of lymphokines. The cultures were incubated for
  48 hours, washed, and the percent of macrophages expressing I-A
  determined immediately or after 3 days culture.

Expression of I-A by Macrophages from Bcg^r Mice Does Not Require Its Continued Synthesis.

We have previously reported that treatment of macrophages with cyclohexamide or hydrocortisone for as little as 4 hours reduced the expression of I-A by macrophages from Bcg^s mice but did not affect I-A expression by macrophages from Bcg^r mice (Vespa et al, 1987; Zwilling et al, 1987). This suggested that macrophages from Bcg^r mice continued to express I-A without continued synthesis. We tested this possibility by metabolically labeling cells with ^{35}S-methionine and immunoprecipitating the class II MHC glycoproteins with monoclonal anti I-A antibody as well as by determining the presence of class II mRNA by slot blot analysis. The results in Figure 2 indicate that the class II mRNA was reduced by 70% and the synthesis of class II glycoprotein was not detected by metabolic labeling and immunoprecipitation.

DISCUSSION

Macrophages can constitutively or transiently express class II MHC glycoproteins (Beller and Unanue, 1980; Johnson and Zwilling, 1985; Zwilling et al 1987). Constitutive expression occurs following injection of certain strains of mice with BCG and correlates with the expression of the Bcg^r phenotype (Johnson and Zwilling, 1985; Zwilling et al, 1987). Macrophages from Bcg^s mice cannot be induced to constitutively express the class II MHC glycoproteins. The linkage of this trait to the Bcg gene was established by showing that macrophages from C.D2Bcg^r mice, which are congenic with Bcg^s BALB/c mice except for 30 centimorgans on chromosome 1 derived from Bcg^r DBA/2 mice, will also constitutively express I-A (Zwilling et al 1987). The macrophages from the congenic mice do not differ in their ability to bind to IFN-gamma nor in the number and affinity of their IFN-gamma receptors.

The constitutive expression is independent of the continued presence of IFN-gamma. Neutralization of IFN-gamma with monoclonal antibody following the in vitro induction of I-A did not affect class II MHC glycoprotein expression by macrophages from Bcg^r mice. In contrast macrophages from Bcg^s mice no longer expressed I-A following removal of the IFN-gamma (Zwilling et al, 1987). The regulation of continuous expression of I-A is at the level of the macrophage and does not correlate with the T cell response to BCG antigens. T cells from strains of mice that are resistant or susceptible to BCG can induce continuous expression by macrophages from Bcg^r mice. T cells from BALB/c background mice produce less IFN-gamma than T cells from other strains. Our observations indicate that other cytokines (IL-2 and IL-4) can act synergisti-cally with low levels of IFN-gamma to induce continuous I-A expression.

The relationship of constitutive expression of I-A to resistance to microorganisms regulated by the Bcg/Ity/Lsh gene remains unknown. Skamene and Blackwell (this publication) have reported that macrophages from mice expressing the resistant phenotype present antigen better than macrophages from susceptible mice. They also report that resistant macrophages are more activated than susceptible macrophages as judged by anti-Listerial or anti-Leishmanial activity. This innate activity of the macrophages is clearly different than the differences in I-A expression that we have described. I-A expression is inducible with IFN-gamma. The macrophages, like those

A. Immunoprecipitation

LANE   1   2

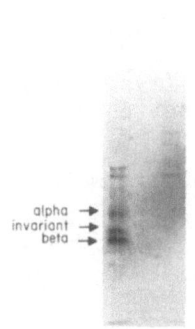

alpha →
invariant →
beta →

B. Northern Blot Analysis

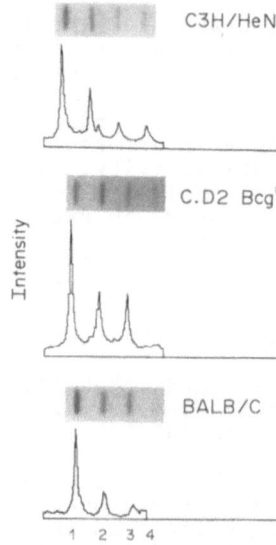

C3H/HeN

C.D2 Bcg^r

BALB/C

1 2 3 4

Time (Days) After I-A Induction

Figure 2.   Continuous Expression of I-A Does Not Require Its
            Continued Synthesis.

A. Cells were metabolically labeled with ^{35}S methionine initially
   after purification (lane 1) and after 4 days of in vitro culture
   (lane 2).   I-A was precipitated with anti I-A monoclonal antibody
   and protein-A sepharose.
B. Northern blot analysis was done with purified RNA obtained from
   $5x10^6$ macrophages cultured for 1 thru 4 days.   The RNA was im-
   mobilized onto nitrocellulose using a slot blot and an I-Aα
   genomic probe was used for hybridization.

from susceptible mice, will only transiently express I-A unless
stimulated with sufficient quantities of IFN-gamma or with combinations of IFN-gamma and IL-2 or IL-4 to induce continuous expression.   We interpret this to mean that the expression of this trait
is inducible and therefore different than the Bcg gene effect.   It
is possible therefore that the effect on I-A expression that we
observe is the result of the activation of a different gene that is
very closely linked to the Bcg gene.

REFERENCES

Beller DI, Unanue ER (1980) Regulation of macrophage populations. II Synthesis and expression of Ia antigens by peritoneal exudate macrophages is a transient event. J Immunol 126: 263-269

Celada A, Gray PW, Rinderknecht E and Schreiber RD (1984) Evidence for a gamma-interferon receptor that regulates macrophage tumoricidal activity. J Exp Med 160:55-74

Davis L, Dibner M and Battley J (1986) Basic Methods in Molecular Biology, Elsevier, New York pp.129-156

Johnson SC and Zwilling BS (1985) Continuous expression of I-A antigen by peritoneal macrophages from mice resistant to <u>Mycobacterium bovis</u> (strain BCG). J Leuk Biol 38:635-645

Munson PJ and Rodbard D (1980) LIGAND: A versatile computerized approach for the charazcterization of ligand binding systems. Anal Biochem 107:220-239

Steinmetz M, Minard K, Horath S, McNicholas J, Frelinger J, Wake C, Long E, Mach B and Hood L (1982) A molecular map of the immune response region from the major histocompatibility complex of the mouse. Nature 300:35-38

Tyring SK and Lefkowitz SS (1980) Strain differences in production of murine interferons. Proc Soc Exper Biol Med 164:519-521

Unanue ER (1985) Antigen presenting function of the macrophage. Annu Rev Immunol 2:395-428

Vespa L, Johnson SC, Aldrich WA and Zwilling BS (1987) Modulation of macrophage I-A expression: Lack of effect of prostaglandins and glucocorticoids on macrophages that continuously express I-A. J. Leuk Biol 41:47-54

Zwilling BS, Vespa L and Massie M (1987) Regulation of I-A expression by murine peritoneal macrophages: Differences linked to the Bcg gene. J Immunol 136:1372-1376

Chromosomal Location of the Gene Determining Resistance to *Plasmodium chabaudi* AS

M. M. Stevenson[1], M. N. Nesbitt[2], and E. Skamene[1]

Plasmodium chabaudi AS (P. chabaudi) is one of four rodent Plasmodium species which causes acute malaria in mice. Differences among inbred strains of mice in the level of resistance to infection with P. chabaudi were initially described by Eugui and Allison (1980). These investigators demonstrated that resistant and susceptible strains could be clearly distinguished based on the outcome of infection. Results from our laboratory confirmed and extended these findings in a survey of 11 inbred strains of mice (Stevenson, Lyanga and Skamene, 1982). Infection with P. chabaudi was shown to result in fulminant parasitemia and death within 10 days in susceptible strains of mice, whereas resistant strains were found to exhibit mild parasitemia and to survive indefinitely.

Genetic analysis of hybrid and backcross progeny derived from the strain combination of C57BL/6 (B) mice, one of the most resistant strains, and A/J (A), the most susceptible strain, allowed us to demonstrate that the level of resistance to infection with P. chabaudi is genetically determined by a major, dominant, non H-2 linked gene. The gene has been designated Pchr for resistance to P. chabaudi (Stevenson, 1985). Pchr was found to be an autosomal gene but its expression is influenced by the sex of the host with female mice exhibiting a superior resistance, evidenced as increased survival. Two allelic forms of the gene exist, designated Pchr^r (resistant) and Pchr^s (susceptible). We have hypothesized that resistance to P. chabaudi, which is determined by Pchr and is apparent within one week of infection, is due to an innate or natural resistance mechanism. This mechanism is not yet defined.

Analysis of the level of resistance to P. chabaudi of the AXB/BXA series of recombinant inbred (RI) mouse strains derived from resistant B (Pchr^r) and susceptible A (Pchr^s) progenitor mice confirmed unigenic control of resistance (Stevenson and Skamene, 1985). Animals of 23 AXB/BXA RI strains have now been typed for the level of resistance to P. chabaudi using three criteria, namely, mean survival time (MST), peak parasitemia level and the magnitude of splenomegaly on day 9 post intraperitoneal infection with 10^6 parasitized erythrocytes (PRBC). These criteria were chosen because expression of these traits is associated with resistance or susceptibility. Progenitor B and A mice exhibit significant differences in these traits (Table 1).

[1] The Montreal General Hospital Research Institute, Montreal, Quebec, H3G 1A4, CANADA
[2] Department of Biology, University of California, La Jolla California, 92093, USA

Table 1. Phenotypic Expression of Traits Associated with Inheritance
of $Pchr^r$ or $Pchr^s$ in Progenitor C57BL/6 and A/J mice

Mouse Strain	MST (Days)[a] Mean ± SEM	% Peak Parasitemia[a] Mean PRBC ± SEM	Spleen Weight[a] (mg) Mean ± SEM	Pchr[b] Typing
C57BL/6	> 14	37.3 ± 1.7	637 ± 25	b
A/J	9.8 ± 0.3	53.4 ± 1.5	360 ± 16	a

[a] $P < 0.001$.
[b] $Pchr^r$ = b; $Pchr^s$ = a.

Table 2. Typing of AXB/BXA Recombinant Inbred Mice for Resistance
to Plasmodium chabaudi

AXB/BXA RI Strain	MST (Days) Mean ± SEM	% Peak Parasitemia Mean PRBC ± SEM	Spleen Weight (mg) Mean ± SEM	Pchr Typing
AXB-1	10.6 ± 0.6	52.5 ± 1.1	310 ± 21	a
AXB-2	> 14	40.3 ± 1.5	587 ± 33	b
AXB-3	> 14	37.2 ± 2.5	604 ± 62	b
AXB-4	10.1 ± 0.4	55.7 ± 1.4	263 ± 45	a
AXB-5	> 14	40.8 ± 1.8	525 ± 22	b
AXB-6	> 14	38.5 ± 0.9	547 ± 42	b
AXB-7	> 14	35.8 ± 2.2	584 ± 19	b
AXB-8	> 14	39.5 ± 1.5	495 ± 12	b
AXB-9	7.0 ± 0.1	52.5 ± 1.2	390 ± 30	a
AXB-10	> 14	38.0 ± 0.7	637 ± 15	b
AXB-12	7.7 ± 0.7	55.8 ± 1.8	426 ± 33	a
AXB-17	> 14	38.2 ± 1.5	594 ± 23	b
AXB-20	> 14	43.0 ± 0.6	585 ± 25	b
BXA-1	> 14	38.8 ± 2.0	811 ± 34	b
BXA-2	8.7 ± 0.1	55.1 ± 0.7	-	a
BXA-6	9.7 ± 0.2	63.1 ± 0.8	339 ± 28	a
BXA-8	> 14	35.1 ± 1.5	510 ± 20	b
BXA-10	> 14	38.2 ± 0.9	606 ± 25	b
BXA-12	8.6 ± 0.2	55.0 ± 1.9	408 ± 30	a
BXA-13	> 14	34.3 ± 2.9	555 ± 74	b
BXA-14	> 14	38.6 ± 1.6	540 ± 57	b
BXA-23	> 14	40.3 ± 2.6	625 ± 29	b
BXA-25	8.6 ± 0.1	50.0 ± 0.6	420	a

As demonstrated in Table 2, the expression of these traits can be
used to predict if an RI strain has inherited the resistant or
susceptible allele of Pchr. RI strains which exhibit a peak
parasitemia of less than 40% and a spleen weight of greater than 450
mg as well as an MST of greater than 14 days are considered to have
inherited the resistant allele. RI strains which exhibit a peak
parasitemia of greater than 50% and a spleen weight of less than 450
mg as well as an MST of less than 10 days are considered to have
inherited the susceptible allele.

In concordance with the results obtained in the segregating populations, female mice of some RI strains were found to be more resistant than their male counterpart when survival was used as the criterion of resistance. Therefore, the data presented in Table 2 for the MST is that derived from male mice only. Results from both male and female mice are presented for the peak parasitemia and spleen weight since there were no significant differences between the sexes in these traits. It is of interest to point out that typing of the AXB/BXA RI strains allowed us not only to confirm unigenic control of resistance to P. chabaudi in this particular strain combination but also to demonstrate genetic linkage between the traits of resistance (defined as prolonged survival and moderate peak parasitemia) and the magnitude of splenomegaly.

Comparison of the strain distribution pattern (SDP) in the AXB/BXA RI strains for inheritance of Pchr with inheritance of known genetic loci showed linkage between Pchr and three different loci (Table 3).

Table 3.   Strain Distribution Pattern of Inheritance of Allelic
           Forms of Mapped Loci Showing Linkage with Pchr

RI Strain	Pchr	Pep-3	Odc-2	Gi
AXB-1	a	b	a	a
AXB-2	b	b	b	a
AXB-3	b	b	b	o
AXB-4	a	b	a	a
AXB-5	b	b	b	b
AXB-6	b	b	a	b
AXB-7	b	b	b	b
AXB-8	b	b	b	b
AXB-9	a	a	a	b
AXB-10	b	b	b	b
AXB-12	a	a	a	a
AXB-17	b	b	a	b
AXB-20	b	b	o	a
BXA-1	b	b	o	b
BXA-2	a	a	o	a
BXA-6	a	a	o	a
BXA-8	b	a	b	b
BXA-10	b	b	o	b
BXA-12	a	b	a	a
BXA-13	b	b	b	a
BXA-14	b	b	b	b
BXA-23	b	b	b	b
BXA-25	a	a	o	a

These are peptidase-3 (Pep-3) which has been mapped to chromosome 1 (Lewis and Trustlove, 1969), ornithine decarboxylase-2 (Odc-2) which has been mapped to chromosome 2 (Nesbitt, unpublished observation) and intestinal G protein (Gi) which has been mapped to chromosome 9 (Cohen, unpublished observation). Allelic diffferences at Odc-2 and Gi are determined by DNA polymorphisms while allelic differences at Pep-3 are determined by electrophoretic heterogeneity of the enzyme.

A summary of the data obtained from comparison of the SDPs of Pchr and Pep-3, Odc-2 and Gi is presented in Table 4. For each of these 3 loci, evidence for linkage, which is based on the 95% confidence limit for recombination between Pchr and the particular genetic locus, is significant.

Table 4. Linkage Data Obtained From Comparison of Strain
          Distribution Pattern of Pchr, Pep-3, Odc-2 and Gi

Gene	Chromosome	Matches	Mismatches	Total	Linkage[a,b]
Pep-3	01	19	4	23	0.23
Odc-2	02	15	2	17	0.21
Gi	09	18	4	22	0.25

[a] Upper limit for 95% confidence limit for recombination frequency
    between Pchr and gene indicated.
[b] Significant if value is <0.50.

The chromosomal location of Pchr can now be mapped using the tool of
linkage analysis by typing animals of the susceptible backcross and
F2 hybrid generations derived from B and A progenitors for the
cosegregation of inheritance of Pchr and of the allelic forms of the
marker genes, Pep-3, Odc-2 and Gi. Determination of the exact
chromosomal location of Pchr may be useful in defining the phenotypic
expression and, consequently, the mechanism whereby this gene
regulates host resistance to acute malaria.

REFERENCES

Eugui, EM, Allison, AC (1980) Differences in susceptibility of
    various mouse strains to haemoprotozoan infections: possible
    correlation with natural killer cell activity. Parasite Immunol 2:
    277-292
Cohen, V Unpublished observation
Lewis, WH, Truslove, GM (1969) Electrophoretic heterogeneity of
    mouse erythrocyte peptidase. Biochem Genet 3: 493-498
Nesbitt, MN Unpublished observation
Stevenson, MM, Lyanga, JJ, Skamene, E (1982) Murine malaria: genetic
    control of resistance to Plasmodium chabaudi. Infect Immun 38:
    80-88
Stevenson, MM, Skamene, E (1985) Murine malaria: resistance of
    AXB/BXA recombinant inbred mice to Plasmodium chabaudi. Infect
    Immun 47: 452-456
Stevenson, MM (1985) Genetic control of resistance in mice to
    Plasmodium chabaudi. Prog Leuk Biol 3: 531-543

ACKNOWLEDGMENT

This work was supported by grants MA7785 and MA6431 from the Medical
Research Council of Canada.

Summary

From Phenotype to Gene: A Molecular Analysis of Complex Loci Involved in Developmental and Immunological Dysregulation

B. Mock[1], S.D.M. Brown[2], C. Janeway[3], H.C. Morse III[1], and M. Potter[1]

I. Localizing and Cloning Genes

The first session of the workshop devoted itself almost entirely to the localization of mammalian genes, particularly those genes identified by mutation but
where nothing is known about the underlying gene product. The isolation of such
genes must necessarily be indirect and the various speakers discussed the prevailing
paradigm for an oblique approach to genes of known phenotype but unknown gene
product. The basic approach discussed by all speakers is, firstly, to construct a
detailed genetic map of DNA probes in the region of the mutation to identify sequences closely-linked to the mutation. These sequences can be used as start-points
for a more detailed mapping analysis in the region of the mutation utilising techniques such as pulse field gel electrophoresis and chromosome jumping.

As regards the first step in this process, J-L. Guenet (Inst. Pasteur, Paris)
described the use of interspecific backcrosses between the species Mus domesticus
and Mus spretus which has greatly aided the genetic mapping of DNA probes on mouse
chromosomes. S. Grant (RPMI, Buffalo) reported that the genetic maps of a number
of X-linked loci spanning some 50cM of the mouse X chromosome were virtually identical in intra and interspecific crosses confirming the veracity of the interspecific
cross system. In contrast, the use of recombinant inbred strains for mapping has
long been established as a classical tool for mouse gene mapping and B. Taylor
(Jackson Labs, Bar Harbor) discussed some of their current limitations, particularly
the inability to map newly arisen mutations. However, Taylor described the construction of a new stock (MEV) containing a large number of endogenous ecotropic
murine leukemia proviruses and visible dominant markers that should allow the
mapping of newly arisen mutations in a single cross. The presence of conserved
linkage groups between mouse and man has always been a useful guide to gene mapping
in both species. Improvements in the rat gene map reported by C. Szpirer (Univer-
ite Libre de Bruxelles) should greatly aid this comparative side of gene mapping.

S. Brown (St. Mary's, London) demonstrated the power of interspecific crosses
applied to the genetic mapping of microclone probes on the mouse X chromosome
and mouse chromosome 7. Between St. Mary's, London and the Institut Pasteur, Paris
some 50 clones have been mapped to the mouse X chromosome making this the best
mapped mouse chromosome so far and providing many start points for the more detailed
mapping of such elusive X-linked loci as Xce and mdx. H. Winking also illustrated
the usefulness of microdissection and microcloning as a technique to recover clones
from specific regions of the genome by microdissection of a large homogeneously
staining region found in chromosome 1 of some populations of the house mouse. The

NCI and [1]NIAID, NIH, Bethesda, MD; [2]St. Mary's Hospital Medical School, London,
[3]Yale University School of Medicine, New Haven, CT

Immunoregulatory Genes Workshop Summary

A workshop devoted to examining reverse genetic approaches at localizing, cloning
and characterizing genes involved in a variety of developmental, autoimmune,
neoplastic and infectious disease processes was sponsored by the National Cancer
Institute, NIH in Bethesda, MD from 27-29 October 1987.

microclones recovered should provide useful tools to understand both the mechanisms
of sequence amplification in such regions and the genetic consequences for chromosme
behavior in pairing, segregation and recombination.

It is clear that the recovery of DNA probes from specific regions and their mapping
have proceeded apace and construction of fairly detailed genetic maps of DNA probes
on many mouse chromosomes is now well-advanced. However, less progress has been
made in the area of proceeding from the many start-points provided by such probes to
the ultimate genetic locus of interest. L. Stubbs (ICRF, London) described a 10:17
translocation which brings the steel mutation in close juxtaposition to DNA marker
probes on mouse chromosome 17. The combined use of chromosome jumping from these
probes and pulse field gel electrophoresis has enabled her to detect the chromosome
breakpoint in the neighborhood of the steel locus. However, final identification of
the gene remains for the future. So too, is the case, for the Wilms Tumour-aniridia
locus on human chromosome 11 discussed by N. Hastie (MRC, Edinburgh). A number of
probes from human chromosome 11 derived by chromosome mediated gene transfer are
closely-linked to the locus and have been used to detect large restriction fragments
on pulse-field gels that appear to cross chromosomal breakpoints associated with
mutations at this particular locus.

Undoubtedly, the presence of chromosomal breakpoints associated with mutation
in any gene will be a powerful indicator for gene localization on the fine molecular
map; the assumption being that often the breakpoint will interrupt the gene itself.
However, in many areas such a strategy will not be available and the ultimate
identification of the gene may depend on more sophisticated biological assays of
sequence function that were barely touched on at this workshop. These may include
the use of transgenic mice in complementation assays or the new and exciting technologies of sequence-directed mutagenesis.

II. A Molecular Analysis of Complex Loci

The following sessions of the workshop were devoted to the molecular analysis
of loci involved in specific developmental and immunological processes. Sessions
on t complex loci, homeo boxes, major urinary protein genes, α-interferon genes
and various genes in the immunoglobulin superfamily provided an examination of
complex gene families consisting of clusters of tightly linked loci.

t Complex Loci

Since the 1932 discovery of a mutation within the t complex of mice, this cluster
of 30 different genes located both proximal to and interspersed with loci in the MHC,
has provided a model system for studying genomic organization and evolution as well as
genetic control of embryonic development, sex determination and spermatogenesis of
mammals. J. Klein (Tubingen) reported on the isolation of 3 molecular clones from
within the t complex by the clever screening of libraries generated from somatic-cell
hybrids specific for chromosomes 17 and 18. He has concluded from the geographical
distribution of RFLP patterns, as defined by hybridization with one of these clones
(Tul, proximal to the t complex), that European wild mice have not contributed significantly to the derivation of the laboratory mouse. L. Silver (Princeton) presented
a historical perspective of t haplotypes and also pointed to the role of molecular
probes as tools in their dissection. He has concluded from his own work and that of
others that all t haplotypes present in mice today are descendents of a single ancestral chromosome which had evolved apart from the wild-type form of mouse chromosme 17
by the generation of several large non-overlapping inversions. Recent comparisons of
the proximal and distal inversions which occur within the t complex have revealed
several interesting features. By analyzing 100 wild-derived chromosomes with several
DNA markers from within the t complex, M. Erhart (The Jackson Lab, Bar Harbor)
suggested that segmental exchange rather than single crossovers is the predominant

means of recombination between t̲ haplotype and wild-type homologues in the region
distal to the proximal inversion. Bernhard Herrman (NIMR, London) has focused his
attention on cloning genes in the proximal region of the t̲ complex which contains
the brachyury (T) locus involved in the formation of the embryonic body axis.
Through the varied uses of classical genetic crosses involving mice which carry
mutant T̲ alleles, the generation of random DNA probes from microdissected chromosomes, the examination of sequences homologous to other vertebrates and the screening
of cDNA libraries, he has cloned a gene (T119II) which is in linkage disequilibrium
with the T̲ mutation suggesting it is very close to the T̲ gene.

Homeo Box Genes

The following session was devoted to an examination of murine homeo box genes.
Homeotic genes were first described in Drosophila and belong to either the engrailed gene complex or the antennapedia and bithorax complex. These genes contain
a 180 bp conserved region, the "homeo box" which codes for a protein domain similar
to DNA-binding domains. More than 20 homeo box genes have been mapped on the murine
genome. F. Ruddle (Yale U., New Haven), B. Hogan (NIMR, London) and M. Fibi (Max
Planck Institute, Gottingen) discussed structural and functional aspects of the
antennapedia-like genes (Hox) of the mouse which are arranged in clusters and
located on different chromosomes (chrs 6,11,12,15). Fibi pointed to the structural
similarity of Hox and Ig genes, both of which have variable and constant region
domains. Ruddle discussed the similarities in linkage of human and mouse Hox
sequences. Both he and Hogan pointed to the similarities in Hox-1 and Hox-2 gene
clusters. It seems likely that the genes within these clusters have evolved via
duplication and divergence of an ancestral gene. All three investigators examined
the spatial and temporal expression of homeo box genes in embryonic and adult mice.
Fibi concentrated on Hox gene expression in adult mice; there are genes only expressed
in one organ, such as Hox-1.3 in adult liver and Hox-2.1 in adult lung and there
are tissues in which a combination of Hox genes seems to be expressed simultaneously.
Via the use of in situ hybridization techniques with RNA probes, Hogan found that
both Hox-2.1 and 2.6 were expressed in embryonic regions of the central nervous
system, peripheral nervous system and in the mesodermal component of several visceral
organs. A member of the murine engrailed complex (En-1) which resides in the
vicinity of the Dominant hemimelia (Dh) mutation was discussed by Michael Frohman
(UCSF, San Francisco). His immunohistochemical studies, utilizing antisera to an
En-1 fusion protein, reveal nuclear protein expression in the mesencephalon and
myelencephalon, restricted portions of the spinal column and in many spinal and
cranial granglia of mid-gestation embryos.

Major Urinary Protein Genes

Mouse major urinary proteins are encoded by a cluster of 30-40 genes. These
proteins are synthesized in the liver, and in submaxillary, sublingual, parotid,
lachrymal and mammary glands. Eva Derman (PHRI, New York) sequenced cDNA clones
from all six of these tissues and found that each gene exhibited a distinct tissue
specific pattern of expression. These differentially expressed genes differ primarily by single nucleotide substitutions, both in the flanking and in the intervening sequences, suggesting that they are regulatory variants of the same ancestral
gene. Bill Held (RPMI, Buffalo) discussed the identification of cis-regulatory
sequences conferring tissue-specific expression of transgenes composed of Mup structural gene sequences fused to the SV40 T antigen. Robert Duncan (NIH, Bethesda)
identified two novel MUP phenotypes in BALB/cJ mice, one of which is controlled by a
gene (Mupm-1) on chromosome 15.

α-Interferon Genes

The interferons are proteins that induce resistance to viral infection in cells.
The α-interferons are a family of 9 genes on chromosome 4 in the mouse. P. Pitha
(Johns Hopkins, Baltimore) has examined the expression of individual members of
the α-interferon gene family in different cell types induced with different
activators, and finds that individual members of the gene family are selectively
activated in different cell types. In this context, S. Vogel (USUHS, Bethesda) has
observed that the failure of the mutant C3H/HeJ mouse to respond to LPS, which maps
to chromosome 4, correlates with a failure of macrophages to produce α-interferon
upon LPS activation. In addition, using Pitha's α-interferon probes, a polymorphism in at least one α-interferon gene was detected in this strain as compared to
all other, LPS-responsive, C3H sublines. This finding lends further weight to the
notion that the multiplicity of α-interferon genes relates to their specificity of
expression. What do the α-interferons do? O. Haller (Zurich) has identified a
gene called Mx on chromosome 16 that is activated by α-interferon, and whose
product specifically protects cells from influenza virus infection. The product of
the Mx gene is probably a DNA binding protein that blocks transcription of influenza
virus. A polymorphism in this gene radically alters susceptibility to influenza
virus, but not to other viruses thus far detected. The existence of this polymorphism in wild as well as laboratory mice is puzzling; mice are not normally hosts
for influenza virus, and a selective advantage of either allele of this gene has
not yet been identified.

Immunoglobulin Superfamily Genes

The immunoglobulin (Ig) superfamily is composed of such functionally important
members as immunoglobulin, major histocompatiblity complex (MHC) class I and II
and T-cell receptor molecules. These molecules share key structural features with
either the variable or constant region immunoglobulin domains. Many of these
molecules are membrane-bound and expressed on lymphocytes where they are capable
of interacting with each other. As such, they play an important role in cell-cell
recognition.

During B cell development, both immunoglobulin heavy chain (IgH) and light
chain (Igk or Igλ) genes rearrange allowing for the expression of membrane
immunoglobulin tetramers which function as antigen receptors. Mechanisms of and
controlling elements involved in Ig rearrangement and expression are largely
unclear. In this session, K. Calame (UCLA, CA) analyzed functional properties of
the IgH enhancer via site-directed mutagenesis and demonstrated that four (E, B, C1
and C2) of eight known protein binding sites are required for optimal enhancer
function in vivo. In addition, she and C. Peterson (UCLA) have purified and partially characterized proteins which bind to sites E and C2.

During rearrangement, the heavy-chain variable region is constructed by joining
three distinct DNA segments: a V (variable segment), a D (diversity) segment and a
J (joining) segment. The mechanism and regulation of VDJ recombination was examined
by M. Lieber (NIH, Bethesda). His studies of 30 murine cell lines, utilizing
extrachromosomal substrates (a plasmid containing heptamer/nonamer joining signals)
which could be recovered and analyzed for recombination within 1-2 days after transfection into cell lines, revealed major changes in the level of recombination
activity during B cell development. Recombination rates were low in pro-GMB cell
lines. However, the highest recombination frequencies were seen in pro-B cells.
From this stage on, activity levels declined progressively, with pre-B cells at the
stage of heavy chain rearrangement generally higher than those that are rearranging
their light chains and with mature B cells showing even lower or zero activity.

The selective and neutral evolution of 8 different Vh gene families within the Igh-V locus was discussed by A. Tutter (MBI, LaJolla). Her RFLP analyses of Mus, Rattus, Peromyscus, Marmota and Oryctolagus Vh families revealed that Vh copy number has evolved via small, random duplication/deletion events and that group III Vh families have been conserved across widely separated mammalian lineages, while group I and II families have evolved more freely. P. D'Eustachio (Rockefeller, NY) presented a multilocus linkage map of the area surrounding the IgH locus on mouse chromosome 12.

Heavy chains by themselves are lacking in functionality. During B cell differentiation, light chains (either κ or λ) must associate with heavy chains to form functional Ig molecules. L. D'Hoostelaere's (NIH, Bethesda) RFLP analysis of 12 Vk families among 55 inbred strains revealed that DNA probes for 12 of the 18 Vk protein groups detect non-overlapping sets of restriction fragments and that at least 7 haplotypes exist among inbred strains. His predicted gene order of Vk loci will be useful in examining the hypothesis of ordered rearrangement during B cell ontogeny.

Yet another group of genes, Igλ, also encode immunoglobulin light chains during B cell development. These λ genes are expressed at low frequency in the mouse compared with κ gene expression. Recently, investigators at the Basel Institute for Immunology isolated 3 pre-B specific genes (λ5, VpreB1, VpreB2) from a pre-B minus B subtractive cDNA library. These pre-B specific genes are found on the same linkage group (mouse chr 16) as the λ genes and they share significant regions of homology with them. S. Bauer (Basel Institute) found that the specific organization of both coding and non-coding DNA sequences in the λ5-VpreB region is highly conserved across Mus subgenera which were separated at least 9-12 mya. This is in marked contrast to the RFLPs and gene amplification found among the Igλ genes. S. Pillai's (Whitehead Institute) immunoprecipitation studies involving pre-B and B cells have revealed that pre-B cells synthesize either or both of two surrogate Ig light chains (designated omega and iota). Preliminary sequence analysis of the omega chain suggests that it is the product of the λ5 gene. Pillai hypothesizes that IgMm and Ig omega or iota tetramers function from an intracellular transmembrane location as a ligand-independent "activated receptor" to provide signals for further differentiation.

MHC Class I molecules are also members of the immunoglobulin superfamily. They are composed of a heavy glycoprotein chain (which is highly polymorphic among both humans and inbred strains of mice and is encoded by H-2K, D and L loci) and a non-covalently associated β2M molecule. Recognition of class I molecules by receptors on cytotoxic T cells determines tissue compatibility and incompatibility. G. Jay (NIH, Bethesda) presented evidence from a number of experiments which suggest that tumor formation in mice varies inversely with the expression of class I antigens. In a typical example, expression of a transfected class I gene (H-2K^b), introduced by DNA-mediated gene transfer, in B16 melanoma cells markedly reduced their tumorigenicity.

The precise molecular mechanisms which regulate class I expression are not known. Recently, an enhancer element in the murine K^b gene was identified. In addition, a 30 bp sequence (the interferon consensus sequence) 5' of the class I transcriptional promoter appears to respond to α- or γ-interferon by increasing the transcription of class I genes. D. Singer (NIH, Bethesda) has identified regulatory elements associated with PD1, a class I MHC gene of the swine which is preferentially expressed in B cells. Analysis of a series of deletion mutants constructed within the 5' end of PD1 revealed that the interferon response element (IRE) was associated with the PD1 promoter. In addition two other regulatory elements were identified -- a positive element which increases the activity of an SV40 promoter and appears to be a classical enhancer and a negative element which reduces the activity of the homologous PD1 promoter.

III. A Molecular Analysis of Mutant Phenotypes

The final sessions of the workshop were devoted entirely to the identification and characterization of specific aberrant or mutant phenotypes/alleles associated with immunological, autoimmune, neoplastic and infectious disease processes.

One of the most mysterious of immunoregulatory loci was described about twenty years ago by Festenstein, who termed it the Mls (mixed lymphocyte stimulating) locus. Disparity at Mls stimulates more potent T cell responses than disparity at the major histocompatibility complex (MHC). The response has been shown to involve CD4[+] T lymphocytes, and the involvement of class II MHC molecules, CD4 and the T cell receptor has been inferred from genetic and antibody inhibition experiments (Janeway, Yale). How does Mls disparity lead to the activation of so many T cells? Janeway has proposed that Mls encodes a quantitative polymorphism in an antigen presenting cell molecule that enhances T cell receptor interactions with class II MHC molecules. Hammerling (SKI, New York) proposes that Mls encodes an inhibitory signal that is more powerful in non-stimulatory than in stimulatory alleles. A third possibility, raised by Janeway, is that Mls encodes a nearly universal T cell receptor and class II MHC-binding peptide. A clear answer awaits identification of the molecular product that varies in Mls disparate strains. Originally, Festenstein defined 4 alleles of Mls, and mapped one such allele (Mls[a]) to chromosme 1. Work of Abe and Hodes (NIH, Bethesda) clearly indicates that Mls[c] is not allelic with Mls[a], and that Mls[d] consists of Mls[a] and Mls[c] expressed together in an inbred strain. A new nomenclature awaits detailed genetic analysis and an agreement among workers in the field. However, it is important to be aware that there are two independent loci encoding this trait, each with at least one stimulatory and one non-stimulatory (responder) allele.

A variety of autosomal recessive mutations associated with the development of autoimmunity (gld,lpr,me,me[v]) and immunodeficiency (me alleles, scid) were discussed. A gene first approach to defining the gld mutation was described by Seldin (NIH). Using interspecific backcross mice, a molecular map of distal chromosome 1 was constructed that places gld in very close proximity to At-3. The data also showed that the synteny between mouse chromosome 1 and human chromosome 1 q covers approximately 30 cM. Shultz (Jackson Laboratory) and Sidman (Jackson Laboratory) demonstrated that the me[v] mutation has multiple effects on the hematopoietic system. Homozygotes exhibit dysfunctions of multiple hematopoietic lineages that reflect abnormalities of precursor cells as well as the microenvironment in which they develop. Within the B cell lineage alone, these defects are characterized by a unique expansion of Ly-1[+] B cells and the development of Mott cells ("constipated" plasma cells). Bosma (Fox Chase) reported the mapping of the scid mutation to chromosome 16 in close linkage to md. Data strongly suggestive that the mutation may affect recombinases was presented by Marcu (Stony Brook) and Bosma. Sidman showed that mice from his scid colony could develop functional T cells and B cells although scids from other colonies do not exhibit this phenotype (Bosma). Teuscher (U.Penn) showed that genetic determinants of susceptibility and resistance to experimental allergic orchitis or encephalitis did not segregate in association with low and high levels of alphafetoprotein.

Finally, Chapman (Roswell Park) and Ansell (U. of Edinburg) described how germline mutations induced by ethyl nitrosourea can be used to study functions encoded by the X chromosome. Nine mutants affecting normal mosaicism were detected and three examined in some detail. One behaves like a cell autonomous lethal while the others are transmissable with selective expression in different cell lineages. One of the latter mutants clearly affects T cell differentiation and may affect other lineages as well.

Infectious and Neoplastic Diseases

Inbred strains of mice often respond differently to infectious agents indicating that underlying genetic differences determine susceptibility(S) or resistance (R). The response of mice to agents that are ingested by macrophages (Leishmania donovani, Salmonella typhimurium, and Mycobacterium bovis (strain BCG)) provides a model system that has been studied for over ten years. A gene that determines the early responses of infected mice influences the ultimate fate of the infection. This gene, located on chromosome 1, has been called Lsh, Ity, and Bcg depending upon the organism studied. The exact location of the gene(s) is still being determined. New closely linked markers Fn (fibronectin), glutaminase and bcl-2, have been found by Schurr (McGill Univ., Montreal) and Mock (NIH), but even closer markers are needed. The function of Lsh is still unresolved but studies by Skamene (MGH, Montreal) and Blackwell (LSTMH, London) suggest that differences exist between R and S macrophages with respect to their priming for activation and that the Lsh-Ity-Bcg gene may possibly code for some type of macrophage receptor. The association of fibronectin and complement receptor genes close to Lsh may be of special importance. Lsh congenic mice are particularly helpful in supplying S and R macrophages for analysis and for searching for relevant pheno-types (as discussed by Blackwell, Skamene and Zwilling (Ohio State)). A dif-ference in expression of class II (Ia) molecules on macrophage cell surfaces of R and S mice has been found by Zwilling and Skamene. Interestingly, the Pchr resistance gene determining the outcome of infection with Plasmodium chabaudi may also be linked to this region on chromosome 1. Stevenson's (MGH, Montreal) studies on the genetic control of P. chabaudi in the AXB/BXA recombinant inbred strains have suggested that the Pchr gene may either be linked to Pep-3 (chr 1), Odc-2 (chr 2) or Gi (chr 9).

Resistance and susceptibility to leukemia and lymphoma development presents com-plex problems. Meruelo (NYU) has identified a locus, Ril, linked to Ly-6 on chr 15 that determines susceptibility to fractionated x-irradiation induced leukemia. Using the congenic pair, C57BL/6 and B6.C-H-30^C, relevant phenotypic differences are being sought that will help in identifying Ril-1. Kozak's (NIAID, NIH) studies on the Gv-1 locus (which suppresses transcription of Moloney ecotropic murine leukemia viruses) indicate that Mus spretus mice exhibit a reduced number of germline retroviral genes compared to most inbred strains. Therefore, these mice may provide better models for the study of viral leukemogenesis. Ishizaka and Lilly (Albert Einstein College of Med.) have found a gene that determines susceptibility to methylcholanthrene induced leukemogenesis that is independent of the Ah locus. The gene is not mapped nor is the phenotype it governs established, however, the gene appears to be expressed in bone marrow cells. Susceptibility and resistance patterns in BALB/c and C.D2 congenic strains to pristane induced plasma cell tumor formation indicate at least 3 genes linked to the Fv-1 (chr 4), Qa2 (chr 17) and Ly-6 (chr 15) markers determine partial resistance to this form of tumor development. One of these genes appears to be linked with a deficiency to repair x-ray induced double stranded breaks incurred during the G2 phase of the cell cycle. In addition, the BALB/cJ subline is re-sistant to plasma cell tumor induction and thus genetic differences that distin-guish BALB/cAn(S) and BALB/cJ (R) potentially provide clues for identifying R genes. Blankenhorn has mapped the Afr-1 gene that regulates serum alphafetopro-tein levels to chr 15 near the Ly-6 locus. This is one of the striking genetic differences between these two strains.

Acknowledgments

We sincerely appreciate all of the efforts of the participants who made this workshop possible.